Perioperative Quality Improvement

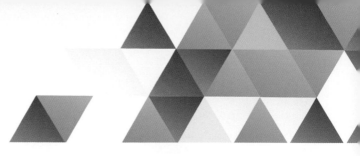

Perioperative Quality Improvement

Carol J. Peden, MB ChB, **MD, FRCA, FFICM, MPH**

Adjunct Professor
Anesthesiology
Keck School of Medicine of USC
Los Angeles, CA
USA;
Adjunct Professor
Anesthesiology
Perelman School of Medicine
University of Pennsylvania
Philadelphia, PA
USA;
Visiting Professor
Centre for Healthcare Innovation
and Improvement
University of Bath
Bath, Somerset
UK

Lee A. Fleisher, MD

Professor of Anesthesiology and Critical Care
Professor of Medicine
Perelman School of Medicine, University of
Pennsylvania
Philadelphia, PA
USA

Michael Englesbe, MD

Cyrenus G. Darling Sr., MD and
Cyrenus G. Darling Jr., MD
Professor of Surgery
Section of Transplantation Surgery
Michigan Medicine
University of Michigan
Ann Arbor, MI
USA

ELSEVIER

Elsevier
1600 John F. Kennedy Blvd.
Suite 1800
Philadelphia, PA 19103-2899

PERIOPERATIVE QUALITY IMPROVEMENT ISBN: 978-0-323-83399-8

Content Development Manager: Kathryn DeFrancesco
Senior Content Strategist: Kayla Wolfe
Senior Content Development Specialist: Ann Anderson
Publishing Services Manager: Shereen Jameel
Project Manager: Janish Paul/Manikandan Chandrasekaran
Design Direction: Renee Duenow

Printed in India

Last digit is the print number: 9 8 7 6 5 4 3 2 1

Working together
to grow libraries in
developing countries

www.elsevier.com • www.bookaid.org

Geeta Aggarwal, MBBS, MRCP, FRCA
Consultant
Anaesthetics and Intensive Care
Royal Surrey County Hospital
Guildford, Surrey, UK

Venkata Andukuri, MD, MPH
Assistant Professor
Internal Medicine
Creighton University
Omaha, NE, USA

Susan LaFollette Arnold, BS
Managing Director
Content Strategy Partners,
    LLC
Estes Park, CO, USA

Alexander F. Arriaga, MD, MPH, ScD
Anesthesiologist
Department of Anesthesiology
Perioperative and Pain Medicine
Brigham and Women's Hospital/Harvard
    Medical School
Boston, MA, USA;
Associate Faculty
Ariadne Labs
Boston, MA, USA

Angela M. Bader, MD, MPH
Professor of Anaesthesia
Department of Anesthesiology
Perioperative and Pain Medicine
Brigham and Women's Hospital/Harvard
Medical School
Boston, MA, USA

Angie Balfour, RN, MSc
Senior ERAS Nurse
    Specialist
Surgical Services
NHS Lothian
Edinburgh, Scotland, UK

Elizabeth R. Berger, MD, MS
Assistant Professor
Surgery
Yale University
New Haven, CT, USA

Nicholas L. Berlin, MD, MPH, MS
House Officer
Department of Surgery
University of Michigan
Ann Arbor, MI, USA

Jeanna D. Blitz, MD, FASA, DFPM
Associate Professor
Anesthesiology
Duke University School of Medicine
Durham, NC, USA;
Medical Director
Preoperative Anesthesia and Surgical
    Screening Clinic
Duke University
Durham, NC, USA;
Director
Perioperative Medicine Fellowship
Duke University School of Medicine
Durham, NC, USA

Alexander Booth, MD
Resident
Department of Surgery
Medical University of South Carolina
Charleston, SC, USA

Laura K. Botwinick, MS
Director
Graduate Program in Health Administration
    and Policy
University of Chicago
Chicago, IL, USA;
Fellow and Faculty
Institute for Healthcare Improvement
Boston, MA, USA

Kevin Bozic, MD, MBA
Professor & Chair
Department of Surgery and
  Perioperative Care
Dell Medical School at UT Austin
Austin, TX, USA

Kate Buehler, MS, RN
Clinical Program Manager
Department of Anesthesiology
University of Michigan
Ann Arbor, MI, USA

Desiree Chappell, MSNA, CRNA
Vice President
Clinical Quality
NorthStar Anesthesia
Irving, TX, USA;
Co-Editor in Chief
TopMedTalk
Louisville, KY, USA

Yun-Yun K. Chen, MD
Instructor in Anaesthesia
Department of Anesthesiology
Perioperative and Pain Medicine
Brigham and Women's Hospital
Boston, MA, USA

Maria Chereshneva, BSc, MBBS, FRCA, PG Dip
Consultant Anaesthetist
Associate Medical Director
  for Quality Improvement,
Department of Anaesthesia
Croydon University Hospital
London, UK

Justin T. Clapp, PhD, MPH
Assistant Professor
Department of Anesthesiology &
  Critical Care
University of Pennsylvania
Philadelphia, PA, USA

Benjamin H. Cloyd, MD, MIPH
Assistant Professor
Anesthesiology
University of Colorado
Aurora, CO, USA

Claire Cruikshanks, MB ChB, FRCA
Consultant Anaesthetist
Anaesthetic and Operating Services
Sheffield Teaching Hospitals Foundation
  Trust
Sheffield, UK

Casey A. Dauw, MD
Associate Professor
Urology
University of Michigan
Ann Arbor, MI, USA

Jugdeep Dhesi, FRCP, PhD
Consultant Geriatrician
Ageing and Health
Guy's and St Thomas' NHS Trust
London, UK;
Honorary Reader
Faculty of Life Sciences and Medicine
King's College London
London, UK;
Honorary Associate Professor
Division of Surgery and Interventional
  Science
University College London
London, UK

John Michael DiBianco, MD
Clinical Instructor
Urology
The University of Michigan
Ann Arbor, MI, USA

Mary Dixon-Woods, BA, DipStat, MSc, DPhil
Health Foundation Professor of Healthcare
  Improvement Studies
THIS Institute
Department of Public Health and
  Primary Care
University of Cambridge
Cambridge, UK

Caoimhe C. Duffy, MD, MSc, CPPS, FCAI
Assistant Professor, Anesthesiology and
  Critical Care
Perelman School of Medicine University of
  Pennsylvania
Philadelphia, PA, USA;
Senior Fellow
Leonard Davis Institute of Health Economics
University of Pennsylvania
Philadelphia, PA, USA

Angela F. Edwards, MD, FASA, DFPM
Associate Professor
Section Head Perioperative Medicine
Vice Chair Professional Affairs
Wake Forest University School of Medicine
Atrium Health Wake Forest Baptist
Winston Salem, NC, USA

Kylie-Ellen Edwards, MB ChB
Centre for Perioperative Medicine Research
Department for Targeted Intervention
University College London Division of Surgery
  and Interventional Science;
Health Services Research Centre
Royal College of Anaesthetists
London, UK

Sally El-Ghazali, MBBS, MSc, FRCA, FFICM
Post CCT Anaesthetic Fellow
Department of Theatres, Anaesthesia and
  Perioperative Care
Guy's and St Thomas' NHS Foundation Trust
London, UK

Michael Englesbe, MD
Professor of Surgery
Department of Surgery—Transplantation
University of Michigan
Ann Arbor, MI, USA

Stephen A. Esper, MD, MBA
Assistant Professor of Anesthesiology
Chief, Perioperative Services
Director, UPMC Center for Perioperative
  Care
UPMC Department of Anesthesiology
Cardiovascular and Thoracic Division
University of Pittsburgh Medical Center
  (UPMC)
Pittsburgh, PA, USA

Scott Falk, MD
Associate Professor of Clinical Anesthesiology
  and Critical Care
Anesthesiology and Critical Care
University of Pennsylvania
Philadelphia, PA, USA

Chelsea P. Fischer, MD, MS
Department of Surgery
Loyola University Medical Center
Chicago, IL, USA

Lee A. Fleisher, MD
Professor of Anesthesiology and
  Critical Care
Professor of Medicine
Perelman School of Medicine
University of Pennsylvania
Philadelphia, PA, USA

Robert L. Fogerty, MD, MPH, SFHM
Director, Bed Resources
Yale New Haven Health
Associate Clinical Professor
Yale School of Medicine
New Haven, CT, USA

Aidan Fowler, MBBS, FRCS
National Director Patient Safety
NHS England
London, UK

Amber Franz, MD, MEng
Assistant Professor
Anesthesiology and Pain Medicine
University of Washington
Seattle, WA, USA

Khurshid R. Ghani, MB ChB, MS, FRCS (Urol)
Professor
Department of Urology
University of Michigan;
Director
Michigan Urological Surgical Improvement
  Collaborative (MUSIC)
Ann Arbor, MI, USA

Michael P.W. Grocott, MBBS, MD, FRCA, FRCP, FFICM
Director Designate
Southampton NIHR Biomedical Research
  Centre
University Hospital Southampton NHS
  Foundation Trust/University of
  Southampton
Wootton, New Milton, UK;
Head
Anaesthesia, Perioperative and Critical Care
  Medicine Research Unit
University Hospital Southampton NHS
  Foundation Trust
Wootton, New Milton, UK;
Professor
School of Clinical and Experimental
  Sciences
University of Southampton
Southampton, New Milton, UK

Lawrence V. Gulotta, MD
Associate Professor of Orthopedic Surgery
Sports Medicine and Shoulder Service
Hospital for Special Surgery
New York, NY, USA

Alexander Hallway, BA
Research Area Specialist
Department of Surgery
University of Michigan
Ann Arbor, MI, USA;
Special Projects Lead
Michigan Surgical Quality Collaborative
Ann Arbor, MI, USA;
Pain Control Optimization Pathway Program
  Lead
Michigan Opioid Prescribing Engagement
  Network
Ann Arbor, MI, USA

Jennifer Harpe-Bates, DNAP, APRN, CRNA
CRNA Quality Director
Anesthesia
Northstar Anesthesia
Louisville, KY, USA;
Adjunct Faculty
Nurse Anesthesia Program
Northern Kentucky University
Highland Heights, KY, USA

Frances Healey, PhD, RN, RN-MH
Deputy Director of Patient Safety
National Patient Safety Team
NHS England
London, UK

Kaveh Houshmand Azad, MSc
Director
Value Improvement Office
Keck Medicine of USC
Los Angeles, CA, USA

Ryan Howard, MD
Surgery Resident
Department of Surgery
University of Michigan
Ann Arbor, MI, USA

Joseph Incorvia, MS
Quality Improvement Consultant
Plastic and Oral Surgery
Boston Children's Hospital
Boston, MA, USA

Thomas E. Jackiewicz, MPH
President
University of Chicago Medical Center
Chicago, IL, USA

Allison Janda, MD
Assistant Professor
Department of Anesthesiology
University of Michigan
Ann Arbor, MI, USA

Emily H. Johnson, MD, MS
Surgery Resident
Department of Surgery
University of Colorado
Aurora, CO, USA

Carolyn Johnston, BM BCh, MA (Oxon), FRCA
Consultant Anaesthetist
Deputy Chief Medical Officer
Department of Anaesthesia
St. Georges University Hospitals
London, UK

Lesley Jordan, MB ChB, FRCA
Consultant Anaesthetist
Trust Patient Safety Lead
Department of Anaesthesia
Royal United Hospitals Bath NHSFT
Bath, Somerset, UK

Rachel R. Kelz, MD, MSCE, MBA
William Maul Measey Professor
  of Surgery
Hospital of the University of Pennsylvania
Philadelphia, PA, USA

Maria Khan, MBBS, FRCA
Consultant Anaesthetist
Department of Anaesthesia and Perioperative
  Medicine
Ashford and St. Peter's Hospitals NHS
  Foundation Trust
Surrey, UK

Sachin Kheterpal, MD, MBA
Professor
Department of Anesthesiology
University of Michigan
Ann Arbor, MI, USA

Christopher J. King, MD
Associate Professor
Department of Medicine
Division of Hospital Medicine
University of Colorado School of Medicine
Aurora, CO, USA

Clifford Y. Ko, MD, MS, MSHS
Director
Division of Research and Optimal Patient
  Care
American College of Surgeons
Chicago, IL, USA;
Professor of Surgery and Health Services
UCLA Schools of Medicine and Public Health
Los Angeles, CA, USA

Meghan B. Lane-Fall, MD, MSHP, FCCM
Vice Chair of Inclusion, Diversity, and Equity
David E. Longnecker Associate Professor
Department of Anesthesiology and Critical Care;
Associate Professor of Epidemiology
University of Pennsylvania;
Vice President
Anesthesia Patient Safety Foundation
Philadelphia, PA, USA

Thomas H. Lee, MD
Chief Medical Officer
Press Ganey Associates, Inc.;
Senior Physician
Brigham and Women's Hospital
Boston, MA, USA

Denny Z.H. Levett, BM BCh, PhD, MRCP, FRCA
Consultant in Critical Care and Perioperative
  Medicine, University Hospital
  Southampton
Southampton, UK;
Honorary Lecturer in Physiology, UCL
London, UK

Della M. Lin, MS, MD, FASA
Department of Surgery
John A Burns School of Medicine, Honolulu
Honolulu, HI, USA

Robert Lloyd, PhD
Vice President
Improvement Science
Institute for Healthcare Improvement
Boston, MA, USA;
Senior Improvement Advisor
Improvement Science
Institute for Healthcare Improvement
Boston, MA, USA

Mark Lockett, MD
Professor
Department of Surgery
Medical University of South Carolina
Charleston, SC, USA

Daniel Low, BMedSci, BM, BS, MRCPCH, FRCA
Associate Professor of Anesthesiology
Anesthesiology and Pain Medicine
University of Washington
Seattle, WA, USA

Aman Mahajan, MD, PhD, MBA
Professor of Anesthesiology and Perioperative
    Medicine
University of Pittsburgh School of Medicine
Pittsburgh, PA, USA

Chris Mainey, PhD
Head of Patient Safety Measurement for
    Improvement
Patient Safety, Medical Directorate
NHS England
London, UK

Michael W. Manning, MD, PhD
Associate Professor
Anesthesiology
Duke University Medical Center
Durham, NC, USA

Graham P. Martin, MA(Oxon), MSc, PhD
Director of Research
Department of Public Health and Primary
    Care
University of Cambridge
Cambridge, UK

Lynn D. Martin, MD, MBA
Professor
Anesthesiology and Pain Medicine
University of Washington
Seattle, WA, USA;
Adjunct Professor
Pediatrics
University of Washington
Seattle, WA, USA

Michael Mathis, MD
Assistant Professor
Department of Anesthesiology
University of Michigan
Ann Arbor, MI, USA

**Peter McCulloch, MB ChB, MA, MD, FCRSEd,
FRCS**
Professor of Surgical Science & Practice
University of Oxford;
Nuffield Department of Surgical Sciences
    (Level 6)
John Radcliffe Hospital
Headington
Oxford, UK

**S. Ramani Moonesinghe, OBE, MD(Res),
FRCA, FFICM, FRCP**
Professor
Perioperative Medicine, Division of Targeted
    Intervention
University College London
London, UK

Dave Murray, MBBS, BSc, FRCA, MMed
Consultant Anaesthetist
Anesthetic Department
James Cook University Hospital
Middlesbrough, UK

**Paul S. Myles, MBBS, MPH, MD, DSc, FCAI,
FANZCA, FAHMS**
Professor/Director
Anaesthesiology and Perioperative Medicine
Alfred Hospital and Monash University
Melbourne, Victoria, Australia

**Monty G. Mythen, MBBS, MD, FRCA, FFICM,
FCAI (Hon)**
Professor of Anaesthesia and Critical Care
Centre for Perioperative Medicine
University College London
London, UK

Wendy Odell, DNP, CRNA
Clinical Leadership Executive
Adjunct Faculty
Texas Christian University
Sothlake, TX, USA

Anaeze C. Offodile II, MD, MPH
Assistant Professor
Department of Plastic and Reconstructive
　Surgery
UT MD Anderson Cancer Center
Houston, TX, USA;
Assistant Professor
Department of Health Services Research
UT MD Anderson Cancer Center
Houston, TX, USA

Gareth Parry, BSc, MSc, PhD
Biostatistician
Cambridge Health Alliance
Cambridge, MA, USA;
Member of Faculty
Harvard Medical School
Boston, MA, USA

Judith Partridge, FRCP, PhD
Consultant Geriatrician
Perioperative Medicine for Older People
　Undergoing Surgery
Guy's and St Thomas'
NHS Foundation Trust;
Honorary Senior Lecturer
King's College London
London, UK

Carol J. Peden, MB ChB, MD, FRCA, FFICM, MPH
Adjunct Professor
Anesthesiology
Keck School of Medicine of USC
Los Angeles, CA, USA;
Adjunct Professor
Anesthesiology
University of Pennsylvania
Perelman School of Medicine, PA, USA;
Visiting Professor
Centre for Healthcare Innovation and
　Improvement
University of Bath
Bath, Somerset, UK

Nial Quiney, MBBS, FRCA
Consultant
Department of Anaesthesia
Royal Surrey Hospital
Guildford, UK

Jacqueline W. Ragheb, MD
Assistant Professor
Anesthesiology
University of Michigan
Ann Arbor, MI, USA

Steven E. Raper, MD, JD
Vice Chairman for Quality and Risk
　Management
Associate Professor of Surgery
University of Pennsylvania Perelman School of
　Medicine
Philadelphia, PA, USA

Andrew Rogerson, MB ChB, MRCP
Specialist Registrar
Geriatric Medicine
Royal Infirmary of Edinburgh
Edinburgh, UK

Kevin Rooney, MB ChB, FRCA, FFICM, FRCP Edin
Clinical Director for Critical Care
Consultant in Anaesthesia and Intensive Care
　Medicine
Department of Anaesthesia
Royal Alexandra Hospital
Paisley, Scotland, UK

Madeleine Roper, MB ChB, FRCA
Specialty Trainee in Anaesthesia
Royal Alexandra Hospital
Department of Anaesthesia
Paisley, Scotland, UK

Ramai Santhirapala, MBBS, FRCA, FFICM, FHEA
Honorary Associate Professor
University College London
London, UK;
Consultant Anaesthetist
Perioperative Medicine Lead
Department of Theatres
Anaesthesia and Perioperative Care
Guy's and St Thomas'
NHS Foundation Trust, London, UK

Michael Scott, MB ChB, FRCP, FRCA, FFICM
Professor
Anesthesiology & Critical Care Medicine
University of Pennsylvania
Philadelphia, PA, USA;
Senior Fellow
Leonard Davis Institute of Health Economics
Philadelphia, PA, USA

Nirav Shah, MD
Associate Professor
Anesthesiology
University of Michigan
Ann Arbor, MI, USA

Georgina F. Singleton, MB ChB
Department for Targeted Intervention
UCL/UCLH Surgical Outcomes Research
    Centre
Centre for Perioperative Medicine University
    College London;
Health Services Research Centre
National Institute for Academic Anaesthesia
Royal College of Anaesthetists
London, UK

Harry Soar, MB ChB, FRCA
Specialty Registrar
Department of Anaesthesia
Sheffield Teaching Hospitals NHS
    Foundation Trust
Sheffield, UK;
Leadership and Quality Improvement Fellow
Future Leaders Programme
Health Education
Yorkshire and Humber, UK,

Paula Spencer, MSHA, PMP, CPHIMS
Director
Office of Clinical Effectiveness
Adjunct Professor
Department of Health Administration Virginia
    Commonwealth University
Richmond, VA, USA

Timothy J. Stephens, RGN, BA (Hons), MSc, PhD
Clinical Lecturer/Implementation Scientist
Critical Care and Perioperative Medicine
    Research Group
Queen Mary, University of London
London, UK

Emma Stevens, MB BChir, FRCA
Quality Improvement Fellow
National Emergency Laparotomy Audit
Specialty Registrar
University College London Hospitals NHS
    Foundation Trust
London, UK

BobbieJean Sweitzer, MD, FACP, SAMBA-F, FASA
Professor
Medical Education
University of Virginia
Charlottesville, VA, USA;
Systems Director
Inova Health
Falls Church, VA, USA

Jason Tong, MD, MSHP
Resident Physician
General Surgery
Hospital of the University of Pennsylvania
Philadelphia, PA, USA;
Veterans Affairs Fellow
National Clinician Scholars Program
Philadelphia, PA, USA

Alan Tung, MD, FRCPC
Clinical Lecturer
Department of Anesthesiology
Pharmacology & Therapeutics
University of British Columbia
Vancouver, BC, Canada

Thomas R. Vetter, MD, MPH
Professor and Chief of Anesthesiology and
    Perioperative Medicine
Department of Surgery and Perioperative Care
Dell Medical School at the University of Texas
    at Austin
Austin, TX, USA

Phillip E. Vlisides, MD
Assistant Professor
Department of Anesthesiology
Michigan Medicine
Ann Arbor, MI, USA

Hester Wain, PhD
Head of Patient Safety Policy
Patient Safety, Medical Directorate
NHS England
London, UK

Elizabeth C. Wick, MD
Professor
Division of General Surgery
University of California San Francisco
San Francisco, CA, USA

Christopher L. Wu, MD
Clinical Professor of Anesthesiology
Anesthesiology
Hospital for Special Surgery
New York, NY, USA;
Clinical Professor of Anesthesiology
Anesthesiology
Weill Cornell Medicine
New York, NY, USA

Ronald Wyatt, MD, MHA
Vice President and Patient Safety Officer
Patient Safety and Loss Prevention
MCIC Vermont
New York, NY, USA

Jacques T. YaDeau, MD, PhD
Associate Attending
Department of Anesthesiology
Critical Care and Pain Management
Hospital for Special Surgery
New York, NY, USA;
Clinical Associate Professor
Department of Anesthesia
Weill Medical College of Cornell University
New York, NY, USA

Most books on clinical medicine focus on establishing the current standard of care; this book has the more ambitious aim of helping clinicians improve. It provides efficient summaries of the state of the science for clinical issues that arise every day for clinicians caring for patients undergoing procedures, but its more remarkable undertaking is preparing those clinicians to keep improving, even after the current state of the science starts to show its age.

To that end, *Perioperative Quality Improvement* has clear and concise chapters that provide support for clinicians with an orientation toward perpetual improvement (i.e., a "growth mindset"). It addresses topics beyond reducing the rate of perioperative complications, embracing modern concepts of safety that focus on the prevention of four major types of harm: physical harm, emotional harm, financial harm, and socio-behavioral harm.

To prevent those four types of harm, clinicians must learn to work in highly effective teams. Thus several chapters are aimed at creating the "social capital" that allows clinicians to work together reliably and effectively. Readers will also learn about how to measure and analyze the data needed to drive improvement.

The bottom line is that this book should not be seen as a guide for "How to Be Excellent." Instead, it should be appreciated as a guide for "How to Get Better." That is a noble aspiration for clinicians in any area of medicine and most valuable in an area where so many clinicians with so many backgrounds must work reliably and effectively together to deliver care to patients at moments of high risk and stress.

Thomas H. Lee, MD
Senior Physician, Brigham and Women's
Hospital, Boston, MA, USA.
Chief Medical Officer, Press Ganey Associates, Inc.

Perioperative medicine is a relatively new specialty that encompasses the care of the surgical patient from the time that surgery is considered to full recovery. As patients traverse the perioperative pathway, they will be in contact with many diverse professionals whose skills are essential to their successful surgical outcome. This book is therefore written for all members of that multidisciplinary perioperative care team, whether they be surgeons, nurses, anesthesiologists, hospitalists, administrators, or any other partners who deliver perioperative care. As Editors of this book, we have a deep knowledge of the anesthetic and surgical skills required to deliver excellent care during surgery, but we also understand that for the patient the actual operation is only a small component of their journey back to health. In the increasingly complex world of perioperative medicine, knowing the evidence and being a skillful clinician are not enough to deliver safe, effective, patient-centered, efficient, and equitable care to every surgical patient every day. We require tools and techniques for improvement and an understanding of implementation science to ensure that evidence-based care is delivered to our patients as intended. In addition, as we work in multidisciplinary teams within complex hospital systems, we need some understanding of how to make change happen, how to work effectively together, how to understand a system, and how to measure and manage improvement work.

The aim of this book is to provide an easy-to-access resource with short chapters providing key messages, essential references, and further reading on each topic. We wanted each chapter to stand alone and to be succinct enough that it could perhaps be read while waiting on a patient between surgical cases. The book is divided into 3 sections containing 62 chapters. The first section provides background to perioperative medicine and covers essential subjects such as safety, equity, and the concepts of patient-centered care and shared decision making. Importantly, we also include advice on how to develop, report, and publish improvement and implementation work, acknowledging that more high-quality research is needed in this area. The second section of the book provides the tools and techniques to make change happen, and in the third section, we provide clinical examples of improvement projects and the results, including lessons learned, from leading organizations.

We would like to thank all our authors who represent many of the world's leading experts in perioperative medicine. We know that writing a chapter requires precious time that must be found in busy lives, and we are grateful for their generosity and expertise. Although the Editors are based in the United States, for our authors we reached out to friends and colleagues from around the world. We aimed to ensure that the best subject experts were involved and to provide guidance that transcends any one healthcare delivery system to be of use to clinicians trying to improve the delivery of surgical care anywhere in the world.

We must acknowledge the fact that the approach we used, of brief chapters with a practical bent directed at busy clinicians, was inspired to some degree by the UK Royal College of Anesthetists Quality Improvement Compendium. The Compendium, now in its 4th edition, edited by Professor Carol Peden and colleagues, has provided practical guidance for UK anesthetists for over 20 years, since its first release. We have further developed the idea of an easy-access resource into a textbook of perioperative care for a multidisciplinary international audience and hope that our book stands the test of time as well as the Compendium.

This book would not have been possible without the dedicated input of the Elsevier team and particularly Sarah Barth, Kayla Wolfe, Ann Anderson, Janish Paul, and Manikandan

Chandrasekaran. Of course, as always, writing and editing, in addition to our day jobs, takes time away from our families and we deeply acknowledge their support.

We hope you find this book a useful resource to improve perioperative care and that it inspires you to develop and lead improvement work, with the important goal of delivering personal, safe, efficient, equitable, and effective surgical care to all your patients every day.

Carol J. Peden
Lee A. Fleisher
Michael Englesbe

CONTENTS

SECTION *2*   *Improvement Science Tools for Change*

SECTION 3   *Putting It All Together—Clinical Quality Improvement*
            Examples

Perioperative Quality Improvement

Background

CHAPTER 1

What Is Quality in Medicine and Why Do We Need to Work on It?

Maria Chereshneva, MBBS, FRCA

KEY POINTS

- The ultimate goal for any clinician and healthcare system is to deliver quality care.
- High quality care should be: safe, effective, timely and patient-centred.
- Quality improvement in medicine has proven to be challenging, complex and at times difficult to sustain.
- In order to deliver quality in medicine, a culture shift is needed, along with recognition of time and effort needed for quality initiatives to be successful.
- Collaborative work between healthcare professions, managers, policy makers and patients is needed in order to improve quality.

Defining Quality in Health Care

The ultimate goal for any clinician or healthcare system is to deliver quality care. Although there is no universally accepted definition of "quality," most healthcare systems around the world have made strides in monitoring and continuously improving the care provided.

In the USA, the Institute of Medicine describes high-quality care as care that is[1]:

- Safe,
- Effective,
- Patient-centered,
- Timely,
- Efficient, and
- Equitable.

In the UK, the National Health Service (NHS) is "organising itself around a single definition of quality: care that is effective, safe, and provides as positive experience as possible by being caring, responsive, and personalized"[2] (Fig. 1.1). This definition also emphasizes that care should be well-led, sustainable, and equitable, achieved through providers and commissioners working together and in partnership with and for local people and communities (Box 1.1). Thus any organization that strives to make improvements should consider all the aforementioned elements.

A System of High-Quality Care

Over the last few decades, significant knowledge and experience have been accumulated in enhancing the quality of health care. Nevertheless, despite this, care is often poorly coordinated, with weak systems of communication focused on the individual practitioner and existing organizational structures. Decision makers and planners need to know which quality improvement (QI) strategies will

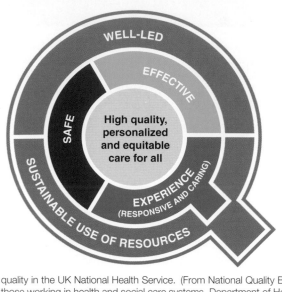

Fig. 1.1 Elements of quality in the UK National Health Service. (From National Quality Board. A shared commitment to quality for those working in health and social care systems. Department of Health and Social Care; 2021. https://www.england.nhs.uk/publication/national-quality-board-shared-commitment-to-quality/.)

BOX 1.1 ■ Elements of Quality in the National Health Service

People working in systems deliver care that is:
1. Safe—avoids harm to people for whom care is intended
2. Effective—providing evidence-based care
3. People centered—providing care that responds to individual preferences, needs and values

Healthcare organizations and systems are:
1. Well-led—driven by collective and compassionate leadership; underpinned by shared vision, values and learning; a just and inclusive culture; and proportionate governance
2. Sustainable resources—centered on delivering optimum outcomes within financial constraints and minimizes impact on public health and the environment
3. Equitable—committed to understanding and reducing variations and inequality to ensure universal access to high-quality care

---

have the greatest impact on the outcomes delivered by their system. We know that even when health systems are well funded, quality is still a major concern, with projected outcomes not reliably achieved and with wide variations in standards of healthcare delivery within and between healthcare systems.[3]

Quality in medicine is an amalgamation of the wider health system environment and the actions of providers and individuals working within the system. To achieve high-quality care, several domains need to be considered.[4]

1. National strategy for quality: National policies are fundamental to improving quality across health care and are ultimately aligned with broader national health planning. The strategy should have a pragmatic approach outlining interventions that improve the system, reduce harm, enhance clinical care, and engage service users and communities.
2. Quality delivered across the health system: Quality must be present across the system with robust governance processes; a skilled, motivated, and supported workforce; financing mechanisms that invest in quality care; information systems that monitor and learn to drive better

care; medicines, devices, and technologies that are available, safe, and appropriately regulated; and accessible and well-equipped healthcare facilities.

3. High-quality primary care: Primary health care is essential to delivering high-quality universal health. In the context of perioperative medicine, this should start at the time of contemplation of surgery.

4. Data collection and assessment: Continuous measurement is needed if improvement is to happen and be sustainable. This requires appropriate and meaningful data to evaluate, transform, and improve services.

5. Dissemination and discovery: Disseminating experiences and lessons both locally and beyond to embed quality and improve learning.

6. Innovation, transformation, and implementation: These are required to improve health, improve health care, and reduce costs. Grassroots innovations are more likely to be successful and sustained, particularly if supported from above.

7. Built-in quality resilience: The recent global pandemic highlighted that for healthcare systems to be resilient, they require quality health services that deliver before, during, and after a health crisis. A resilient, highly skilled, and protected workforce is the key.

Delivering Quality in Health Care

If we want to deliver health care that is fit for the 21st century, QI must be at the heart of it. For example, the growing number of comorbid patients and the challenges of managing them between various groups of professionals requires new ways of working. For the patient to receive optimal care, their management should be organized with harmonious information transfer and delivery, enabling them to smoothly navigate the system.[5] Unfortunately, in practice, care is fragmented, slow, and often leaves patients confused and dissatisfied, and healthcare staff frustrated. Although information sharing can be improved with advances in technologies, much more is needed. Creating health care that is underpinned by a culture of collaboration, flat hierarchy, respect, and better patient outcomes is what is needed. Adopting QI approaches in organizations will involve significant and sustained changes in culture and will require time and resources. QI is neither a "quick fix" in the face of huge operational pressures nor a form of "turnaround" strategy.[6]

Advances in technology, ease of access to information, and shifting cultural views means that patients are no longer passive passengers but active collaborators when it comes to their care. Patients are looking for healthcare staff that are more engaged, listening to their concerns and treating them with empathy, and enabling them to be more proactive in navigating a complicated landscape of health care. Initiatives such as those highlighted in the following points have been gaining recognition to enable this.

1. Shared decision making (SDM) is a process by which both patient and clinicians work together to make evidence-based decisions based on patient preferences and values. There is strong evidence that SDM benefits patients, improves overall experience and satisfaction, and also betters communication with healthcare professionals and adherence to treatments[7] (see also Chapter 11).

2. Experience-based codesign is another important method. Globally, healthcare providers tend to use questionnaire surveys to gain the perspective of patients on how they are performing. Nevertheless, there is evidence that there are shortcomings with existing (largely quantitative) methods of capturing the experiences of patients and what patients really want, so we should look for alternative approaches that help us to understand and improve[8] (see also Chapters 14 and 40).

These collaborative efforts are required to enable change at the local level through use of QI interventions with the explicit aim of improving patient experience. Nevertheless, such "true" engagement with patients is challenging, time consuming, and has been more difficult to deliver than foreseen. This will only be truly possible if organizations value these activities and provide necessary resources to support both patients and staff.

In practice, delivering high-quality care is laborious, complex, and challenging, and at times has proven difficult to sustain. There is also growing concern that quality initiatives have become focused on those aspects of care that are easy to measure, viewing patients as data sources and forgetting the "care" in quality. Top-down driven "quality" initiatives that do not reflect professional views of outstanding care methods or patient concerns, also rarely acknowledge the complexity of delivering quality health care. These top-down initiatives potentially stifle innovative and creative approaches to delivering quality care because the time and space becomes ever more "squeezed" by externally mandated requirements. It is important that healthcare staff are valued and allowed time to reflect together and share their experiences with peers. Critical appraisal, practice reflection, and integrity in actions, should take prominent roles in education activities to facilitate better understanding of how to deliver quality within a service development framework.

In the UK, the Royal College of Anaesthetists (RCOA) is leading a cross-organizational, multidisciplinary initiative called the Center for Perioperative Care (CPOC). This initiative aims to improve the quality of care within perioperative settings by empowering patients, supporting the workforce, influencing policy, leading on innovation and research, and exploiting new technology. This healthcare-wide collaboration will have the right expertise, the ability to test and implement projects across the sector, multidisciplinary professional leadership, and an openness to innovations. It will also allow for better disseminations of ideas to test projects on larger scale, use high-level skills and expertise to develop possible solutions, and support sharing of ideas. This whole sector involvement is what's needed if QI is to improve quality.[9]

References

1. Institute of Medicine (US) Committee on Quality of Health Care in America. *Crossing the Quality Chasm: A New Health System for the 21st Century.* Washington, DC: National Academies Press (US); 2001.
2. National Quality Board. *A shared commitment to quality for those working in health and social care systems.* Department of Health and Social Care; 2021. www.england.nhs.uk/publication/nationa-quality-board-shared-commitment-to-quality.pdf. Accessed 5 May 2022.
3. World Health Organization. *Quality of care: a process for making strategic choices in health systems;* 2016. https://apps.who.int/ iris/handle/10665/43470. Accessed 25 June 2021.
4. World Health Organization. *Fact sheet: quality health services;* 2020. who.int. Accessed 25 June 2021.
5. Mckee M, Merkur S, Edwards N, Nolte E. Conclusions—challenges for hospitals of the future. In: J. North (Author) & M.McKee, S. Merkur, N. Edwards, E. Nolte, eds. *The Changing Role of the Hospital in European Health Systems* (European Observatory on Health Systems and Policies, pp. 288-297). Cambridge: Cambridge University Press.
6. Jabbal J. *Embedding a culture of quality improvement.* London: The Kings Fund; 2017. kingsfund.org.uk. Accessed 25 June 2021.
7. Sturgess J, Clapp JT, Fleisher LA. Shared decision-making in peri-operative medicine: a narrative review. *Anaesthesia.* 2019;74(Suppl 1):13–19.
8. Mohta NS, Prewitt E, Volpp KG, et al. Insights Roundtable Report: measuring what matters and capturing the patient voice. *NEJM Catalyst.* 2017. https://catalyst.nejm.org/doi/full/10.1056/CAT.17.0380. Accessed 21 May 2022.
9. Dixon-Woods M, Martin GP. Does quality improvement improve quality? *Future Hosp J.* 2016;3:191–194.

CHAPTER 2

Where Does Safety Fit In?

Aidan Fowler, MBBS, FRCS ■ Hester Wain, PhD ■
Frances Healey, PhD, RN, RN-MH ■ Chris Mainey, PhD

KEY POINTS

- Psychological safety is essential for learning.
- Safety requires safe systems, not just individuals working safely.
- Involving patients in their own safety improves quality of care.

We are not here to curse the darkness but to light the candle that can guide us through that darkness to a safe and sane future.

JOHN F KENNEDY, 1960

John F Kennedy's quote describes our patient safety journey in the National Health Service (NHS) towards understanding and proactivity, from talking about harm to talking about safer systems that provide the right care, as intended, every time and learning from what works, not just what does not. It also speaks to the idea of doing that in a just culture where psychological safety means we will hear more, learn more, and can act more to improve care.

Since 2009 in the UK, with the publication of the World Health Organization (WHO) Guidelines for Safe Surgery[1] and the launch of the framework for identifying and monitoring "never events,"[2] there has been significant progress, review, and emphasis placed on safety within perioperative medicine. In 2015, this was further supported by the publication of the National Safety Standards for Invasive Procedures (NatSSIPs),[3] which enabled organizations to standardize the key elements of procedural care that lay mostly outside the operating room environment.

National Health Service Patient Safety Strategy

Any health system that wants to become safer needs to move from an approach based on individual effort to a systems-based approach that understands and addresses major patient safety challenges such as healthcare-associated venous thromboembolism and eliminates rare but significant errors such as misconnection of gases. This requires insight from a range of sources, infrastructure, an approach to the involvement of staff and patients, a syllabus and training, and then the development of the improvement capability to bring about the required systematic changes (Fig. 2.1).

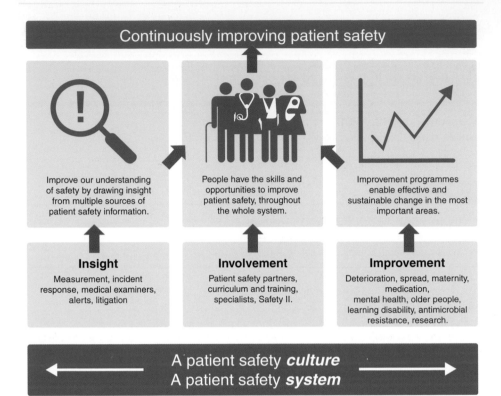

Fig. 2.1 Summary of the National Health Service (NHS) Patient Safety Strategy (From the https://www.england. nhs.uk/wp-content/uploads/2020/08/190708_Patient_Safety_Strategy_for_website_v4.pdf NHS England and NHS Improvement. The NHS patient safety strategy: safer culture, safer systems, safer patients; 2019. https:// www.england.nhs.uk/wp-content/uploads/2020/08/190708_Patient_Safety_Strategy_for_website_v4.pdf. Accessed April 12, 2021.)

The first NHS patient safety strategy[4] was launched in England in 2019 and seeks to continuously improve patient safety by building on the foundations of a patient safety culture and patient safety system.

Patient Safety Culture

Safety culture has been described as a "collective mindfulness" about safety issues, where leadership and frontline staff take a shared responsibility for ensuring care is delivered safely.[5] Unfortunately, in health care, there remains a culture of blame and fear from a mistaken belief that patient safety is about individual effort and that safety will be improved by tackling the performance of individuals,[6] rather than strengthening the systems they work within.

The study by Muensterer et al.[7] supports the concept that it is how systems work alongside how humans behave that creates conditions of failure, not a lack of effort/competence by individuals. This study randomly introduced prearranged errors in 120 cases and showed that errors in the time-out part of the surgical procedure were not recognized by the operating team in 46% of cases. Those errors that were least likely to be detected included age, intervention, allergy, and side/site, with anesthetists being the most likely members of the surgical team to identify errors. To be clear, this study does not propose that the surgical checklist and timeout process are not useful. Furthermore, as is discussed by Weinger,[8] checklists and other safety tools are potentially valuable; however, they need to be implemented in a systems-oriented multimodal approach supported by leadership. If used as a tick box exercise by unengaged staff, a checklist will not add value, whereas if staff use it as a mechanism to reduce hierarchy, encourage all to speak up, foster a culture of focusing on safety issues, and use it as a memory aid, then it will.

All healthcare safety improvement takes place within a highly complex system. Mary Dixon-Woods is articulate on the risk of "cargo cults"[9] where attempts to spread successful safety improvement initiatives focus on a visible tool such as a checklist, without spreading the complex associated leadership, teamwork, attitudes, values, culture, funding, and protected time that accompanied it and underpinned its success. The opposite may also be true; organizations, teams, and leaders who are becoming engaged and knowledgeable in safety science, human factors, and safety improvement may already be creating iterative improvements before adopting a visible tool that is then considered the cause of their safety improvement, rather than the icing on the cake. This might explain why decreases in adjusted in-hospital surgical mortality reported from Scotland[10] and in unadjusted in-hospital mortality from England (Fig. 2.2) appear to begin before the introduction of the WHO checklist and certainly well before its implementation was comprehensive.

Patient Safety Systems

Established patient safety systems sit within each healthcare organization and these encompass reporting, investigating, and acting on incidents and complaints; understanding culture via surveys; training and equipping staff to work safely; monitoring implementation to provide assurance; and developing quality improvement programs. Some of these systems, such as incident reporting, directly feed into national repositories from which information is reviewed and alerts created.

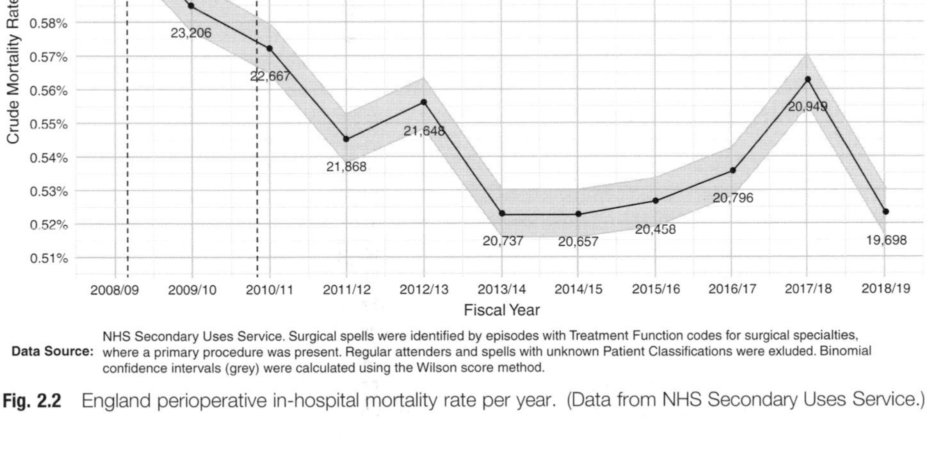

England periopertative in-hospital mortality rate per year

Data Source: NHS Secondary Uses Service. Surgical spells were identified by episodes with Treatment Function codes for surgical specialties, where a primary procedure was present. Regular attenders and spells with unknown Patient Classifications were exluded. Binomial confidence intervals (grey) were calculated using the Wilson score method.

Fig. 2.2 England perioperative in-hospital mortality rate per year. (Data from NHS Secondary Uses Service.)

Insight

In the UK, over 10 million surgical and invasive procedures take place every year.[11] Data from the NHS Secondary Uses Service (see Fig. 2.2) show a reduction over the past decade in absolute numbers of in-hospital deaths in England after surgical procedures per year (4481 fewer per year by 2018/2019) and in the crude mortality rate. This reduction is even more significant considering the greater age and morbidity of patients undergoing surgery, the complexity of surgical interventions that can now be offered, and the proportion of low-mortality procedures that no longer require a hospital spell.

In England, over 2 million patient safety incidents are reported to the NRLS (National Reporting and Learning System) each year, the majority (97%) of which result in no or low harm.[12] Clinical review of these incidents allows the identification of new or underrecognized patient safety issues and finds solutions that will prevent future harm to patients before it occurs in other hospitals.[13] This can include National Patient Safety Alerts that require hospitals to make systemic changes to protect staff from error and patients from harm for risks including foreign body aspiration during intubation[14] or misidentification of orthopedic fracture plates.[15] Various regulators can perform this alerting function but how notification occurs matters and so the NHS has worked on the type, design, and wording of safety alerts to ensure they are as effective as possible.[16]

Typing of incidents, such as never events,[2] can be a helpful way to bring focus in some areas. Nevertheless, there is a cost of potentially drawing attention to incidents with less potential for harm than others, such that death from disconnection of a ventilator might not be a never event but leaving a vaginal swab in situ is. Nevertheless, where strong barriers exist that make incidents preventable, identifying this (as a never event) makes the point that these events should not occur.

Involvement

The importance of the role of patients, their families and carers, and other lay people in improving the quality of health care is increasingly recognized,[17] as is involving patients as partners in their own care. This involvement also includes ensuring that patients and/or their families receive an explanation and apology when things go wrong. In England, this has been codified within law as the "Duty of Candour"[18] and requires a written apology. In the US, some healthcare systems have implemented proactive "Communication and Resolution Programs" (CRP) to promote transparent communication with patients after medical injuries, offering an explanation from the investigations and, when relevant, apologizing and offering compensation.[19]

Nevertheless, more work is needed to support widespread inclusion of patients and their feedback, which is being taken forward by many healthcare systems. Within the NHS, patient safety partners are being developed to act as key patient participants within all areas including the perioperative environment, helping to support and coproduce safety improvements.

Improvement

Continuous and sustainable improvement in patient safety is vital in health care, so that everyone is reliably learning from insights to provide safer care in the future. Quality improvement methodology provides the framework on which successful changes have been built to ensure maximum impact. The collaborative work on the Emergency Laparotomy Pathway Quality Improvement Care bundle,[20] which has been shown to be effective in reducing mortality and length of stay, is a classic example of how this approach to safety works.

Anesthetists have championed human factor approaches to patient safety and, in 2010, the anesthetists' nontechnical skills (ANTS)[21] taxonomy and behavior rating tool was developed, which is used for training, workplace assessment, self-reflection, simulator debriefing, and incident analysis.

The Royal College of Anaesthetists has developed a Quality Improvement Compendium[22] that provides clear, evidence-based practical implementation across 13 areas of care to improve standardization and reduce variation. In addition, human factor ergonomics such as the optimization of the design of processes, equipment, and the environment have been used to improve both the safety and efficiency of surgical and anesthetic care.[23]

Patient safety is multifaceted and is often considered a catch-all concept for anything that involves risk. Nevertheless, it is integral to everything we do for our patients from the decision that surgery is the appropriate treatment to postoperative recovery and rehabilitation. Every step of this pathway has risks and opportunities, and we need to understand that all the improvements we have made in patient safety mean that very few of the millions of surgical patients suffer harm and when they do, we have processes in place to help us continue to improve.

References

1. World Health Organization. WHO guidelines for safe surgery 2009: safe surgery saves lives. https://apps. who.int/iris/bitstream/handle/10665/44185/9789241598552_eng.pdf; jsessionid¼0FACE586F33322FEA2396333C5F88286?sequence¼1. Accessed 12 April 2021.
2. NHS England and NHS Improvement. Never Events policy and framework; 2018. https://www.england. nhs.uk/wp-content/uploads/2020/11/Revised-Never-Events-policy-and-framework-FINAL.pdf. Accessed 11 May 2021.
3. NHS England and NHS Improvement. National safety standards for invasive procedures (NatSSIPs); 2015. https://webarchive.nationalarchives.gov.uk/20160604221242/https:/www.england. nhs.uk/patientsafety/never-events/natssips/. Accessed 12 April 2021.
4. NHS England and NHS Improvement. The NHS patient safety strategy: safer culture, safer systems, safer patients; 2019. https://www.england.nhs.uk/wp-content/uploads/2020/08/190708_Patient_Safety_ Strategy_for_website_v4.pdf. Accessed 12 April 2021.
5. The Health Foundation. Safety culture: what is it and how do we monitor and measure it? 2013. https:// www.health.org.uk/publications/safety-culture-what-is-it-and-how-do-we-monitor-and-measure-it. Accessed 12 April 2021.
6. NHS England and NHS Improvement. Just culture guide; 2018. https://improvement.nhs.uk/documents/ 2490/NHS_0690_IC_A5_web_version.pdf. Accessed 12 April 2021.
7. Muensterer OJ, Kreutz H, Poplawski A, Goedeke J. Timeout procedure in paediatric surgery: effective tool or lip service? A randomised prospective observational study; 2021. https://qualitysafety.bmj.com/content/ qhc/early/2021/02/25/bmjqs-2020-012001.full.pdf. Accessed 21 April 2021.
8. Weinger M. Time out! Rethinking surgical safety: more than just a checklist; 2021. https://qualitysafety. bmj.com/content/qhc/early/2021/03/22/bmjqs-2020-012600.full.pdf. Accessed 21 April 2021.
9. Dixon-Woods M. Perspectives on context: the problem of context in quality improvement. The Health Foundation Inspiring Movement; 2014. https://www.health.org.uk/sites/default/files/PerspectivesOn ContextDixonWoodsTheProblemOfContextInQualityImprovement.pdf. Accessed 10 May 2021.
10. Ramsay G, Haynes AB, Lipsitz SR, et al. Reducing surgical mortality in Scotland by use of the WHO surgical safety checklist. *Br Surg.* 2019;106(8):1005–1011.
11. The King's Fund. Integrating care throughout the patient's surgical journey; 2016. https://www.kingsfund. org.uk/events/integrating-care-throughout-patients-surgical-journey. Accessed 21 April 2021.
12. NHS England and NHS Improvement. NRLS national patient safety incident reports: commentary; 2020. https://www.england.nhs.uk/wp-content/uploads/2020/03/NAPSIR-commentary-Sept-2020-FINAL. pdf. Accessed 11 May 2021.
13. Hibbert PD, Healey F, Lamont T, Marela WM, Warner B, Runciman WB. Patient safety's missing link: using clinical expertise to recognize, respond to and reduce risks at a population level. *Int J Qual Health Care.* 2016;28(1):114–121.
14. National Patient Safety Alert. Foreign body aspiration during intubation, advanced airway management or ventilation; 2020. https://www.england.nhs.uk/wp-content/uploads/2020/09/Foreign-Body-Aspiration-NaPSA-September-2020-v3.pdf. Accessed 21 April 2021.

15. National Patient Safety Alert. Wrong selection of orthopaedic fracture fixation plates; 2019. https://www.england.nhs.uk/wp-content/uploads/2019/12/Patient_Safety_Alert_-_Fracture_fixation_plates_FINAL_v2.pdf. Accessed 28 April 2021.

16. Introducing NHS England and NHS Improvement. Introducing National Patient Safety Alerts and the role of the National Patient Safety Alerting Committee. https://www.england.nhs.uk/patient-safety/national-patientsafety-alerting-committee/. Accessed 11 May 2021.

17. O'Hara JK, Aase K, Waring J. Scaffolding our systems? Patients and families 'reaching in' as a source of healthcare resilience. *BMJ Qual Saf.* 2019;28(1):3–6. https://qualitysafety.bmj.com/content/28/1/3. Accessed 21 April 2021.

18. Care Quality Commission. Regulation 20: duty of candour; 2014. https://www.cqc.org.uk/guidanceproviders/regulations-enforcement/regulation-20-duty-candour. Accessed 28 April 2021.

19. Kachalia A, Sands K, Niel MV, et al. Effects of a communication-and-resolution program on hospitals' malpractice claims and costs. *Health Aff.* 2018;37:1836–1844.

20. Aggarwal G, Peden CJ, Mohammed MA, et al. Evaluation of the collaborative use of an evidence-based care bundle in emergency laparotomy. *JAMA Surg.* 2019;154, e190145.

21. Flin R, Patey R, Glavin R, Maran N. Anaesthetists' non-technical skills. *Br J Anaesth.* 2010;105(1):38–44.

22. Chereshneva M, Johnston C, Colvin J, Peden CJ (eds.). RCoA Quality Improvement Compendium. The Royal College of Anaesthetists, London; 2020. https://rcoa.ac.uk/sites/default/files/documents/2020-08/21075%20RCoA%20Audit%20Recipe%20Book_Combined_Final_25.08.2020_0.pdf. Accessed 6 September 2021.

23. Marshall SD, Touzell A. Human factors and the safety of surgical and anaesthetic care. *Anaesthesia.* 2020;75 (Suppl. 1):e34–e38.

CHAPTER 3

What Is Perioperative Medicine and Why Do We Need It?

Michael P.W. Grocott, MBBS, MD, FRCA, FRCP, FFICM ▪
Denny Z.H. Levett, BM BCh, PhD, MRCP, FRCA

KEY POINTS

- Perioperative medicine is the medical care of patients undergoing surgery from the moment of contemplation of surgery until full recovery.
- The term "perioperative care" is increasingly used instead of perioperative medicine to emphasize the multidisciplinary nature of care across the patient's surgical journey and to acknowledge the role of nonmedical healthcare professionals in delivery.
- Reframing the period before surgery as an active opportunity, rather than a passive delay, is emphasized by the concept of "preparation lists," in contrast to the traditional notion of "waiting lists."
- Comprehensive screening and assessment before surgery enables fully informed shared decision making, targeted preparation for surgery (including management of comorbidities and prehabilitation), and rehabilitation after surgery.

Introduction

The idea that care should be structured around patient need, rather than provider convenience, seems self-evident when we consider ourselves as sometime consumers of health care. In practice, however, this aim is frequently not achieved. Within hospitals, funding is siloed in departments or divisions that are typically identified by clinical activities (e.g., surgery) rather than patient needs (e.g., cancer diagnosis, treatment and management). The integration of primary and secondary care is much talked about but often limited in practice. Specialists practice within a defined workplace environment that rarely maps onto a patients' experience of a pathway of care. At the heart of perioperative medicine is the notion that patient-centered care is by definition pathway-focused, multidisciplinary, and integrated (primary and second care) because that is how patients experience health care.[1]

Perioperative medicine is the medical care of patients undergoing surgery from the moment of contemplation of surgery until full recovery.[2,3] This definition excludes the conduct of the operation/procedure itself but encompasses the medical care of patients before, during, and after the procedure. Of note, the term "perioperative care" is increasingly used instead of perioperative medicine because it emphasizes the multidisciplinary nature of such activities and appropriately acknowledges the role of nonmedical healthcare professionals in care delivery. The temporal scope of this definition is important. The time available between the first contemplation of surgery and the procedure itself is often substantial, whereas the time actively used to prepare for surgery is typically very limited. Taking advantage of the whole pathway from first contemplation of surgery until full recovery offers numerous opportunities to improve clinical outcomes and experience of care both directly, in relation to the surgery, and in relation to health more generally.[4] Reframing of the period before surgery as an active opportunity, rather than a passive delay, is emphasized by the concept of "preparation lists," in contrast to the traditional notion of "waiting lists."[5]

A huge amount of resource is concentrated into a short period of time for the delivery of procedures in secondary care, with a substantial team required to enable the safe and effective delivery of surgery. Nevertheless, although adverse outcomes are, in part, associated with the nature, magnitude, and duration of the surgical procedure, a key determinant is the patients' resilience to the physiological (and psychological) challenge of surgery and anesthesia.[6] The interaction between the operative stress and the patients' resilience to it will determine outcomes from surgery, and characterizing individual patient risks for these outcomes underpins needs-based perioperative care. Comprehensive screening and assessment before surgery can effectively characterize the risks of different types of complications and should be achieved as early in the pathway as possible. This, in turn, enables fully informed shared decision making[7] and targeted preparation for surgery, including management of comorbidities and prehabilitation.[8] Efficient allocation of scarce secondary care resources, including priority operating room slots and critical care beds, benefits from clarity in relation to patient and surgical risk. In a well-managed pathway, all this feeds through to enhanced recovery and supports discharge and rehabilitation plans, maximizing the chance of a rapid and full recovery.[9]

Background

From a public/population health perspective, the consequences of outcomes after surgery are substantial and increasing. The global burden of surgery was estimated at 234 million in 2004,[10] which by 2012 had grown to 312 million procedures.[11] Mortality within 30 days of surgery is recognized as being one of the top three leading causes of death globally,[12] and complications after surgery are a burden on patients, increase costs (two- to threefold),[13] and are associated with increased subsequent mortality.[14,15] There is a clear and present challenge and a solution on offer.

The care of patients around the time of surgery has traditionally been the responsibility of the surgeon, with different individuals and specialties engaging to varying degrees. The integrated preoperative evaluation and optimization of comorbidities, health behaviors (prehabilitation), and rehabilitation have received less attention as greater focus has been placed on the technical aspects of surgical procedures and immediate perioperative care. This tendency has been amplified as healthcare professionals have become increasingly specialized and the integrated care of patients throughout the surgical pathway has been identified as an unmet need. Perioperative care is evolving to fill this gap.

Alongside the changes in individual specialist practice, the scale and scope of surgical activity has dramatically increased because of the evolving nature of the patient population and the innovative nature of surgical practice. Population structure has altered with more older patients[16] and an ever-increasing comorbidity burden[17]: the number of years lived with comorbidities is growing year-on-year. Surgical innovation has developed new procedures with extraordinary adoption and spread. For example, the first modern knee replacement was conducted in 1969,[18] and it is estimated that in 2030 more than 3.4 million knee replacements per year are projected to be conducted in the United States.[19] Moreover, surgeries previously considered to be high-risk, and therefore restricted to younger and healthier patients, are increasingly being safely conducted in older and sicker patients because of advances in perioperative and critical care. The in-hospital mortality rate for major cancer surgical procedures is falling despite considerable expansion of the indications for surgery into older and less healthy patients.[20]

Processes of care have also changed. Same-day admission to hospital became the norm in the late 1990s and early 2000s and yielded substantial savings in terms of bed usage.[21] With this, came the need for outpatient preassessment with dedicated clinics and an increasing focus on preoperative testing and the consent process. The concept of "enhanced recovery" developed over this time period and was probably first adopted on a system level through the National Health Service Enhanced Recovery Partnership Program between 2009 and 2011.[22] The combination of improved preparation through expectation management, minimization of fasting and dehydration before surgery, anesthetic and surgical techniques focused on minimizing physiological disturbance (e.g., minimally invasive and laparoscopic surgery, use of regional/local anesthetic techniques), and early mobilization and resumption of normal diet after surgery have been shown to improve patient experience of care and reduce duration of hospital stay, without any increase in readmissions.[23] Such approaches are now largely accepted as the "new normal."

Perioperative Medicine/Care

Perioperative care has built on these foundations, and the nature of care around the time of surgery is now well-recognized to have a substantial impact on clinical outcomes and patient experience. Much of the focus of perioperative care has been in the preoperative period. As the opportunities for beneficial intervention before surgery have become clear, the notion of pathway redesign has been proposed to highlight the importance of maximizing this opportunity by lengthening the time available for effective intervention. This, in turn, leads directly to the emphasis on engaging with the patient as soon as possible after the "moment of contemplation" of surgery, the first time that an operative solution becomes part of the likely future care of a patient's problem. Early engagement enables early screening, which, in turn, determines the nature of the pathway to surgery and beyond or may result in a nonsurgical pathway. Increasingly, screening processes use the most efficient approach available in a flexible manner, meaning that many patients may complete this process virtually using appropriate technological solutions. Patients who screen as low-risk in terms of health behaviors and morbidity burden may need very little subsequent preparation for surgery and minimal preassessment. Patients who are identified as being possibly or definitely at elevated risk in one or more areas progress to more detailed assessment, which, in turn, dictates which perioperative interventions are needed. Comprehensive screening and assessment should effectively identify and characterize perioperative risks, leading to a structured approach to mitigating these risks through ensuring that the best decisions are made about the subsequent approach to treating the primary pathology (shared decision making) and that physiological and psychological resilience to the surgery are maximized through management of long-term conditions (comorbidity management) and improvement of health behaviors (prehabilitation).

Effective screening and assessment are also fundamental to the delivery of intraoperative and postoperative care. For example, the risk of adverse outcomes during and immediately after surgery determines the level of monitoring during surgery (e.g., arterial and central venous pressure monitoring), the selection of analgesic techniques (e.g., central/peripheral blocks vs. systemic analgesia), and hemodynamic management (e.g., goal-directed therapy, pressor infusions). Postoperative care needs to balance the benefits of early mobilization and resumption of normal diet delivered by enhanced recovery approaches with the need for intensive monitoring and targeted interventions offered by postoperative augmented care environments, including intensive care, high-dependency settings, and overnight extended recovery units. Technology, in the form of wearable monitors and enhanced predictive algorithms, may offer significant benefits in balancing these contrasting approaches. Finally, the journey back to previous normal life, which is what patients expect to experience after surgery, is facilitated by targeted rehabilitation, careful attention to drug management, avoidance where possible of discharge opioids, and early attention to discharge planning, particularly if this requires additional resources such as care in the home or discharge to a care facility.

Conclusion

Perioperative care meets the aims of the Institute of Healthcare Improvement (IHI) "triple aim" to optimize health system performance[24] by improving the patient experience of care (quality and satisfaction), improving the health of the population, and reducing the per capita cost of health care. The challenge now is to reliably and effectively deliver perioperative care to all of our surgical patients all of the time.

References

1. Grocott MP. Pathway redesign: putting patients ahead of professionals. *Clin Med (Lond).* 2019;19 (6):468–547.
2. The Royal College of Anaesthetists. *Perioperative medicine. The pathway to better surgical care.* London: RCoA; 2015. https://www.rcoa.ac.uk/sites/default/files/documents/2019-08/Perioperative%20Medicine%20-%20The%20Pathway%20to%20Better%20Care.pdf. Accessed May 23, 2022.
3. Grocott MPW, Pearse RM. Perioperative medicine: the future of anaesthesia? *BJA.* 2012;108(5):723–726.
4. Grocott MPW, Plumb JOM, Edwards M, Fecher-Jones I, Levett DZH. Re-designing the pathway to surgery: better care and added value. *Perioper Med (Lond).* 2017;6:9.
5. Levy N, Selwyn DA, Lobo DN. Turning 'waiting list' for elective surgery into 'preparation lists'. *Br J Anaesthesia.* 2021;126(1):1–5.
6. Richardson K, Levett DZH, Jack S, Grocott MPW. Fit for surgery? Perspectives on preoperative exercise testing and training. *Br J Anaesth.* 2017;119(suppl 1):i34–i43.
7. Santhirapala R, Fleisher LA, Grocott MPW. Choosing wisely: just because we can, does it mean we should? *Br J Anaesth.* 2019;122(3):306–310.
8. Levett DZ, Edwards M, Grocott M, Mythen M. Preparing the patient for surgery to improve outcomes. *Best Pract Res Clin Anaesthesiol.* 2016;30(2):145–157.
9. Grocott MP, Martin DS, Mythen MG. Enhanced recovery pathways as a way to reduce surgical morbidity. *Curr Opin Crit Care.* 2012;18(4):385–392.
10. Weiser TG, Regenbogen SE, Thompson KD, et al. An estimation of the global volume of surgery: a modelling strategy based on available data. *Lancet.* 2008;372(9633):139–144.
11. Weiser TG, Haynes AB, Molina G, et al. Size and distribution of the global volume of surgery in 2012. *Bull World Health Organ.* 2016;94(3):201–209F.
12. Nepogodiev D, Martin J, Biccard B, et al. Global burden of postoperative death. *Lancet.* 2019;393:401.
13. Eappen S, Lane BH, Rosenberg B, et al. Relationship between occurrence of surgical complications and hospital finances. *JAMA.* 2013;309:1599–1606.
14. Khuri SF, Henderson WG, DePalma RG, et al. Determinants of long-term survival after major surgery and the adverse effect of postoperative complications. *Ann Surg.* 2005;242:326–341, discussion 41–43.
15. Moonesinghe SR, Harris S, Mythen MG, et al. Survival after postoperative morbidity: a longitudinal observational cohort study. *Br J Anaesth.* 2014;113:977–984.
16. Fowler AJ, Abbott TEF, Prowle J, Pearse RM. Age of patients undergoing surgery. *Br J Surg.* 2019;106:1012–1018.
17. Barnett K, Mercer SW, Norbury M, et al. Epidemiology of multimorbidity and implications for health care, research, and medical education: a cross-sectional study. *Lancet.* 2012;380(9836):37–43.
18. Walker PS. Requirements for successful total knee replacements. *Design considerations Orthop Clin North Am.* 1989;20(1):15–29.
19. Kurtz S, Ong K, Lau E, Mowat F, Halpern M. Projections of primary and revision hip and knee arthroplasty in the United States from 2005 to 2030. *J Bone Joint Surg Am.* 2007;89(4):780–785.
20. Learn PA, Bach PB. A decade of mortality reductions in major oncologic surgery: the impact of centralization and quality improvement. *Med Care.* 2010;48(12):1041–1049.
21. Kerridge R, Lee A, Latchford E, Beehan SJ, Hillman KM. The perioperative system: a new approach to managing elective surgery. *Anaesth Intensive Care.* 1995;23(5):591–596.

22. Simpson JC, Moonesinghe SR, Grocott MP, et al. Enhanced recovery from surgery in the UK: an audit of the enhanced recovery partnership programme 2009–2012. *Br J Anaesth.* 2015;115(4):560–568.
23. Levy N, Mills P, Mythen M. Is the pursuit of DREAMing (drinking, eating and mobilising) the ultimate goal of anaesthesia? *Anaesthesia.* 2016;71(9):1008–1012.
24. Grocott MPW, Edwards M, Mythen MG, Aronson S. Peri-operative care pathways: re-engineering care to achieve the 'triple aim'. *Anaesthesia.* 2019;74(suppl 1):90–99.

CHAPTER 4

The Case for Improvement in Perioperative Medicine

Aman Mahajan, MD, PhD, MBA ■ Stephen A. Esper, MD, MBA

KEY POINTS

- Despite enormous strides in the reduction of intraoperative risk, the incidence of postoperative complications remains high and perioperative care is frequently fragmented.
- Significant variability in healthcare outcomes across different hospitals and hospital systems exists.
- Relatively new tools of improvement science, implementation science, and safety science should be accelerators of change and integrate into evidence-based pathways of care.
- Fundamental interventions include:
  - proactive engagement in a patient's health and optimization for surgery
  - segmenting patients based on complexity and risk
  - implementation of data-driven and evidence-based perioperative pathways
  - positively affecting population health by using the surgical experience to reengage patients in their own health care

Introduction

Health care in the United States (US) is in the midst of a momentous change with an imperative to refocus our approaches on the best care for patients within a value-based framework.[1,2] The dawn of new payment models and care delivery pathways serves as the agent of change to drive for value-based care. There are high expectations from patients, hospital services, and insurance payors for physicians to develop clinical programs and pathways that improve outcomes and reduce costs. Although anesthesiologists have made enormous strides over the past decades in reducing intraoperative risk, the incidence of postoperative complications remains high and perioperative care continues to be fragmented. The opportunity exists for anesthesiologists to advance perioperative care and impact the long-term health of surgical patients. The ongoing novel coronavirus (COVID-19) pandemic and its associated shutdown of surgical care in the year 2020 exposed the vulnerabilities of our hospital systems that largely rely on the fee-for-service model (focusing on volume over value) to generate revenue. It further established the need for acceleration of value-based care with the Centers for Medicare and Medicaid Services (CMS) providing guidance so that Medicare, Medicaid, and private insurance payers can work in tandem with one another and also calling on the state healthcare services to advance value-based care payment models.[3] The impact of the COVID-19 pandemic on surgical practices further highlights the urgency and need for anesthesiologists to expand their role in perioperative care.

Increasing Healthcare Costs and Poor Outcomes

Healthcare spending in the US has reached approximately $11,559 USD per person for a total of $3.81trillion USD in 2019,[4] which is actually projected to nearly double over the next 10 years to over $6.2 trillion USD. Despite these increased costs, it has not translated to an improvement in health and health care. To assess population health, the members of the Organisation for Economic Co-Operation and Development (OECD) use life expectancy. In spite of its increased spend, the US life expectancy remains low compared with the other countries that make up the OECD.[5–10]

Perioperative mortality and morbidity status after surgery remain a key concern despite the significant technological advancements and abundant new treatments in surgical and anesthesia care. For example, of the annual approximately 60 million mortal events worldwide, around 25% are caused by heart attack and stroke (the two leading causes).[11] Shockingly, the third leading cause is 30-day postoperative mortality, laying infamous claim to 4.2 million, or approximately 8%, of all global deaths.[11] Indeed, in the US, 30-day postoperative mortality is third behind heart disease and cancer.[12] There is significant variability in healthcare outcomes across different hospitals and hospital systems, which accounts for the high incidence of postoperative complications and mortality.[13,14] Additionally, many surgical procedures that were performed may not be associated with improved quality of life or quantity in life years and, as a result, may be of low or no value.[15]

There are many reasons for poor outcomes. Traditional perioperative care focuses on the short episode of the surgical event; fragmented, siloed, and idiosyncratic, much of it is driven by the culture of a physician/institution or by focus on reimbursement. Consider two examples. In the first, the surgeon operates on a patient because they do not want to lose referrals from a specific practice. In the second, the surgical team refers the patient to multiple specialists but perhaps not to an anesthesiologist, in which case those referrals may not be very effective if they do not optimally prepare the patient for the surgery. Perioperative care is frequently marred by avoidable and costly events—patients do not receive the right care, their care is not coordinated (leading to dissatisfaction), procedures/tests of questionable benefit are performed, prolonged hospital stays are caused by complications, or unnecessary readmissions and reinterventions occur, which may cause further complications and even mortality. The lack of standardization and high variability of routine clinical practice that repeatedly occurs within the realm of perioperative medicine has been shown to negatively affect both outcomes and costs.[16–21] In truth, the perioperative period sees care providers acting independently and without coordination or best evidence for practice, which incurs expenses and inefficiencies because of poor coordination of care and the subsequent avoidable errors that are introduced into the system. This deficiency results in increased hospital-acquired conditions, hospital readmissions, added costs, and increased patient mortality, all of which both put an unnecessary strain on scarce health resources and, even more importantly, on the single patient.

Variability in health care is strongly associated with poor outcomes and perioperative care is significantly burdened by lack of consistency and standardization.[20,22] An interinstitutional difference in failure to rescue from complications after surgery has been cited as a major reason for poor postoperative outcomes in some hospitals. Among nearly 4500 US hospitals, although types and rates of postsurgical complications were similar (24%–26%), mortality rates ranged from 12.5% to 21.4%.[22] There are other barriers to practice that may account for such variability, found by comparing safety profiles of surgical procedures and anesthesia to other unrelated medical fields. For example, cardiac surgery in an American Society of Anesthesiology (ASA) Class III-V is only slightly safer than Himalayan mountaineering above 8000 meters, but it is less safe than traveling by planes, trains, and automobiles, and is over 1000-fold less safe than the nuclear industry.[23] An important role for anesthesiologists going forward is to try to address the variability in perioperative practices and partner with the other stakeholders to reduce the overall risk for the patients. Relatively new tools of improvement science, implementation science, and safety science should be accelerators of change and integrate into evidence-based pathways of care for medical and surgical conditions.

Addressing the Gap Through Innovations in Perioperative Care

Through a few key approaches in the perioperative period, anesthesiologists can make a significant impact on the health of their surgical patients. Some of the fundamental interventions effectively instituted by the anesthesiologists include proactively engaging in a patient's health and optimization for surgery; segmenting patients based on complexity and risk, thereby personalizing and standardizing care delivery; implementing data-driven and evidence-based perioperative pathways to allow for best recovery, not only through the immediate postoperative period but also beyond; and positively affecting population health by using the surgical experience to effectively reengage patients in their own health care through education. Through collaborative relationships with other perioperative stakeholders, anesthesiologists can consolidate their role as clinical leaders driving value-based care and healthcare transformation for the surgical patients.

First, and importantly, is the ability to practice population health via perioperative medicine and to encourage patients to take responsibility for their own health as they engage in a perioperative care processes. Many surgeries are life-altering experiences for patients; it may be the first experience patients have of grappling with their own health. We can use that sentinel surgical experience as a touchpoint to proactively improve patient health to not only improve the short-term surgical episode but also prevent another disease or more serious procedure from occurring. This is in opposition to the largely practiced reactive medicine, which uses the preoperative encounter to only gather information and perform laboratory testing to prevent same-day delay or cancellation. Second, segmenting patients based on risk (low vs. high) not only helps to personalize care but also improves hospital efficiencies and can lower healthcare costs. Finally, for the patient to have the best recovery possible, an evidence-based approach to the standardization of processes for routine care and implementation of in-hospital and value-based perioperative pathways should be implemented, guided by processes of facilitated data gathering and analysis. By using intensive clinical databases to stratify risk, reduce silo-driven care, and coordinate the entire perioperative process while proactively helping the patient move in a positive direction for their health, the focus becomes the longitudinal episode of care, over years, as opposed to the short, immediate perioperative episode, which ends at discharge. This may even start before the final decision to undergo surgery, and we must be able to provide the patient with resources to understand the perioperative journey from best case to worse case.[24]

Only by understanding the patient's goals, needs, values, and lifestyle can we make their health care work within a value-based framework. Many elements of perioperative medicine have been implemented at different institutions, and those that have employed comprehensive approaches to perioperative health have garnered success.[25–27] As an example, at the University of Pittsburgh Medical Center's Center for Perioperative Care, which encompasses outpatient clinics and in-patient perioperative services, the care for the surgical patient includes taking a holistic view of the patient, modifying risk and lifestyle, and reengaging the patient in their community care[2,28] (Fig. 4.1). Using machine-learning predictive algorithms and protocol-driven care, the program's goals are to: (1) identify patients who are at high risk for poor surgical outcomes, encouraging a "surgical pause" for the opportunity to mitigate risk; (2) provide a comprehensive menu of services aimed at improving both physiologic and psychosocial conditions that contribute to vulnerability of high risk before their nonurgent or even urgent surgical procedure (e.g., comprehensive medical assessment, measurement of frailty and cognitive status, nutrition and weight management, cardiopulmonary rehabilitation, chronic pain and opioid management, substance use, mental health evaluation, and supportive care [finances, transportation, and postoperative planning]); (3) provide at-risk patients with a supportive "surgery coach," who guides patients, readying them for their surgical episode; and (4) engage an anesthesiologist-directed multidisciplinary team to work in concert with the patient in a shared decision-making approach. In the intraoperative and postoperative

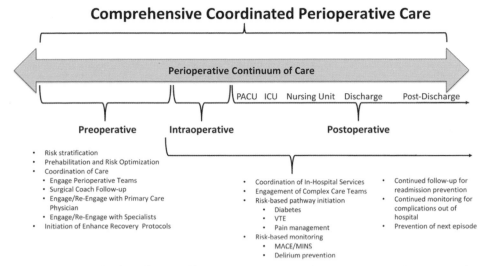

Fig. 4.1 Coordinated perioperative care with targeted population health interventions and risk-based care pathways during the surgical episode of care that can improve patient outcomes.

period, tailored clinical pathways and enhanced recovery protocols instituted on patients help with reduction of stress through the surgical episode and improvement of outcomes. This has led to reduction in postoperative complications, length of stay, 30-day mortality, and 1-year mortality and an improvement in discharge to home compared with a long-term care facility.[26]

Conclusion

Perioperative care for surgical patients needs to get better in US healthcare systems to improve outcomes. Anesthesiologists have much to contribute to the health of surgical patients because their focus extends from the operating room to the expanded continuum of care. Targeted strategies for enhancing perioperative value-based care through coordinated preoperative and postoperative interventions have shown that surgical outcomes can be improved. Meanwhile, the drivers for change in US health care continue to move the delivery systems to payment models with increased value-base care, alternative payment, and risk-based models in nearly every US market. The case for advancing perioperative medicine is as strong as it has ever been.

References

1. Fleisher LA, Lee TH. Anesthesiology and anesthesiologists in the era of value-driven health care. *Healthc (Amst).* 2015;3(2):63–66.
2. Mahajan A, Esper SA, Cole DJ, Fleisher LA. Anesthesiologists' role in value-based perioperative care and healthcare transformation. *Anesthesiology.* 2021;134(4):526–540.
3. Centers for Medicare & Medicaid Services. CMS issues new roadmap for states to accelerate adoption of value-based care to improve quality of care for Medicaid beneficiaries; 2020. https://www.cms.gov/newsroom/press-releases/cms-issues-new-roadmap-states-accelerate-adoption-value-based-care-improve-quality-care-medicaid. Accessed December 7, 2020.
4. Centers for Medicare & Medicaid Services. National health expenditure data; 2020. https://www.cms.gov/Research-Statistics-Data-and-Systems/Statistics-Trends-and-Reports/NationalHealthExpendData/NHE-Fact-Sheet. Updated March 24, 2020. Accessed March 29, 2020.
5. Adedeji WA. The Treasure called antibiotics. *Ann Ib Postgrad Med.* 2016;14(2):56–57.

6. Cutler D, Miller G. The role of public health improvements in health advances: The twentieth-century United States. *Demography.* 2005;42(1):1–22.

7. Department of Health and Human Services NCfHS. National Vital Statistics Reports. In: Prevention CfDCa, ed2012.

8. Kontis V, Bennett JE, Mathers CD, Li G, Foreman K, Ezzati M. Future life expectancy in 35 industrialised countries: projections with a Bayesian model ensemble. *Lancet.* 2017;389(10076):1323–1335.

9. Rappuoli R, Pizza M, Del Giudice G, De Gregorio E. Vaccines, new opportunities for a new society. *Proc Natl Acad Sci U S A.* 2014;111(34):12288–12293.

10. Roser M, Ortiz-Ospina E, Ritchie H. Life expectancy; 2020. https://ourworldindata.org/life-expectancy#what-drives-improvements-in-life-expectancy. Accessed April 2, 2020.

11. Nepogodiev D, Martin J, Biccard B, Makupe A, Bhangu A. National Institute for Health Research Global Health Research Unit on Global Surgery. Global burden of postoperative death. *Lancet.* 2019;393 (10170):401.

12. Bartels K, Karhausen J, Clambey ET, Grenz A, Eltzschig HK. Perioperative organ injury. *Anesthesiology.* 2013;119(6):1474–1489.

13. Fry BT, Smith ME, Thumma JR, Ghaferi AA, Dimick JB. Ten-year trends in surgical mortality, complications, and failure to rescue in Medicare beneficiaries. *Ann Surg.* 2020;271(5):855–861.

14. Pearse RM, Moreno RP, Bauer P, et al. Mortality after surgery in Europe: a 7 day cohort study. *Lancet.* 2012;380(9847):1059–1065.

15. Shrank WH, Rogstad TL, Parekh N. Waste in the US health care system: estimated costs and potential for savings. *JAMA.* 2019;322(15):1501–1509. https://doi.org/10.1001/jama.2019.13978.

16. Kwon MA. Perioperative surgical home: a new scope for future anesthesiology. *Korean J Anesthesiol.* 2018;71(3):175–181.

17. McCulloch P, Nagendran M, Campbell WB, et al. Strategies to reduce variation in the use of surgery. *Lancet.* 2013;382(9898):1130–1139.

18. Fleischut PM, Eskreis-Winkler JM, Gaber-Baylis LK, et al. Variability in anesthetic care for total knee arthroplasty: an analysis from the anesthesia quality institute. *Am J Med Qual.* 2015;30(2):172–179.

19. Ladha KS, Bateman BT, Houle TT, et al. Variability in the use of protective mechanical ventilation during general anesthesia. *Anesth Analg.* 2018;126(2):503–512.

20. Lilot M, Ehrenfeld JM, Lee C, Harrington B, Cannesson M, Rinehart J. Variability in practice and factors predictive of total crystalloid administration during abdominal surgery: retrospective two-centre analysis. *Br J Anaesth.* 2015;114(5):767–776.

21. Sessler DI. Implications of practice variability. *Anesthesiology.* 2020;132(4):606–608.

22. Ghaferi AA, Birkmeyer JD, Dimick JB. Variation in hospital mortality associated with inpatient surgery. *N Engl J Med.* 2009;361(14):1368–1375.

23. Amalberti R, Auroy Y, Berwick D, Barach P. Five system barriers to achieving ultrasafe health care. *Ann Intern Med.* 2005;142(9):756–764.

24. Taylor LJ, Nabozny MJ, Steffens NM, et al. A framework to improve surgeon communication in high-stakes surgical decisions: best case/worst case. *JAMA Surg.* 2017;152(6):531–538.

25. Aronson S, Westover J, Guinn N, et al. A perioperative medicine model for population health: an integrated approach for an evolving clinical science. *Anesth Analg.* 2018;126(2):682–690.

26. Esper SA, Holder-Murray J, Subramaniam K, et al. Enhanced recovery protocols reduce mortality across eight surgical specialties at academic and university-affiliated community hospitals. *Ann Surg.* 2020. https://doi.org/10.1097/SLA.0000000000004642.

27. Brigham and Women's Hospital, Department of Anesthesiology, Perioperative and Pain Medicine. Anesthesiology, perioperative, and pain medicine; 2020. https://www.brighamandwomens.org/anesthesiology-perioperative-and-pain-medicine. Accessed June 13, 2020.

28. Varley PR, Borrebach JD, Arya S, et al. Clinical utility of the risk analysis index as a prospective frailty screening tool within a multi-practice, multi-hospital integrated healthcare system. *Ann Surg.* 2021;274 (6):e1230–e1237. https://doi.org/10.1097/SLA.0000000000003808.

CHAPTER 5

The Promise and Pitfalls of Big Data Studies in Perioperative Medicine

Michael Mathis, MD ■ Allison Janda, MD ■ Sachin Kheterpal, MD, MBA

KEY POINTS

- Because of a paucity of randomized controlled trial (RCT) literature in perioperative medicine, well-designed "big data" studies can fill an important void.
- Robust, validated perioperative registries can be the foundation of research to inform perioperative practice patterns in clinical areas for which equipoise currently exists.
- Consensus reporting guidelines offer a structured method to assess the quality of research and quality improvement (QI) studies using big data.
- Novel analytic techniques combined with diverse health data sets present unique insights as to how perioperative care can be individualized and optimized.
- Platform prospective pragmatic trials offer a unique way to advance perioperative medicine decision making.

"Big Data" Studies and Perioperative Clinical Equipoise

Although the quantity and quality of randomized controlled trials (RCTs) in perioperative medicine continues to rise, many fundamental clinical decisions continue to lack a robust evidence base. For example, inhaled volatile versus total intravenous (IV) general anesthesia remains a controversial clinical decision without large-scale RCTs. In the surgical realm, the choice between laparoscopic versus robot-assisted minimally invasive surgery continues to challenge consensus. In addition, the limited number of high-quality, reproducible clinical trials in perioperative medicine often lack the generalizability to inform the care of most patients or focus on the average treatment effects, which may hide risks to individual patients.

In the perioperative setting, big data studies can offer three forms of value: (1) describing clinical care variation; (2) forming hypothesis-generating inferences to inform the design of clinical trials; and (3) providing incremental evidence when prospective RCTs are infeasible or impractical. Simply describing national, regional, or clinician variation in care can provide vital knowledge and be the first step to reliable evidence. A given clinician may not realize that their own practice varies from local, regional, or national standards of care; however, clinician-specific feedback combined with peer-reviewed studies of variation in care can inform and improve clinician adherence to accepted standards of care.[1,2] Additionally, as clinical care evolves over time, clinician feedback and high-quality studies with recent and longitudinal data provide insight into dynamic rather than static care patterns as new evidence is applied. Next, observational research using large national databases can identify possible areas for future prospective trials. The field of "failure to rescue" research was inspired by rigorous observational analyses of administrative data[3] and surgical registries.[4] Since these seminal hypothesis-generating papers identifying the concept of failure to rescue, many interventions have been proposed and are undergoing rigorous prospective testing. Finally, some processes of care are difficult or prohibitively costly to evaluate using prospective clinical trials. For example, the relationship between overlapping surgery and postoperative adverse events remains unclear; there are ethical and practical challenges in randomizing patients to receive care from a surgeon involved in two overlapping procedures. As a result, research using data from millions of patients[5] has provided some evidence to guide the vigorously debated topic.

Perioperative Medicine Registries, Big Data, and Future Directions

Clearly, the use of big data in perioperative medicine assumes the availability of representative, validated, and analyzable big data sources. There is no clear, accepted consensus of what qualifies as a big data analysis. It could be based on a large number of patients included in the analysis (e.g., millions of patients), the sheer number of data elements evaluated (e.g., every 15 second intraoperative blood pressure values), or the diversity of data (e.g., national databases including hundreds of hospitals or clinics). Regardless of the definition, many of the challenges are similar. It is important to consider the variety of big data sources commonly used in perioperative medicine research: administrative, prospective registry, or electronic health records (EHRs; Table 5.1).

TABLE 5.1 ■ Examples of Big Data Sources in Perioperative Medicine Research

Name	Type
Society of Thoracic Surgeons–National Database (STS)	Registry
American College of Surgeons–National Surgical Quality Improvement Program (ACS-NSQIP)	Registry
American Academy of Orthopedic Surgeons–American Joint Replacement Registry (AJRR)	Registry
Scientific Registry of Transplant Recipients (SRTR)	Registry
American College of Surgeons National Trauma Data Bank (ACS-NTDB)	Registry
Surveillance, Epidemiology, and End Results Program (National Cancer Institute)	Registry
Danish National Patient Register (and associated databases)	Registry + Administrative
Swedish National Patient Register (and associated databases)	Registry + Administrative
UK National Audit Projects (NAP)	Registry
Center for Medicare and Medicaid Services Databases	Administrative
Marketscan (IBM)	Administrative
Premier Healthcare Database (Premier)	Administrative
Optum Research Database (United Health)	Administrative
Healthcare Cost and Utilization Project databases (AHRQ)	Administrative
ICES (Ontario Health Insurance Plan, formerly Institute for Clinical Evaluative Sciences)	Administrative
Patient Centered Outcomes Research Network	Administrative + Electronic Health Record
United Kingdom Biobank Multicenter Perioperative Outcomes Group	Electronic Health Record + Registry Electronic Health Record + Registry + Administrative

Administrative big data sources typically build on billing, compliance, reporting, or other administrative processes, which then generate data regarding patients, procedures, processes of care, and outcomes. Government or private payer databases such as those provided by the United States (US) Centers for Medicare & Medicaid Services (CMS), Canadian provincial health insurance plans, and United Healthcare (Optum) can provide long-term data regarding an individual's use of healthcare resources over time. Although these data are not generated for the purposes of clinical research, detailed diagnoses and procedure codes, prescription fulfillment, outpatient and inpatient acute care services, and mortality are valuable for clinical and health services research. The strengths and weaknesses of these administrative data sources are typically similar. Strengths include longitudinal data across multiple centers and clinicians and include excellent documentation of resource-intensive, expensive therapies (e.g., renal replacement therapy). Nevertheless, the administrative databases often fail to capture patient symptoms, severity of disease, or subtle nuances driving clinical decision-making (e.g., surgical complexity). The data are generated by administrative personnel based on clinical processes, but there is rarely adjudication or prospective validation of the data against "gold standard" truths such as clinician documentation.

Prospective clinical registries can range from the society-specific (e.g., American Joint Replacement Registry, National Surgical Quality Improvement Program [NSQIP],[6] or Society of Thoracic Surgeons) to the national condition specific (e.g., American Heart Association Get With the Guidelines, Danish Clinical Quality Program & National Clinical Registries[7]). These prospective registries are often driven by a shared epidemiology, quality improvement (QI), and research mission. These registries offer significant advantages over administrative databases: typically, some data validation and curation is performed and reported; data collection processes can be modified over time to enable research activities; and disease- or hypothesis-specific detailed information is included. Nevertheless, several challenges are also present. First, the significant resources required for data collection and validation may limit adoption of the registry to a sampling of facilities, clinicians, or patients. Second, financial costs are often prohibitive for many specialties or conditions. Third, the abstraction of detailed data into analyzable concepts (e.g. "acute renal failure" rather than individual serum creatinine values) prevents many analyses, or adaptation to evolving clinical definitions.

Finally, the widespread adoption of EHRs has enabled the creation of detailed big data resources. Granular, structured, searchable data elements offer researchers the flexibility to address many different clinical questions using EHRs. These databases can be single or multicenter. Many single-center EHR databases could be considered big data but do not offer the diversity of patients, care processes, or clinicians necessary for definitive generalizable conclusions. Within perioperative medicine, there are few multicenter EHR databases. The Patient-Centered Outcomes Research Institute-funded PCORnet has been used for surgical comparative effectiveness research[8] and the Multicenter Perioperative Outcomes Group (MPOG) database of more than 17 million patients has been used for a variety of anesthesiology, surgical, and health services research projects.[5,9,10] EHR-based big data research allows the consideration of a wide range of questions and can adapt to evolving clinical definitions and standards. There are many challenges as well. For multicenter databases, harmonizing variant documentation processes across centers is challenging and requires significant coordination. Although there are emerging EHR standards for the use of specific lexicons (e.g., ICD 10, RxNorm [https://www.nlm.nih.gov/research/umls/rxnorm/index.html], LOINC [https://loinc.org/get-started/what-loinc-is/]) and data structures for interoperability, individual hospitals, specialties, and clinicians have a variety of documentation standards. For example, although a bariatric surgery patient's history and physical may have detailed information regarding gastroesophageal reflux symptoms, a total joint arthroplasty patient's EHR may be focused on osteoarthritis symptoms. In addition, the widespread use of unstructured data (images, free text notes, or dictations) presents challenges to extracting consistent, meaningful information from the EHR for research.

Assessing the Quality of Big Data Research

Although large sample sizes may allow for well-powered statistical analyses, consumers of big data research should not be focused on statistical significance alone. Hypothesis-driven research with causal inferences based on directed acyclic graphs and a priori specified statistical analysis plans are the hallmark of reproducible and reliable research that may be clinically actionable (Fig. 5.1).[11,12] Hypothesis-generating research is also a valuable output of big data but requires appropriate, measured interpretations that drive future research efforts rather than clinical recommendations.

One challenge of big data analyses can be the proliferation of "statistically significant" associations lacking any biological plausibility, mechanistic insight, or clinical significance. Although complex statistical modeling may be possible because of large sample size, the interpretation of such models is fraught with challenges. Interpretation must be based on clear modeling goals: prediction, risk adjustment, or causal inference. The terms are often misused interchangeably and result in inappropriate conclusions. Recent work in epidemiology has advanced the standard that observational research must clearly define primary exposures of interest (e.g., potential causal factors) versus secondary exposures or confounders and then reporting must focus on these primary exposures.[13] Otherwise, confounders found to have statistical or effect size significance (e.g., association of vasopressors with adverse outcomes) may be incorrectly asserted to have a causal effect on the outcome of interest.

Finally, consumers of big data research should expect the use of industry standard reporting guidelines. Many are advanced by the EQUATOR (Enhancing the QUAlity and Transparency Of health Research) network, which previously published and implemented the CONSORT requirements for RCTs. Many readers are already familiar with the broadly applicable STROBE (The STrengthening the Reporting of OBservational studies in Epidemiology) guidelines, which provide specific recommendations for conduct, reporting, and interpretation. For example, disclosing the handling of missing data is an important aspect of observational big data research, which requires adherence to statistically accepted processes and transparent reporting. Increasingly, the STROBE guidelines are augmented by specific checklists for analyses using routinely collected data (RECORD [https://www.record-statement.org]), prediction analyses (TRIPOD [https://www.tripod-statement.org]), and QI (SQUIRE) (see Chapter 16 for more information on the SQUIRE guidelines). Consensus guidelines regarding the conduct and reporting of machine learning analyses are emerging.[14]

Machine Learning as a Powerful Tool, Not a Panacea

Although big data research is often assumed to use "machine learning" or "artificial intelligence," these are related but not synonymous domains. In many ways, even the concept of "machine

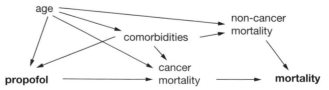

Fig. 5.1 An example of causal structure of a purported relationship between total intravenous anesthesia using propofol and postoperative mortality. There may be confounders such as age and comorbidities, which may affect mortality via mediators along the pathway of interest (cancer mortality) or by alternative pathways to the outcome (noncancer mortality). (Adapted from Gaskell AL, Sleigh JW. An introduction to causal diagrams for anesthesiology research. *Anesthesiology*. 2020;132(5):951–967.)

learning" as a novel technique is mistaken. Logistic and linear regression techniques, which can be computationally intensive, have been used for decades and are a form of machine learning. Nevertheless, the use of classification modeling techniques, deep learning, which creates new "features" from existing variables, natural language processing, and ensemble analytical techniques, which combine several models into a single "super model," are relatively new to clinical medicine. Enabled by rapid increases in computing power, these machine learning techniques can go beyond classic linear and logistic regressions to model unique, patient-specific associations including millions of variables. Recent perioperative machine learning success stories include intraoperative hypotension prediction and identifying which patients are most likely to benefit from a preoperative type and screen. Nevertheless, machine learning is just a tool and must be interpreted cautiously. In many cases, novel machine learning algorithms offer no incremental value over classic modeling techniques. Underlying data quality or missingness issues affect machine learning, similar to other techniques. And just like other prediction efforts, machine learning techniques should be validated in specific populations of interest before being deployed for widespread clinical use.[15] By modeling existing processes and outcome, these models can exacerbate existing systemic racism and bias in health care.[16]

The Emerging Future of Perioperative Medicine Integrates Big Data and Prospective Trials

Although big data research is often considered to focus on retrospective observational research, the advent of interoperable EHRs, adaptive clinical trial designs, and pragmatic cluster design trials opens up a new frontier integrating big data and prospective clinical trials. Several such registry-based prospective trial examples already exist in perioperative medicine. In the Flexibility in Duty Hour Requirements for Surgical Trainees (FIRST) trial, researchers used the NSQIP data collection infrastructure as the foundation for a cluster RCT of surgical resident work hours.[17] In a trial of surgical versus medical management of acute appendicitis, NSQIP definitions and processes were used to assess postoperative complications. Finally, in the recently announced THRIVE (Trajectories of Recovery after Intravenous Propofol vs inhaled VolatilE anesthesia) trial, the MPOG EHR data collection infrastructure will be used to assess patient-centered outcomes after two different general anesthesia options.

Many lessons have been learned in such platform-embedded trials.[18] First, big data information collection strategies can enable research into structures and processes of care that were previously considered beyond the realm of prospective, interventional research. Next, more patient-reported and patient-centered outcomes are essential to create evidence that impacts clinical decision making. Large-scale studies that include patient-reported outcomes using smartphones rather than researcher-mediated interviews, home healthcare devices such as ambulatory blood pressure monitors or continuous glucose monitors, ecological momentary assessments, and wearables may reflect a participant's experience before and after surgery far more closely than the occasional postoperative clinic visit.[19,20]

Conclusion

Big data resources are already widely available in perioperative medicine and research based on them is impacting daily care. Going forward, advances in EHRs, novel analytic techniques, patient-centered data, and integration with existing prospective research techniques will create new big data opportunities.

References

1. McCormick PJ, Yeoh C, Vicario-Feliciano RM, et al. Improved compliance with anesthesia quality measures after implementation of automated monthly feedback. *J Oncol Pract.* 2019;15(6):e583–e592.
2. Bender SP, Paganelli WC, Gerety LP, et al. Intraoperative lung-protective ventilation trends and practice patterns: a report from the multicenter perioperative outcomes group. *Anesth Analg.* 2015;121:1231–1239.
3. Silber JH, Williams SV, Krakauer H, Schwartz JS. Hospital and patient characteristics associated with death after surgery. A study of adverse occurrence and failure to rescue. *Med Care.* 1992;30(7):615–629.
4. Ghaferi AA, Birkmeyer JD, Dimick JB. Variation in hospital mortality associated with inpatient surgery. *N Engl J Med.* 2009;361(14):1368–1375.
5. Sun E, Mello MM, Rishel CA, et al, Multicenter Perioperative Outcomes Group (MPOG). Association of overlapping surgery with perioperative outcomes. *JAMA.* 2019;321:762–772.
6. Khuri SF, Henderson WG, Daley J, et al. Successful implementation of the department of veterans affairs' national surgical quality improvement program in the private sector: the patient safety in surgery study. *Ann Surg.* 2008;248(2):329–336.
7. Epidemiology Frank L. When an entire country is a cohort. *Science.* 2000;287(5462):2398–2399.
8. McTigue KM, Wellman R, Nauman E, et al. Comparing the 5-year diabetes outcomes of sleeve gastrectomy and gastric bypass: the national patient-centered clinical research network (PCORNet) bariatric study. *JAMA Surg.* 2020;155(5), e200087.
9. Colquhoun DA, Shanks AM, Kapeles SR, et al. Considerations for integration of perioperative electronic health records across institutions for research and quality improvement: the approach taken by the multicenter perioperative outcomes group. *Anesth Analg.* 2020;130(5):1133–1146.
10. Kheterpal S, Vaughn MT, Dubovoy TZ, et al. Sugammadex versus neostigmine for reversal of neuromuscular blockade and postoperative pulmonary complications (STRONGER) a multicenter matched cohort analysis. *Anesthesiology.* 2020;132(6):1371–1381.
11. Thomas L, Peterson ED. The value of statistical analysis plans in observational research: defining high-quality research from the start. *JAMA.* 2012;308(8):773–774.
12. Gaskell AL, Sleigh JW. An introduction to causal diagrams for anesthesiology research. *Anesthesiology.* 2020;132(5):951–967.
13. Westreich D, Greenland S. The table 2 fallacy: presenting and interpreting confounder and modifier coefficients. *Am J Epidemiol.* 2013;177(4):292–298.
14. Stevens LM, Mortazavi BJ, Deo RC, Curtis L, Kao DP. Recommendations for reporting machine learning analyses in clinical research. *Circ Cardiovasc Qual Outcomes.* 2020;13(10), e006556.
15. Paulus JK, Kent DM. Predictably unequal: understanding and addressing concerns that algorithmic clinical prediction may increase health disparities. *NPJ Digit Med.* 2020;3:99.
16. Obermeyer Z, Powers B, Vogeli C, Mullainathan S. Dissecting racial bias in an algorithm used to manage the health of populations. *Science.* 2019;366(6464):447–453.
17. Bilimoria KY, Chung JW, Hedges LV, et al. National cluster-randomized trial of duty-hour flexibility in surgical training. *N Engl J Med.* 2016;374(8):713–727.
18. Richesson RL, Marsolo KS, Douthit BJ, et al. Enhancing the use of EHR systems for pragmatic embedded research: lessons from the NIH health care systems research collaboratory. *J Am Med Inform Assoc.* 2021; 28(12):2626–2640.
19. Golbus JR, Pescatore NA, Nallamothu BK, Shah N, Kheterpal S. Wearable device signals and home blood pressure data across age, sex, race, ethnicity, and clinical phenotypes in the michigan predictive activity & clinical trajectories in health (MIPACT) study: a prospective, community-based observational study. *Lancet Digit Health.* 2021;3(11):e707–e715.
20. Karas M, Marinsek N, Goldhahn J, Foschini L, Ramirez E, Clay I. Predicting subjective recovery from lower limb surgery using consumer wearables. *Digit Biomark.* 2020;4(suppl 1):73–86.

CHAPTER 6

Clinical Trials in Perioperative Medicine

Paul S. Myles, MBBS, MPH, MD, DSc, FCAI, FANZCA, FAHMS

KEY POINTS

- Because most improvements in perioperative care are incremental, large numbers of patients need to be studied to have adequate statistical power to detect a clinically important difference.
- Large, pragmatic, multicenter, randomized trials are more reliable because they provide an unbiased evaluation of specific interventions delivered across a range of healthcare settings.
- Large pragmatic trials therefore test for effectiveness in routine clinical practice; their results are more generalizable.
- Examples of practice-improving clinical trials are outlined.

The Importance of Clinical Trials

Advances in anesthesia, surgery, and other perioperative practices over recent decades have led to amazing improvements in patient experience and outcomes in the days, weeks, and months after surgery. How and why do these improvements come about? The history of medicine has mostly been founded on accruing experience, often as trial and error, whereby obviously harmful therapies are discarded and more effective therapies are eventually taken up by clinicians. Most of these changes, however, happen too slowly or there is too much inexplicable variation in care, such that optimal care is not delivered to many patients.

Our patients are older and sicker, and increasingly complex surgical procedures are being done more often. The risks of adverse perioperative outcomes are greater. We need to reliably identify effective treatments to optimize care.

Training and experience are essential to good practice, but quality improvement demands evaluation and research. Genuine improvements in care, and the reasons for these, can be difficult to identify. Audit is important but accurate and complete data collection of all relevant variables, especially patient outcomes, can often miss important information. Single-center studies may not accrue enough cases, and their results may not apply to other centers. Large observational (nonrandomized) studies can collect extensive data from many centers, but these are prone to numerous biases that can result in misleading conclusions.[1] This perpetuates uncertainty and helps explain why variations in practice are so common.

Research as Evidence

Observational studies, often derived from large electronic patient databases, are sometimes promoted as "real-world evidence."[2] Observational studies have their strengths but also have important limitations.[2,3] Observational studies are particularly prone to selection bias (who gets what treatment and why) and confounding factors (other factors associated with an outcome that have not been fully accounted for).

The randomized controlled trial is universally accepted as being the best method to properly evaluate the effects of any intervention.[4] Random assignment to treatment groups minimizes bias, and if the trial is large (e.g., >500 participants), it will balance both known and unknown confounding factors. Large randomized trials are therefore more reliable and because they are typically multicentered (i.e., involving different healthcare settings and clinicians), their results are more generalizable.[5,6]

Most randomized trials are too small to detect clinically important effects.[4,7] Severe complications and death are rare after most types of surgery. Because most improvements in perioperative care are modest and incremental, large numbers of patients need to be studied to have adequate statistical power to detect a clinically important difference.[4-6] Statistical power refers to the probability that a true effect can be detected by the size of the study population, given some basic assumptions. Adequately powered clinical trials in perioperative medicine need to enroll thousands of patients to achieve reliable results.

Useful Clinical Trials: When to Change Practice

Outcomes that matter to patients are those that meaningfully affect their comfort, well-being, and quality of life. In the perioperative setting, this obviously includes the prevention of serious complications and death after surgery but also includes freedom from pain, postoperative nausea and vomiting (PONV), and sleep disturbance.[8] Patient-centered outcomes also include quality of recovery,[9-11] more days at home after surgery,[12] patient satisfaction, and disability-free survival.[13]

The use of surrogate, or intermediate, outcome measures in clinical research is widespread.[4,14] Many are not reflected in the patient's actual experience. For example, too many perioperative clinical studies report morphine consumption rather than opioid-related side effects, laboratory measurements rather than actual complications, and hypotension rather than organ failure.

Thankfully, most patients undergoing surgery have a complication-free recovery. Because serious complications occur infrequently, large randomized trials are needed in anesthesia and surgery to reliably identify useful advances in care. The good news is that there are many excellent examples of practice-improving clinical trials.

Real-World Examples

1. Perioperative beta-blockade: the POISE (Perioperative Ischemic Evaluation) trial[15]— Treatment guidelines previously recommended perioperative beta-blockade in patients undergoing noncardiac surgery. This randomized trial was conducted across 190 hospitals in 23 countries and enrolled 8351 at-risk surgical patients to receive extended-release metoprolol or placebo. The primary endpoint of the trial was a composite of cardiovascular death, nonfatal myocardial infarction, and nonfatal cardiac arrest. Although less patients in the metoprolol group had a myocardial infarction (4.2% vs. 5.7%, $P = .0017$), there were also more deaths (3.1% vs. 2.3%, $P = .0317$) and more strokes (1.0% vs. 0.5%, $P = .0053$) in the metoprolol group. The sensible interpretation of this trial is that perioperative beta-blockade should not be routinely adopted in patients undergoing noncardiac surgery. That is, the relevant guidelines needed to be heavily modified. This trial offers many insights into why large trials are needed before developing and implementing guidelines or considering changes in practice. A smaller trial would not have identified the more serious but less common complications of stroke or death. A consideration of the net benefit needed relevant, additional data that could only come from a large, multicenter trial.[16]

2. Prevention of PONV: the IMPACT trial[17]—This randomized trial was conducted across 28 hospitals in 5 countries and enrolled 5199 patients at high risk for PONV. The factorial design allowed 64 possible combinations of six prophylactic interventions to be compared. Ondansetron, dexamethasone, and droperidol were similarly effective at reducing the risk of PONV, each by approximately 26%. Combination treatment was additive. This was a definitive result that has reliably informed clinical practice up to this day.[18]

3. The safety of dexamethasone in noncardiac surgery: the PADDI (Perioperative Administration of Dexamethasone and Infection) trial[19]—There has been ongoing concern that dexamethasone, a glucocorticoid, may increase the risk of surgical site infection. This has limited its use in many surgical settings, particularly in patients with diabetes. Dexamethasone, a highly effective prophylactic and treatment for PONV, was being denied to a sizeable proportion of surgical patients because of a genuine safety concern that had not been resolved. This randomized trial was conducted across 55 hospitals in 4 countries and enrolled 8725 patients undergoing major noncardiac surgery. It was a noninferiority design, meaning it was designed to demonstrate that dexamethasone was at least as safe as placebo in a broad range of patients (including those with diabetes) and surgeries. The incidence of surgical site infection was less in the dexamethasone group (8.1% vs. 9.1%) and noninferiority was clearly demonstrated ($P < .001$). Results were similar in patients with diabetes. As expected, the incidence of PONV was reduced in the dexamethasone group (42% vs. 54%, $P < .001$). This compelling evidence of safety and effectiveness should markedly increase the use of dexamethasone in a broader range of surgical patients.

4. Tight glucose control in critical care: the NICE SUGAR (Normoglycemia in Intensive Care Evaluation–Survival Using Glucose Algorithm Regulation) trial[20]—A previous small trial had suggested that "tighter" control of blood glucose concentration could reduce some complications in critical care patients. This randomized trial was conducted across 42 hospitals in 3 countries and enrolled 6104 patients admitted to an intensive care unit. Patients were randomly assigned to intensive glucose control (target blood glucose 81–108 mg/dL) or conventional glucose control (target 180 mg/dL or less). Unexpectedly, more patients in the intensive-control group (27.5% vs. 24.9%, $P = .02$) died. Severe hypoglycemia was also far more common (6.8% vs. 0.5%, $P < .001$). The results of this trial also offer important insights. Serious complications, typically rare, require a large sample size to be detected. Like the POISE trial,[15] unexpected harms can be detected that would otherwise be missed.

5. Preoperative physiotherapy to prevent postoperative respiratory complications: the LIPPSMAck-POP (Lung Infection Prevention Post Surgery-Major Abdominal-with Pre-Operative Physiotherapy) trial[21]—This randomized trial was conducted across 3 hospitals in Tasmania and enrolled 441 patients within 6 weeks of elective abdominal surgery. Patients were randomly assigned to receive either an information booklet (control) or preoperative physiotherapy that consisted of an additional 30-minute physiotherapy education and breathing exercise training session. The incidence of postoperative pulmonary complications was more than halved in the physiotherapy group (12% vs. 27%, $P < .001$). These findings are compelling, but should the physiotherapy intervention be introduced elsewhere? There are some aspects of the trial that require further consideration. These include that the effect size was surprisingly large (a 56% relative risk reduction), the trial was relatively small so that randomization could not ensure a balance of risk, patients in the intervention group had better physical function, the trial only included three centers in a single state of Australia, and there was likely to be a high level of motivation in the physiotherapy (intervention) teams. Nevertheless, the intervention is simple and inexpensive, and the findings would be very important if they can be replicated.[22]

Conclusions

Large pragmatic trials test for effectiveness in routine clinical practice.[2,6,23] They include large numbers of patients, are done in a variety of settings (usually multicenter), and test simple interventions used by clinicians who may or may not have research expertise. They, therefore, represent "real-world" patients and clinical practice.[5,6,23] Large trials can also measure outcomes that matter to patients, such as potential adverse effects of the intervention. If clinical research in perioperative medicine is to provide more reliable and valid evidence to inform therapeutic decision making in the future, it is clear that a greater proportion of such research needs to be large, high-quality, multicenter randomized trials.[5,6,24]

References

1. Sackett DL. Bias in analytic research. *J Chronic Dis.* 1979;32:51–63.
2. Collins R, Bowman L, Landray M, Peto R. The magic of randomization versus the myth of real-world evidence. *N Engl J Med.* 2020;382:674–678.
3. MacMahon S, Collins R. Reliable assessment of the effects of treatment on mortality and major morbidity, II: observational studies. *Lancet.* 2001;357:455–462.
4. Rigg J, Jamrozik K, Clarke M. How can we demonstrate that new developments in anesthesia are of real clinical importance? *Anesthesiology.* 1997;86:1008–1010.
5. Yusuf S, Collins R, Peto R. Why do we need some large simple randomized trials? *Statistics in Medicine.* 1984;3:409–420.
6. Myles PS. Why we need large randomized studies in anaesthesia. *Br J Anaesth.* 1999;83:833–834.
7. Kelly MJ, Wadsworth J. What price inconclusive clinical trials? *Ann R Coll Surg Engl.* 1993;75:145–146.
8. Myles PS, Boney O, Botti M, et al. Systematic review and consensus definitions for the Standardised Endpoints in Perioperative Medicine (StEP) initiative: patient comfort. *Br J Anaesth.* 2018;120:705–711.
9. Myles P, Hunt J, Nightingale C, et al. Development and psychometric testing of a quality of recovery score after general anesthesia and surgery in adults. *Anesth Analg.* 1999;88:83–90.
10. Myles P, Weitkamp B, Jones K, et al. Validity and reliability of a post-operative quality of recovery score: the QoR-40. *Br J Anaesth.* 2000;84:11–15.
11. Stark PA, Myles PS, Burke JA. Development and psychometric evaluation of a postoperative quality of recovery score: the QoR-15. *Anesthesiology.* 2013;118:1332–1340.
12. Myles PS, Shulman M, Heritier S, et al. Validation of days at home as an outcome measure after surgery: a prospective cohort study in Australia. *BMJ Open.* 2017. https://doi.org/10.1136/bmjopen-2017-015828.
13. Shulman MA, Myles PS, Chan MT, et al. Measurement of disability-free survival after surgery. *Anesthesiology.* 2015;122:524–536.
14. Fisher D. Surrogate outcomes: they don't get it. *Anesth Analg.* 2009;109:994. author reply 994-5.
15. The POISE Study Group. Effects of extended-release metoprolol succinate in patients undergoing non-cardiac surgery (POISE trial): a randomised controlled trial. *The Lancet.* 2008;371:1839–1847.
16. Nishikawa G, Prasad V. Diagnostic expansion in clinical trials: myocardial infarction, stroke, cancer recurrence, and metastases may not be the hard endpoints you thought they were. *BMJ.* 2018;362, k3783.
17. Apfel C, Korttila K, Abdalla M, et al. A factorial trial of six interventions for the prevention of postoperative nausea and vomiting. *N Engl J Med.* 2004;350:2441–2451.
18. Gan TJ, Diemunsch P, Habib AS, et al. Consensus guidelines for the management of postoperative nausea and vomiting. *Anesth Analg.* 2014;118:85–113.
19. Corcoran T, Myles PS, Forbes AF, et al. Dexamethasone and surgical site infection. *N Engl J Med.* 2021.
20. Finfer S, Chittock DR, Su SY, et al. Intensive versus conventional glucose control in critically ill patients. *N Engl J Med.* 2009;360:1283–1297.
21. Boden I, Skinner EH, Browning L, et al. Preoperative physiotherapy for the prevention of respiratory complications after upper abdominal surgery: pragmatic, double blinded, multicentre randomised controlled trial. *BMJ.* 2018;360, j5916.
22. Ioannidis JPA. Contradicted and initially stronger effects in highly cited clinical research. *JAMA.* 2005;294:218–228.

23. Tunis SR, Stryer DB, Clancy CM. Practical clinical trials: increasing the value of clinical research for decision making in clinical and health policy. *JAMA*. 2003;290:1624–1632.
24. Saag KG, Mohr PE, Esmail L, et al. Improving the efficiency and effectiveness of pragmatic clinical trials in older adults in the United States. *Contemp Clin Trials*. 2012;33:1211–1216.

CHAPTER 7

Large-Scale Audits: Using Citizen Science to Gather High-Quality "Big Data"

S. Ramani Moonesinghe, OBE, MD(Res), FRCA, FFICM, FRCP

KEY POINTS

- Large-scale audits have been hugely successful in gathering large volumes of data in short spaces of time to inform research and quality improvement (QI) endeavors and policy development.
- Built on the model of "citizen science," they harness the efforts of thousands of collaborators to approach a specific challenge, using a collaborative and cost-effective approach.
- Key points for success include choosing topics that are important to collaborators, establishing networks that enable delivery, and keeping the data set as small as possible.

Why Is This Important in Perioperative Medicine?

While we wait for electronic health records to be ubiquitous, interoperable, and provide accessible data for audit and research, we need to harness alternative methods to collect large volumes of high-quality risk, process, and outcome data to inform both research and quality improvement (QI) endeavors. In the United Kingdom (UK) and internationally, perioperative clinicians have applied the principles of "citizen science" to support these types of endeavors.

What Is Citizen Science?

Citizen science is also known as "crowd science," "crowd-sourced science," or "volunteer monitoring." Its essence is that it uses the collective efforts of large numbers of nonscientists to create or analyze so-called "big data." Multiple citizen science platforms exist, some generic (e.g., Zooniverse—www.zooniverse.org) and some linked to familiar organizations (e.g., the GLOBE [Global Learning and Observations to Benefit the Environment] program hosted by the National Aeronautics and Space Administration [NASA]—https://www.nasa.gov/solve/feature/globe) These platforms provide a staggering diversity of opportunities, from mapping satellite images to helping understand seasonality on the south pole of Mars to transcribing historical papers (including Shakespearean scribblings!).

How Has Citizen Science Been Applied in Health Care?

Anesthesia, perioperative care, and critical care have a proud pedigree in delivering clinically impactful citizen science projects. In the UK, many of the long-running national audits and QI programs, such as the National Emergency Laparotomy Audit and the Perioperative Quality Improvement Programme, both discussed elsewhere in this text, are delivered using a combination of career research staff and clinicians with variable research experience. The UK's National Confidential Enquiry into Patient Outcome and Death (NCEPOD; https://www.ncepod.org.uk) conducts mixed method evaluations of specific services, conditions, or interventions; in recent years, these have included the inpatient care of patients who have had out-of-hospital cardiac arrests and the quality of care afforded to patients with Parkinson's disease and dysphagia who were admitted acutely unwell. These enquiries usually take the form of a national audit to establish denominator numbers and basic demographics about the population of interest, accompanied by a deep dive into the care of a random sample of patients. In 2011 NCEPOD led an evaluation of inpatient surgical care and outcomes, leading to a report titled "Knowing the Risk."[1] This yielded important data about the quality of risk assessment before surgery and how a failure to appreciate an individual patient's risk of poor outcomes was associated with subsequent challenges in recognizing and managing deterioration. A key recommendation was the development of a national system for risk prediction, which was duly delivered a few years later.[2] The study set the scene for many future programs of work, which focused on risk prediction, implementation of risk assessment, and failure to rescue.

The first international citizen science project in perioperative care was the European Surgical Outcomes Study, involving 28 European nations and 498 hospitals and recruiting 46,539 patients.[3] Remarkable for its efficiency and the quality of the data captured, it demonstrated not just that this type of research was possible, but that it could be achieved cost effectively and to a high standard. The key findings (that inpatient surgery was associated with substantially higher mortality within 60 days than might have previously been anticipated) prompted international discussion and renewed focus on the challenge of perioperative care. The same leadership team later went a step further and conducted the International Surgical Outcomes Study (ISOS), which invited participation from anywhere in the world.[4] Aiming to define complication and failure to rescue rates in patients having inpatient elective surgery, it highlighted the stark disparity in clinical outcomes between high- and low/middle-income nations. Although this was another remarkable feat of citizen science in perioperative medicine in some respects, ISOS findings were limited by the substantially higher participation from high-income countries. This challenge was comprehensively addressed by the African Surgical Outcomes Study (ASOS), which recruited 11,422 patients from 247 hospitals across the African continent.[5] Their key finding (that postoperative mortality was twice that of high-income countries, despite patients being younger and having a generally lower risk profile) prompted international attention and subsequent studies to develop risk-prediction models[6] and complex interventions aimed at reducing failure to rescue after surgery.[7]

All of these projects have been remarkable for their agility, cost-effectiveness, engagement, and impact. Challenges include the potential for bias in results where convenience sampling is used to recruit participating institutions. The aim of the UK's National Audit Projects (NAPs) and Sprint National Anaesthesia Projects (SNAPs) is to overcome this problem by engaging as close to 100% of eligible public hospitals as possible. There have been seven NAPs in total to date (https://www.rcoa.ac.uk/research/research-projects/national-audit-projects-naps), which use mixed methods (qualitative evaluation of structured reports and quantitative analyses of activity data) to evaluate rare but potentially catastrophic events in anaesthesia and perioperative care, such as death or serious harm associated with airway management or anaphylaxis, and perioperative cardiac arrest. Qualitative data collection usually takes place over a year, with a confidential structured reporting system being made available to participating centers, and an independent panel reviewing fully anonymized data. A shorter (up to 7-day) snapshot of activity helps determine the denominator (i.e., enables the total number of anesthetics or procedures of interest to be mathematically modeled), and therefore the incidence of these rare events can be estimated. This has provided key information of value to clinicians and patients alike (e.g., the incidence of paralysis after neuraxial block;

https://www.nationalauditprojects.org.uk/NAP3_home?newsid=464#pt). The SNAPs take almost the opposite approach to the NAPs, a short-term snapshot to evaluate a common challenge or dilemma. SNAP1 focused on patient-reported outcomes after anesthesia, recruiting 15,010 patients in 2 days from 97% of UK hospitals.[8,9] SNAP2 evaluated issues around critical care admission after surgery and is informing public policy in the UK.[10–13] SNAP3 will take place in 2023 and evaluate risk factors for, and the management of, perioperative frailty and postoperative delirium.

Two features common to all of these endeavors are their low cost and high value, given the academic and clinical outcomes, and the fact that dissemination and clinical impact of findings is enhanced because of the community engagement, which supported the projects in the first place. So, what are the enablers that support delivery of these ambitious collaborative efforts?

Practical Guidance

- First and foremost, the research or audit question must appeal to frontline clinicians because they will be doing much of the hard work. Ideally, the community helps to choose the research or audit questions, as has latterly been the case for the NAPs and SNAPs. A process that involves surveying the community, followed by a smaller group of experienced academics deciding which of the topics suggested is amenable to the particular methodology of a large-scale audit, has worked well.
- Second, it is important to resist the temptation to "boil the ocean." Keeping the list of specific research or audit questions as trim as possible is the key to local engagement and generating high-quality data.
- Third, piloting the approach is critical. A handful of institutions should be approached for the task of doing a "dry run" of the audit, ideally representing a diversity of size and type (rural vs. urban, academic vs. community, small vs. large, and so on). The pilot should ideally appraise every aspect of the process, including online data entry portals where they are being used, obtaining research or information governance permissions, and so on.
- Fourth, the proposed analysis should be sensitive to the hopes and fears of local investigators and the strengths and limitations of the likely sampling approach. For example, unless a NAP- or SNAP-type approach is planned, where the aim is to gather data from as close to 100% of eligible institutions as possible, there is likely to be little benefit in presenting results that compare institutions against each other; the results will be disputed on the basis of sampling bias and potentially undermine other findings.
- Finally, and most importantly, establishing your network is the key to success.

In the UK, the Health Services Research Centre at the Royal College of Anaesthetists has established a network of "Quality Audit and Research Coordinators" or "QuARCs" who are the "go-to" individuals in each department of anesthesia and perioperative medicine, who are responsible for delivering NAPs and SNAPs on the ground. The individual QuARCs do not have to locally lead every project, but they are responsible for finding someone in their department who has enough interest in the proposed project to lead it. The local leads get experience in leading and supporting a major collaborative effort, which is good for personal development. Many of these projects name every local lead and all local collaborators who have made a significant contribution in publications as coauthors or collaborators; this provides much needed reward for hard work and time invested. There are challenges associated with creating and maintaining such networks, which have been well described by others, but for QI, five key characteristics have been identified: common purpose, a cooperative structure, critical mass, collective intelligence, and community building.[14] Although large-scale audits and research projects of the nature described do not initially fulfill the criteria of a QI project, it is likely that the audit would identify areas requiring attention, which an improvement network could then support. This has certainly been the case for the NAPs, which have led to development of national guidelines and requirements for named local leads to support improvement in key challenges (e.g., airway management or the immediate management and longer-term follow-up of anaphylaxis or accidental awareness during general anesthesia).

In conclusion, large-scale projects that use citizen science methods can present a relatively cost-effective means of gathering large volumes of high-quality data to support audit, QI, and research. The time and energy needed to establish the networks required to successfully deliver these types of endeavor should not be underestimated, but the rewards can be significant and lead to practice- and policy-influencing outputs.

References

1. Findlay GP, Goodwin APL, Protopapa K, Smith NCE, Mason M. Knowing the risk: a review of the perioperative care of surgical patients. National Confidential Enquiry into Patient Outcome and Death; 2011. https://www.ncepod.org.uk/2011report2/downloads/POC_fullreport.pdf.
2. Protopapa KL, Simpson JC, Smith NC, Moonesinghe SR. Development and validation of the surgical outcome risk tool (SORT). *Br J Surg.* 2014;101:1774–1783.
3. Pearse RM, Moreno RP, Bauer P, et al. Mortality after surgery in Europe: a 7 day cohort study. *Lancet.* 2012;380:1059–1065.
4. International SOSG. Global patient outcomes after elective surgery: prospective cohort study in 27 low-, middle- and high-income countries. *Br J Anaesth.* 2016;117:601–609.
5. Biccard BM, Madiba TE, Kluyts HL, et al. Perioperative patient outcomes in the African Surgical Outcomes Study: a 7-day prospective observational cohort study. *Lancet.* 2018;391:1589–1598.
6. Kluyts HL, le Manach Y, Munlemvo DM, et al. The ASOS Risk Calculator: development and validation of a preoperative risk stratification tool for identifying African surgical patients at risk of severe postoperative complications. *Br J Anaes.* 2018;121(6):1357–1363.
7. ASOS-2 I. Enhanced postoperative surveillance versus standard of care to reduce mortality among adult surgical patients in Africa (ASOS-2): a cluster-randomised controlled trial. *Lancet Glob Health.* 2021;9: e1391–e1401.
8. Moonesinghe SR, Walker EM, Bell M. Design and methodology of SNAP-1: a Sprint National Anaesthesia Project to measure patient reported outcome after anaesthesia. *Perioper Med (Lond).* 2015;4:4.
9. Walker EM, Bell M, Cook TM, Grocott MP, Moonesinghe SR. SNAP-1 IG. Patient reported outcome of adult perioperative anaesthesia in the United Kingdom: a cross-sectional observational study. *Br J Anaesth.* 2016;117:758–766.
10. Moonesinghe SR, Wong DJN, Farmer L, et al. SNAP-2 EPICCS: the second Sprint National Anaesthesia Project-EPIdemiology of Critical Care after Surgery: protocol for an international observational cohort study. *BMJ Open.* 2017;7, e017690.
11. Wong DJN, Harris SK, Moonesinghe SR, et al. Cancelled operations: a 7-day cohort study of planned adult inpatient surgery in 245 UK National Health Service hospitals. *Br J Anaesth.* 2018;121:730–738.
12. Wong DJN, Popham S, Wilson AM, et al. Postoperative critical care and high-acuity care provision in the United Kingdom, Australia, and New Zealand. *Br J Anaesth.* 2019;122:460–469.
13. Wong DJN, Harris S, Sahni A, et al. Developing and validating subjective and objective risk-assessment measures for predicting mortality after major surgery: an international prospective cohort study. *PLoS Med.* 2020;17, e1003253.
14. The Health Foundation. *Effective networks for improvement*; 2014. https://www.health.org.uk/publications/effective-networks-for-improvement.

CHAPTER 8

Education in Perioperative Medicine

Jeanna D. Blitz, MD, FASA, DFPM ■ Angela F. Edwards, MD, FASA, DFPM ■
BobbieJean Sweitzer, MD, FACP, SAMBA-F, FASA

KEY POINTS

- The proficient perioperative medicine specialist is skilled in managing patient complexities across the entire surgical continuum to care for patients at all stages of life, with a focus on improving patient comfort, safety, and perioperative outcomes.
- The foundation of an educational curriculum includes elements of medicine, surgery, anesthesiology, geriatrics, psychometrics, care coordination, business management, and principles of clinical quality.
- Delivery of high-quality perioperative care requires excellence in six equally important domains: safety, timeliness, effectiveness, efficiency, equity, and patient-centeredness.
- A nuanced appreciation of system-based resources within various surgical settings is integral to any curriculum.

Perioperative medicine (POM) is a distinct medical discipline with a unique focus on mitigating the physiological and psychological stress responses associated with procedures, anesthesia, and recovery. Expertise in this area requires extensive knowledge of medicine, anesthesiology, pharmacology, surgery, geriatrics, pain management, and psychometrics. Thus the foundation of any educational curriculum includes elements of intraoperative management, preoperative and postoperative care, care coordination, business management, and key principles of clinical quality.[1] The aim is to develop our clinicians' abilities to create efficient and effective preoperative processes, implement perioperative optimization protocols, and streamline perioperative care transitions to improve the health of the patient and the population at a lower cost.[1-3] Scaling current POM programs and maximizing access to the content will ultimately result in a generation of perioperative specialists equipped to lead proficient multidisciplinary teams.

The transformation toward value-based care and population health management requires that we provide trainees with a deep understanding of the factors that challenge the clinical microsystems in which care is delivered.[4] The Institute of Medicine's (IOM) conceptual framework for high-quality care delivery includes six equally important domains: safety, timeliness, effectiveness, efficiency, equity, and patient-centeredness (Table 8.1).[5] Framing clinical medicine concepts around the opportunity to improve the six domains of quality care will elucidate for trainees how to use improvement science tools and engage interdisciplinary teams to achieve peak performance within their own institutions.[2,3,6]

Table 8.2 and other chapters in this book provide the framework for using quality improvement techniques to enhance patient care.

TABLE 8.1 ■ Opportunities to Enhance the Six Domains of Quality Care Within Perioperative Medicine

Six Domains of Quality Care	Perioperative Medicine–Specific Examples and Opportunities
Safe: Minimizes risk and harm[17,18]	• Confirm accuracy of reported allergies and medications • Create accurate medical histories • Ensure administration of first-line antibiotic therapy via penicillin allergy testing • Optimize blood management • Decrease surgical site infections • Impact unanticipated ICU admission • Reduce in-hospital mortality
Efficient: Maximizes resource use, avoids waste[22,23]	• Decrease length of hospitalization • Lower day of surgery case cancellation rates • Identify appropriate candidacy for venues of care or same-day discharge • Reduce inappropriate and unnecessary testing and consults • Decrease costs of care • Enhance access to care via telemedicine
Effective: Based on evidence and results in improved outcomes[7,24–26]	• Development of evidence-based protocols: anemia management, glycemic control, DAPT and anticoagulation management, CIED recommendations • OSA screening, diagnosis, and PAP initiation • Smoking cessation • Nutritional optimization • ERAS pathways • Well-trained staff
Timely: Delivery of well-coordinated, accessible care[27]	• Telemedicine visits for patient convenience • Streamlined, coordinated care to reduce the number of appointments • Same-day appointments
Equity: Race, gender, ethnicity, socioeconomic status, and other patient demographic factors are not barriers to receipt of high-quality care[28,29]	• Address social determinants of health • Case management and discharge planning • Leverage telemedicine to reduce barriers to care
Patient-Centered: Based on patient's individual preferences and culture[16,30]	• Anemia management for patients who refuse blood • Use of preferred pronouns • Access to interpretation services • Education and instructions in patient's preferred format (videos, diagrams, pamphlets) • Provision of procedural and sensory information

CIED, Cardiovascular implantable electronic device; DAPT, dual antiplatelet therapy; ERAS, enhanced recovery after surgery; ICU, intensive care unit; OSA, obstructive sleep apnea; PAP, positive airway pressure.

TABLE 8.2 ■ Key Quality Improvement Tools and Concepts[6]

Problem Identification Tools
- Ishikawa (fishbone) diagrams
- Pareto analysis
- Affinity diagrams
- 5 Why's

Project Definition
- Determine the scope of the project
- Identify key stakeholders
- Determine key metrics, objectives, and timeframe
- Charter creation

Process Mapping
- Document the process in its current state
- Label value-added and nonvalue-added steps
- Identify areas of waste that can be removed to streamline the process
- Clearly outline roles and responsibilities for members of the team
- Highlight needed resources

Data Collection and Tracking
- Process metrics
- Outcome metrics
- Run charts and Control charts

Change Management and Communication of Success
Plan Do Study Act (PDSA) Cycles
Root Cause Analysis
Failure Mode Effects Analysis

Preoperative Clinical Vignette

A 48-year-old woman with fibroids and dysfunctional uterine bleeding presents to the preoperative evaluation clinic in preparation for a hysterectomy in 2 weeks. Laboratory testing reveals a hemoglobin of 7.5 g/dL. Reflex iron studies confirm iron deficiency anemia (transferrin saturation [TSAT]: 7%, ferritin: 5 ng/mL). The surgery is not without risk of significant blood loss, and this patient has little reserve. The surgeon asks you whether the patient should undergo preoperative blood transfusion. After discussion with the patient and her surgeon, surgery is deferred for two additional weeks so that she may receive treatment for her iron deficiency anemia. The patient is scheduled for intravenous (IV) iron therapy and erythropoietin injections before her procedure. After treatment, her preoperative hemoglobin improves to 11.8 g/dL. She reports improved energy levels and that she is feeling much better. She is thankful to have avoided a blood transfusion. She proceeds with an uneventful hysterectomy and is discharged home without complications. After this patient encounter, the preoperative assessment team meets with the gynecologists to educate and develop a process for the gynecologists to identify patients with iron deficiency anemia expeditiously with early referral to the preoperative and/or anemia clinic. This is also leveraged across other specialties.

This clinical vignette illustrates how the concepts of quality care may be incorporated into the design of our preoperative processes. Anemia is a known risk multiplier that is associated with increased adverse outcomes in the perioperative period.[19,20] Diagnosis of a previously unrecognized medical condition, and correction before surgery enhances **patient safety**. The creation of a reflex testing algorithm to determine the cause of anemia without delay or additional patient visits or diagnostic testing addresses the principle of **efficiency**.[21] IV iron and erythropoietin therapy are examples of an evidence-based approach, which replace the more costly strategy of blood transfusion, highlighting the principle of **efficacy**. Although the surgery was rescheduled to treat her anemia, the principle of **patient-centeredness** is evident. Correction of her iron deficiency anemia led to an improvement in her energy levels and quality of life, avoided blood transfusions, and minimized her risk of readmission to the hospital. Preoperative anemia management improves **equitable** care delivery for our patients who refuse blood products and quality of postoperative recovery. The collaboration, sharing of knowledge, and development of pathways for primary surgeons to diagnose iron deficiency, recognize associated risks, and understand appropriate alternatives for treatment is an example of effective quality improvement.

For the POM specialist, educational elements include an appreciation for the evidence-based differences in clinical management compared with the nonoperative setting (e.g., glycemic and blood pressure control targets), the accelerated cadence of interventions such as smoking cessation,[7] and the modified approach to managing chronic diseases in the perioperative environment (acceptable blood pressures or glucose control).[8] POM specialists need a working knowledge of common surgical interventions including risks and alternative therapies, risk prediction tools, evidence-based management of conditions common in surgical populations, and options for and implications of anesthetic management. Examples of program components and implementation are available from several institutions.[1,9]

A nuanced appreciation of system-based resources within various surgical settings[10] (ambulatory surgery centers vs. hospital-based locations), quality improvement techniques, patient safety strategies, and interdisciplinary leadership tools are important to any curriculum. Fellowship training programs in POM exist in a growing number of institutions (see Table 8.5). These intend to train physicians across multiple specialties, including anesthesiology, surgery, and hospital medicine. Trainees require skills to develop best practices and implement and execute comprehensive perioperative programs.[11]

The role of the POM specialist is to create and lead a patient-centric, evidence-based process that encompasses the entire perioperative continuum and ensures goals of care are met. At a minimum, the skill set of the POM specialist includes:
- The ability to critically evaluate scientific literature and evidence
- Effective interview and physical examination skills
- Medical knowledge to independently diagnose and treat comorbidities and interpret test results
- Application of evidence-based guidelines to treat a wide variety of diseases
- Effective interdisciplinary communication, care coordination, and problem-solving skills
- Familiarity with telehealth and electronic medical records
- Ability to work with diverse care providers
- Technical and procedural skills, such as point-of-care ultrasound (POCUS)
- Business and healthcare administration aptitude, including:
  - Proficiency with personnel management
  - Budget and financial (including billing) expertise
- Training in quality improvement and implementation science
- Data collection and analysis skills
- Leadership and change management skills

Because POM is a nascent discipline, novel curriculum content is emerging to supplement and build on the traditional topics and concepts taught during residency. Additionally, practitioners in the POM space come from diverse training backgrounds. Because of its multidimensional nature, POM concepts are often best taught via a combination of modalities. Some topics are delivered effectively in a standard didactic format, whereas others require a hands-on, experiential approach. Asynchronous formats allow for remote learning and self-study, whereas group projects facilitate the building of leadership and communication skill sets. Incorporating an asynchronous remote learning component within the curriculum may also improve access to educational content for a wider audience, including more mature practitioners who want to expand their knowledge or transition to POM while still working in traditional healthcare practices. Nevertheless, active participation in perioperative quality improvement initiatives is essential to any clinical POM curriculum or fellowship. Appropriate mentors should be available to guide progress and facilitate learning.

Perioperative Education

Progressive competency in POM can be tracked from beginning through mastery based on The Accreditation Council for Graduate Medical Education (ACGME)'s six core competencies (Table 8.3).[12,13]

With the continued advancement and expansion of knowledge and evidence-based guidelines specific to the perioperative period, POM has become a specialty practice that requires a level of expertise that an average anesthesiologist, surgeon, internal medicine physician, or allied health professional does not inherently possess. Increasing surgical complexity, minimally invasive procedures that allow interventions even in medically fragile patients, an aging population, and advanced anesthesia techniques will continue to drive demand and expansion of procedural services. Nevertheless, significant morbidity, mortality, and costs come with perioperative interventions. Patients should be aware of probable outcomes and risks of postoperative disability.[14] The POM specialist should be skilled in shared decision making using valid, reliable, and responsive patient-reported outcome tools, like the WHODAS 2.0 and American College of Surgeons National Surgical Quality Improvement Program (NSQIP) risk calculator to review patient expectations relative to the degree of preoperative optimization.[14,15] Patient-expected outcomes relative to probable outcomes and intraoperative management should guide shared decision making among the patient, caregivers, surgeon, anesthesiologist, and the POM specialists.[16] This is a unique skill set developed by the POM specialist.

Current evidence supports the fact that care delivered in a dedicated preoperative medicine practice can be cost-effective, can reduce cancellations and delays, and can decrease mortality.[4,17,18,11] Medical practices and providers must be trained in and continually advance POM practices. Clinicians at all levels of training benefit from a commitment to lifelong learning. Easily accessible, high-yield resources and professional collaboration within subspecialty organizations support this practice (Table 8.4).

The practice of POM requires an in-depth understanding not only of the physiological and psychological stress responses to surgery but also of the direct experience and expertise in providing interventions to mitigate those stressors. The value of formal training in POM lies in the ability to develop these skills as a cohesive skill set and the opportunity to perfect them via mentorship by a subject matter expert. A variety of fellowships and other training opportunities exist, with more emerging as the field grows (Table 8.5). Teaching methodology is tailored to suit the learners' needs, clinical duties, and time constraints. Didactics, problem-based learning, and interactive experiential opportunities should accompany more traditional assessments of knowledge. Individual fellowship programs should incorporate certification in one or more directly applicable

TABLE 8.3 ■ Proposed Competencies for the Perioperative Medicine Specialist[28]

American College of Graduate Medical Education Core Competencies With Specific Notations	POM Examples of Subcompetencies
Patient Care Clinicians must be able to provide patient care that is compassionate, appropriate, and effective for the treatment of health problems and the promotion of health	**Evidence-based preoperative risk reduction and optimization strategies** (Beta-blockers, statins, aspirin, antiplatelet, anticoagulant, insulin and glycemic control agents, anemia management, nutrition, prehabilitation) **Evidence-based intraoperative management** (glycemic control, fluid management, blood pressure optimization, regional anesthesia) **Evidence-based postoperative management** (Prevention and mitigation of delirium and postoperative neurocognitive disorders, venous thromboembolism prophylaxis, MINS, MACE prevention, and monitoring), **Mitigating risk of ventilatory compromise** (opioid-induced ventilatory depression, OSA, COPD

Patient Care (technical and interpretation skills)
Clinicians must be able to provide patient care that is compassionate, appropriate, and effective for the treatment of health problems and the promotion of health
	Clinicians must be prepared to be the primary consultant for medical issues commonly seen in the surgical patient.
	• History and physical examination skills pertinent to clinic-based practices
	• Patient education and preparation:
	  ◦ Effective delivery of individualized information
	  ◦ Patient-centered and motivational interviewing
	  ◦ Stress reduction techniques
	• Medication management:
	  ◦ Antithrombotic agents (anticoagulation and dual antiplatelet therapy)
	  ◦ Insulin management
	  ◦ Mixed opioid agonists/antagonists
	• Allergy testing
	• Performance of electrocardiograms and point of care ultrasound (POCUS) examinations
	• CIED management
	• Intrathecal pump management
	• Indications for and interpretation of CPET testing, pulmonary function tests, echocardiograms, biomarkers, and other common tests

Medical Knowledge Clinicians must demonstrate knowledge of established and evolving biomedical, clinical, epidemiological, and social-behavioral sciences, as well as the application of this knowledge to patient care.	**Expertise in major organ disease and management** • Heart, brain, lung, kidney, liver, immune and hematological systems • Anemia evaluation • Nutrition management • Frailty assessment and impact **For example:** Hypertension, heart failure, anticoagulation, diabetes, sleep disordered breathing, pulmonary disorders (COPD, fibrosis, asthma) delirium, POCD, stroke, ischemic and congenital heart disease, (CKD), prevention of failure to rescue, MINS, MACE **Postoperative acute and chronic pain management (including regional techniques)**

Continued on following page

TABLE 8.3 ■ **Proposed Competencies for the Perioperative Medicine Specialist** (Continued)

American College of Graduate Medical Education Core Competencies With Specific Notations	POM Examples of Subcompetencies
Practice-Based Learning and Improvement Clinicians must demonstrate the ability to investigate and evaluate their care of patients, to appraise and assimilate scientific evidence, and to continuously improve patient care based on constant self-evaluation and life-long learning.	• Protocol and pathway development • Competency in systematic quality improvement frameworks such as the Plan Do Study Act, Six Sigma and Lean Methodology • Information technology for process improvement, decision support, and outcome measurement • Routine personal practice review to understand the impact of perioperative decisions and care on patients' longitudinal health trajectory • Participation in education of patients and their families, residents, students and other health professionals
Systems-Based Practice Clinicians must demonstrate an awareness of and responsiveness to the larger context and system of health care, as well as the ability to call effectively on other resources in the system to provide optimal health care.	• Implementation of perioperative initiatives to achieve the Triple Aim: • Improved quality of care and patient experience • Improved population health • Lower cost of care • Value-based strategies to improve short- and long-term patient outcomes ◦ Geriatric Surgical Verification Program (https://www.facs.org/quality-programs/geriatric-surgery) • Familiarity with data collection and analysis, metric selection • Requirements for nonoperating room, ambulatory surgery, office-based, and hybrid environments • Integration of primary care and specialty input • Care coordination and care transitions • Identification of potential system errors (failure mode and effects analysis) and implementation of potential solutions
Communication and Interpersonal Skills Clinicians must demonstrate interpersonal and communication skills that result in the effective exchange of information and collaboration with patients, their families, and health professionals	• Effective communication skills (both verbal and written) • Comfort and skill with shared decision-making discussions and difficult conversations • Provision of compassionate, patient-centric goals of care discussions • Obtaining informed consent • Care planning, including discussions on surgical timing and deferral for optimization • Promoting value-based POM initiatives to stakeholders • Supervision of extended care providers • Appreciation of ethical issues and the ability to manage ethical dilemmas that arise in the perioperative period • Serving as a consultant to other healthcare providers

TABLE 8.3 ■ **Proposed Competencies for the Perioperative Medicine Specialist** (Continued)

American College of Graduate Medical Education Core Competencies With Specific Notations	POM Examples of Subcompetencies
Professionalism Clinicians must demonstrate a commitment to carrying out professional responsibilities and an adherence to ethical principles. Residents are expected to demonstrate:	• Expertise in collaboration and the ability to establish trusting relationships with patients, families, and care providers from all disciplines • Appreciation and cultural sensitivity while caring for a diverse patient population including vulnerable patients with unique care needs • Modeling behaviors and interpersonal skills expected of an interdisciplinary team

CIED, Cardiovascular implantable electronic devices; *CKD*, chronic kidney disease; *COPD*, chronic obstructive pulmonary disease; *CPET*, cardiopulmonary exercise testing; *MACE*, major adverse cardiovascular events; *MINS*, myocardial injury after noncardiac surgery; *OSA*, obstructive sleep apnea; *POCD,* postoperative cognitive dysfunction; *POM*, perioperative medicine.
Based on Six Domains of Health Care Quality. Agency for Healthcare Research and Quality, Rockville, MD. Accessed May 2021. https://www.acgme.org/Portals/0/PDFs/Milestones/AnesthesiologyMilestones2.0.pdf?ver=2020-12-02-125500-287.

TABLE 8.4 ■ **High-Yield Educational Resources, References, and Supplemental Certificate Programs**

Resource	Description
Institute for Healthcare Improvement http://www.ihi.org/ Royal College of Anaesthetists Quality Improvement Compendium. RCoA 2021, Eds Chereshneva, Johnston, Colvin, and Peden. https://www.rcoa.ac.uk/safety-standards-quality/quality-improvement/raising-standards-rcoa-quality-improvement-compendium	Free online courses and quality improvement toolkit. IHI open school basic certificate in quality and safety available. Quality Improvement resources free to download. Short perioperative improvement outlines with key references.
National Health Services Bradford Institute for Health Research Improvement Academy Improvement Academy—Bronze Quality Improvement Training	Free online courses and quality improvement tools.
Perioperative Medicine in Action https://www.futurelearn.com/courses/perioperative-medicine/9/todo/103630	Free online 4-week course through University College London.
Society for Perioperative Assessment and Quality Improvement *Society for Perioperative Assessment and Quality Improvement (spaqi.org)*	Multidisciplinary organization and collaborative forum for delivery of high-value, safe perioperative care. Membership includes access to a discussion forum, business models and high-yield references, and up-to-date clinical practice guidelines (ACC/AHA risk assessment, CIED management, ASRA anticoagulation guidelines).

Continued on following page

TABLE 8.4 ■ **High-Yield Educational Resources, References, and Supplemental Certificate Programs** (Continued)

Resource	Description
The Perioperative Quality Initiative https://thepoqi.org/home	A multidisciplinary organization that organizes consensus conferences on perioperative medicine topics. Free access to publications and consensus statements.
American Society of Anesthesiologists – American College of Healthcare Executives Physician Leadership Development Collaborative	https://www.asahq.org/education-and-career/ leadership-development/ache Free self-assessment and study tool: https://www. ache.org/-/media/ache/career-resource-center/ competencies_booklet.pdf
Evidence-Based Perioperative Medicine https://ebpom.org/	Clinical conferences and podcasts.
Diagnostic POCUS Certificate Program: https://www.asahq.org/education-and-career/ educational-and-cme-offerings/pocus	CME-based certificate program to develop and enhance perioperative point of care ultrasound skill set.
Sweitzer BJ. *Preoperative Assessment and Management.* 3rd ed.	High-yield reference for the management of common clinical conditions and preoperative decision making.
Nelson EC, Batalden PB, Godfrey MM, eds. *Quality by Design: A Clinical Microsystems Approach.*	Effective illustration of key clinical quality principles via case studies.
Trainees interested in Perioperative Medicine: https://tripom.org	Online tutorials, podcasts
American College of Perioperative Medicine https://www.acpm.health/operational.php	Access to publications and concept papers
Perioperative Surgical Home https://www.asahq.org/psh	Access to case studies and relevant literature

ACC/AHA, American College of Cardiology/American Heart Association; *ASRA,* American Society of Regional Anesthesia and Pain Management; *CIED,* cardiovascular implantable electronic devices; *CME,* continued medical education; *IHI,* Institute for Healthcare Improvement; *RCoA,* Royal College of Anaesthetists.

programs. Examples include POCUS expertise, quality improvement, leadership, and patient safety. Several organizations offer directly applicable certification programs to supplement and validate POM fellowship programs.

In summary, the proficient POM specialist is skilled in managing patient complexities across the entire surgical continuum to care for patients at all stages of life. Understanding how comorbidities, the surgical stress response, physiological perturbations of anesthesia and surgery, and patient goals affect preoperative and postoperative management are critical to ensuring an ideal outcome for the patient. Communicating risks and probable outcomes to patients, families, surgeons, and others is a unique skill set substantiated by years of multifaceted training. Preparing a POM specialist requires teaching both how and why we optimize a patient for anesthesia and surgery and providing opportunities for both mentored experiential learning and administrative leadership. Altogether, the focus remains on improving patient comfort, safety, and perioperative outcomes.

TABLE 8.5 ■ **Opportunities for Formal Training in Perioperative Medicine**

In-Person Clinical Perioperative Medicine, Quality and Safety Fellowships in the United States	
Duke University	https://anesthesiology.duke.edu/?page_id=834806
Vanderbilt University	https://www.vumc.org/anesthesiology/perioperative-medicine-fellowship
Brigham and Women's Hospital	https://www.brighamandwomens.org/anesthesiology-and-pain-medicine/clinical-fellowships/perioperative/perioperative-fellowship-landing
Beth Israel Deaconess Medical Center	Anesthesia Fellowships	BIDMC of Boston
Washington University St Louis	https://anesthesiology.wustl.edu/patient-care/perioperative-medicine/#periop
Stanford University	https://surgicalhome.stanford.edu/
University of California, Los Angeles	https://www.uclahealth.org/anes/perioperative-medicine-fellowship
University of California, San Diego	https://medschool.ucsd.edu/som/anesthesia/education/fellowships/Pages/Perioperative-Management-Fellowship.aspx
Wake Forest University	https://school.wakehealth.edu/Departments/Anesthesiology
University of Michigan	Perioperative Medicine Fellowship	Anesthesiology	Michigan Medicine	University of Michigan (*umich.edu*)
University of California Irvine	University of California, Irvine : Department of Anesthesiology & Perioperative Care (*uci.edu*)
University of Washington (UW)	Fellowship in Perioperative Quality & Patient Safety: UW Anesthesiology & Pain Medicine (*washington.edu*)
Tulane University	Fellowships	Medicine (*tulane.edu*)
Virtual Perioperative Medicine Fellowships	
Society for Perioperative Assessment and Quality Improvement www.spaqi.org	Perioperative medicine program combining virtual curriculum with 1-on-1 mentorship toward completion of a capstone quality improvement project within perioperative medicine: 1 year
Morpheus Consortium http://morpheusconsortium.org/	Perioperative care program (Perioperative medicine fellowship- physicians) and certificate program (nonphysicians) online, virtual: 1 year
Comprehensive Virtual Perioperative Medicine Training Program (1–5 years)	
University College London https://www.ucl.ac.uk/prospective-students/graduate/taught-degrees/perioperative-medicine-msc	Postgraduate certificate in Perioperative Medicine (60 credits) 1 year: postgraduate diploma in Perioperative Medicine (120 credits) 2–5 years: Master of Science (MSc) in Perioperative Medicine (180 credits)

References

1. Beutler S, McEvoy MD, Ferrari L, Vetter TR, Bader AM. The future of anesthesia education: developing frameworks for perioperative medicine and population health. *Anesth Analg*. 2020;130(4):1103–1108.
2. Blitz JD, Mabry C. Designing and running a preoperative clinic. *Anesthesiol Clin*. 2018;36(4):479–491.
3. Edwards AF, Slawski B. Preoperative Clinics. *Anesthesiol Clin*. 2016;34(1):1–15.
4. Aronson S, Murray S, Martin G, et al. Roadmap for transforming preoperative assessment to preoperative optimization. *Anesth Analg*. 2020;130(4):811–819.
5. Six Domains of Health Care Quality. https://www.ahrq.gov/talkingquality/measures/six-domains.html Accessed April 2022.
6. Nelson EC, Batalden PB, Godfrey MM. In: *Quality By Design. A Clinical Microsystems Approach*. 1st ed. San Francisco, CA: Jossey-Bass; 2007.
7. Wong J, An D, Urman RD, et al. Society for Perioperative Assessment and Quality Improvement (SPAQI) consensus statement on perioperative smoking cessation. *Anesth Analg*. 2020;131(3):955–968.
8. Joshi GP, Chung F, Vann MA, et al. Society for ambulatory anesthesia consensus statement on perioperative blood glucose management in diabetic patients undergoing ambulatory surgery. *Anesth Analg*. 2010;111(6).
9. Carli F, Awasthi R, Gillis C, et al. Integrating prehabilitation in the preoperative clinic: a paradigm shift in perioperative care. *Anesth Analg*. 2021;132(5):1494–1500.
10. Fleisher LA. Ambulatory anesthesia: the innovating edge of perioperative medicine? *Anesthesiol Clin*. 2019;37(2):xiii–xiv.
11. Gerber AM, Schaff JE. Leading changes in perioperative medicine: beyond length of stay. *Int Anesthesiol Clin*. 2020;58(4):2–6.
12. New England Journal of Medicine Professionalism. https://knowledgeplus.nejm.org/blog/acgme-core-competencies-professionalism/. Accessed May 2021.
13. Anesthesiology Milestones. https://www.acgme.org/Portals/0/PDFs/Milestones/AnesthesiologyMilestones2.0.pdf?ver=2020-12-02-125500-287. Accessed May 2021.
14. Shulman MA, Myles PS, Chan MT, McIlroy DR, Wallace S, Ponsford J. Measurement of disability-free survival after surgery. *Anesthesiology*. 2015;122(3):524–536.
15. Glance LG, Faden E, Dutton RP, et al. Impact of the choice of risk model for identifying low-risk patients using the 2014 American College of Cardiology/American Heart Association perioperative guidelines. *Anesthesiology*. 2018;129(5):889–900.
16. Cooper Z, Sayal P, Abbett SK, Neuman MD, Rickerson EM, Bader AM. A conceptual framework for appropriateness in surgical care: reviewing past approaches and looking ahead to patient-centered shared decision making. *Anesthesiology*. 2015;123(6):1450–1454.
17. Blitz JD, Kendale SM, Jain SK, Cuff GE, Kim JT, Rosenberg AD. Preoperative evaluation clinic visit is associated with decreased risk of in-hospital postoperative mortality. *Anesthesiology*. 2016;125(2):280–294.
18. Bader A, Hepner DL. The role of the preoperative clinic in perioperative risk reduction. *Int Anesthesiol Clin*. 2009;47(4):151–160.
19. Warner MA, Shore-Lesserson L, Shander A, Patel SY, Perelman SI, Guinn NR. Perioperative anemia: prevention, diagnosis, and management throughout the spectrum of perioperative care. *Anesth Analg*. 2020;130(5):1364–1380.
20. Musallam KM, Tamim HM, Richards T, et al. Preoperative anaemia and postoperative outcomes in non-cardiac surgery: a retrospective cohort study. *Lancet*. 2011;378(9800):1396–1407.
21. Okocha O, Dand H, Avram MJ, Sweitzer B. An effective and efficient testing protocol for diagnosing iron-deficiency anemia preoperatively. *Anesthesiology*. 2020;133(1):109–118.
22. Allin O, Urman RD, Edwards AF, et al. Using time-driven activity-based costing to demonstrate value in perioperative care: recommendations and review from the Society for Perioperative Assessment and Quality Improvement (SPAQI). *J Med Syst*. 2019;44(1):25.
23. Callahan KE, Clark CJ, Edwards AF, et al. Automated frailty screening at-scale for pre-operative risk stratification using the electronic frailty index. *J Am Geriatr Soc*. 2021;69(5):1357–1362. May.
24. O'Glasser AY, Pfeifer KJ, Edwards AF, Blitz JD, Urman RD. Striving for evidence-based, patient-centered guidance: the impetus behind the society for perioperative assessment and quality improvement (SPAQI) medication management consensus statements. *Mayo Clinic Proceedings*. 2021.

25. Wischmeyer PE, Carli F, Evans DC, et al. American society for enhanced recovery and perioperativ equality initiative joint consensus statement on nutrition screening and therapy within a surgical enhanced recovery pathway. *Anesth Analg.* 2018;126(6):1883–1895.
26. Cooper L, Abbett SK, Feng A, et al. Launching a geriatric surgery center: recommendations from the society for perioperative assessment and quality improvement. *J Am Geriatr Soc.* 2020;68(9):1941–1946.
27. Correll DJ, Bader AM, Hull MW, Hsu C, Tsen LC, Hepner DL. Value of preoperative clinic visits in identifying issues with potential impact on operating room efficiency. *Anesthesiology.* 2006;105(6):1254–1259. discussion 6A.
28. Blitz J, Swisher J, Sweitzer B. Special considerations related to race, sex, gender, and socioeconomic status in the preoperative evaluation: part 1: race, history of incarceration, and health literacy. *Anesthesiol Clin.* 2020;38(2):247–261.
29. Swisher J, Blitz J, Sweitzer B. Special considerations related to race, sex, gender, and socioeconomicstatus in the preoperative evaluation: part 2: sex considerations and homeless patients. *Anesthesiol Clin.* 2020; 38(2):263–278.
30. Chew LD, Bradley KA, Flum DR, Cornia PB, Koepsell TD. The impact of low health literacy on surgical practice. *Am J Surg.* 2004;188(3):250–253.

CHAPTER 9

System Thinking in Perioperative Medicine

Claire Cruikshanks, MB ChB, FRCA ■ Harry Soar, MB ChB, FRCA ■
Carol J. Peden, MB ChB, MD, FRCA, FFICM, MPH

KEY POINTS

- A healthcare system can be viewed at micro, meso, or macrosystem levels.
- System thinking is a set of skills, behaviors, and tools that enable analysis of the processes interactions, perspectives, and boundaries of the system.
- Adopting a system-thinking approach provides opportunities to improve the processes and outcomes of perioperative care and extend improvement into population health for the surgical population.
- This chapter describes approaches to understanding and analyzing a perioperative system, with case examples of how such an approach has informed perioperative improvement.

Complexity in Medicine

When a frail 80-year-old patient attends for an elective hip replacement, her perioperative care pathway may include interactions with the primary care physician, physiotherapist, occupational therapist, pharmacist, the anesthesiologist and preoperative clinic staff, and eventually the surgeon. She may be brought into hospital by a transport service, be reviewed by geriatricians, pass through the operating department and postanesthesia care unit, and interact with hundreds of staff throughout this journey. Multiple procurement systems, financial systems, information technology (IT) systems, and human resource systems will interact around her care pathway for a successful outcome. The care she receives will be shaped by the culture and context of the organization.

Because of the complexity of the healthcare system, any attempt to improve part of this process in isolation may not result in a predictable improvement in her outcome overall. The usual input-output-result relationship no longer functions. Approaching the complexity in perioperative medicine requires us to apply a system-thinking approach.

What Is a System?

A system is a series of interconnecting components that interact for a common purpose. Health care is very much a system, and an increasingly complex one.

In health care, we can consider care at **micro, meso,** or **macro** system levels. We refer to microsystems as the environment where the patient directly experiences clinical care. At the level of the microsystem, care includes the patient, the clinical team, and their interactions in a defined environment, such as an operating room (OR).[1,2] Mesosystems are collections of interrelated

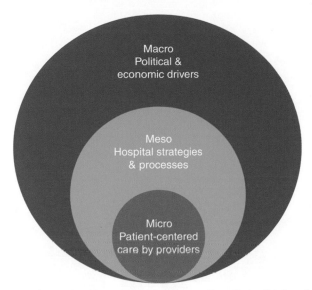

Fig. 9.1 Micro, meso, and macro level framework in health care. (From Peden CJ, Campbell M, Aggarwal G. Quality, safety, and outcomes in anesthesia; what's to be done? An international perspective. *Br J Anaesth.* 2017;119 [S1]:i5–i14.)

microsystems that interact across a care pathway; for example, breast cancer care is delivered in the outpatient clinic, radiology department, OR, and oncology clinic, among other places. Achieving improvements in patient experience and outcome requires an understanding of how the system is integrating and functioning at this mesosystem level. At the macrosystem level, we understand that the hospital is operating with interactions into primary and community services, shaped by economic, political, and wider organizational drivers, and that these interactions need to be mapped and understood to facilitate improvement. System thinking can be applied to each level of these healthcare interactions (Fig. 9.1).

What Is System Thinking?

System thinking has diverse multidiscipline origins, which have resulted in a plethora of terms and methods, the definitions of which can be unclear and daunting to clinicians. After a review of these multiple definitions, Arnold and Wade[3] proposed the following in 2015:

> *Systems thinking is a set of synergistic analytic skills used to improve the capability of identifying and understanding systems, predicting their behaviors, and devising modifications to them in order to produce desired effects. These skills work together as a system.*[3]

Barry Richmond, the originator of the term *system thinking,* stated simply that by system thinking "people see both the forest and the trees; one eye on each."[4] By understanding the complexity, we begin to appreciate that there are no longer any simple solutions, and our mindset must shift, and we must adopt new skills to system think (Fig. 9.2).

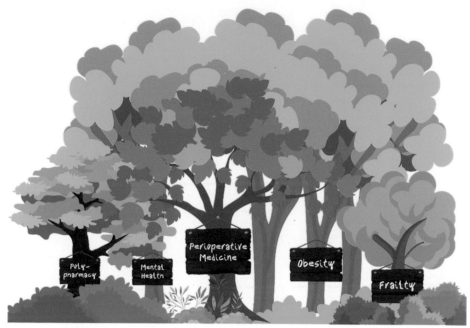

Fig. 9.2 The perioperative medicine forest and trees. (From Richmond B. System dynamics/systems thinking: let's just get on with it. *Syst Dyn Rev.* 1994;10[2–3]:135–157.)

BOX 9.1 ■ Habits of a Systems Thinker

A systems thinker:
- Makes meaningful connections within and between systems
- Seeks to understand the big picture
- Changes perspectives to increase understanding
- Considers how mental models affect current reality and the future
- Observes how elements within systems change over time, generating patterns and trends
- Surfaces and tests assumptions
- Recognizes that a system's structure generates its behavior
- Identifies the circular nature of complex cause and effect relationships
- Recognizes the impact of time delays when exploring cause and effect relationships
- Considers short-term, long-term and unintended consequences of actions
- Considers an issue fully and resists the urge to come to a quick conclusion
- Pays attention to accumulations and their rates of change
- Uses understanding of system structure to identify possible leverage actions

---

System thinking requires a different skill set and approach to thinking about problems (Box 9.1).[5]

Additional information about system thinking approaches can be found in the "Habits of a System Thinker" courses at https://thinkingtoolsstudio.waterscenterst.org/courses/habits, which list 14 considerations, including recognizing the impact of time delays when exploring cause-and-effect relationships and considering the short-term, long-term, and unintended consequences of making changes to a system.

How to Do It: Key Concepts

Williams and Hummelbrunner examined the wide range of system thinking approaches to explore what they had in common. They suggested that there are three core concepts underpinning all system methodologies that are vital for novice system thinkers to consider at the beginning of systems work[6,7]: interrelationships, perspectives, and boundaries.

INTERRELATIONSHIPS

When evaluating a system, the interconnections between components, or microsystems, must be examined. It is important to consider the structural links and the processes and behaviors between them. Interrelationships across systems are often dynamic, affected by feedback into the system, and context sensitive. Techniques to reveal these interrelationships include process and stakeholder mapping (see Chapter 29 on Process Mapping), stock-flow diagrams, and causal loop analysis.

PERSPECTIVES

It is important to understand that underlying these systemic connections are the perspectives that shape human behavior in the system. The mental models in the system can be revealed using techniques such as the ladder of inference (Fig. 9.3) or the iceberg model (Fig. 9.4).

By working at the level of mental models, it is possible to reveal leverage points that could transform care. For example, in the case of the frail 80-year-old discussed earlier, a preoperative therapy service's review for frail patients, as successfully provided by therapists in the Proactive Care of Older People Having Surgery (POPS) program[8] could be useful. The POPS program incorporated a comprehensive geriatric assessment into the preoperative pathway of elective orthopedic patients. In addition, these patients received a preoperative home occupational therapy assessment, which significantly reduced delayed discharges caused by lack of equipment. Such an approach could be trialed in a vulnerable day surgery or ambulatory care population.

BOUNDARIES

It is unavoidable that at some point in the journey of system improvement, a boundary will be set around what will, and what will not, be included. To think systematically requires using a deliberate and critical approach to relationships, connections, and perspectives, and then deciding where the boundaries lie and what will be included or excluded. Boundaries are often adopted for organizational, practical, financial, or political purposes. For example, when purchasing a new hospital IT system, the procurement team may not liaise with primary care providers, despite the need for the new system to work harmoniously with the primary care IT system to provide best patient care; a procurement boundary has been set.

Improvement work, using a system-thinking approach, starts with a diagnostic phase during which the processes, boundaries, and components of the system, the stakeholders, and their interactions and perspectives are explored.

Healthcare Improvements Via System Thinking

HEALTH FOUNDATION: SAFER CLINICAL SYSTEMS

In the Safer Clinical Systems program[9] funded by the Health Foundation in London, clinical teams coupled with engineering, ethnographic, and business researchers to deploy a series of system tools to improve two difficult patient safety issues: handovers and safe medication management. The first

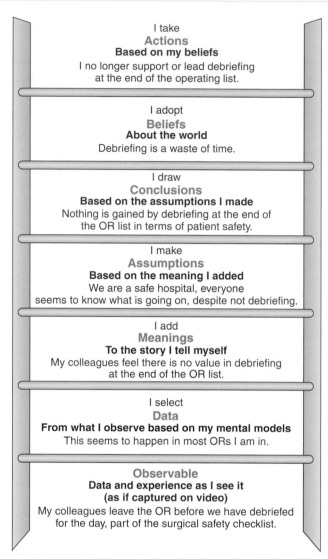

Fig. 9.3 An example of a "ladder of inference" using debriefing at the end of an OR list as an example. *OR*, Operating room. (Adapted from Flow Coaching Academy. Improving communication: the ladder of inference; 2020. https://flowcoaching.academy/news/improving-communication-the-ladder-of-inference, and Senge P. *The Fifth Discipline*. New York: Random House Business, 2006.)

phase of the program was the diagnostic phase of pathway, definition and context (3 months) and system diagnosis (5 months), during which sites sought to define their patient pathways and make visible any weaknesses or flaws. The next two steps of the program were options appraisal (2 months) and planning interventions, and finally there were system improvement cycles (15 months).

The nature of this scheme of work was to examine persistent risks and hazards affecting patient safety. Safety culture index and human factors analysis were undertaken to understand the behavior generated by the system. Subsequently improvements were iteratively trialed via PDSA (Plan-Do-Study-Act) cycles. Although the impact of the program was variable, the diagnostic analysis of the

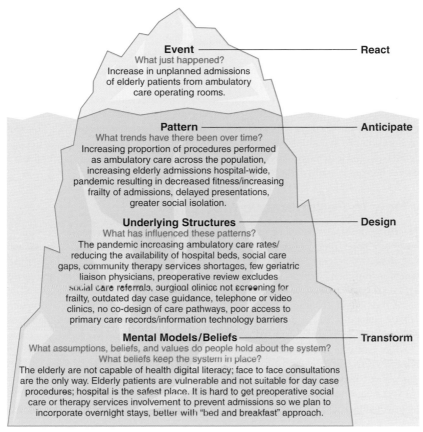

Event ———————————————— **React**
What just happened?
Increase in unplanned admissions
of elderly patients from ambulatory
care operating rooms.

Pattern ———————————————— **Anticipate**
What trends have there been over time?
Increasing proportion of procedures performed
as ambulatory care across the population,
increasing elderly admissions hospital-wide,
pandemic resulting in decreased fitness/increasing
frailty of admissions, delayed presentations,
greater social isolation.

Underlying Structures ———————————————— **Design**
What has influenced these patterns?
The pandemic increasing ambulatory care rates/
reducing the availability of hospital beds, social care
gaps, community therapy services shortages, few geriatric
liaison physicians, preoperative review excludes
social care referrals, surgical clinics not screening for
frailty, outdated day case guidance, telephone or video
clinics, no co-design of care pathways, poor access to
primary care records/information technology barriers

Mental Models/Beliefs ———————————————— **Transform**
What assumptions, beliefs, and values do people hold about the system?
What beliefs keep the system in place?
The elderly are not capable of health digital literacy; face to face consultations
are the only way. Elderly patients are vulnerable and not suitable for day case
procedures. It is hard to get preoperative social
care or therapy services involvement to prevent admissions so we plan to
incorporate overnight stays, better with "bed and breakfast" approach.

Fig. 9.4 An example of the iceberg model. (Adapted from https://www.researchgate.net/figure/The-iceberg-model-as-a-tool-for-guiding-systems-thinking-16_fig1_329324529.)

system was found invaluable by all teams who found it challenged previous assumptions and revealed hidden system weaknesses. The time taken for evaluation and development of solutions was significant (and felt abnormal for busy clinical teams), and although some teams had success, this often did not occur until late into the program.[10] One team produced an 80% reduction in hospital-associated thrombosis after surgery from 0.2% in January 2014 to 0.04% in December 2015, with a reduction in the number of all-hospital–associated venous thromboembolism (VTE; from a baseline median of 9 per month in January 2014 to a median of 1 per month by December 2015).[11] This was achieved by in-depth analysis and improvement of the processes required to effect safe and reliable VTE prescribing and management across the whole system of care.

HEALTH FOUNDATION: FLOW COACHING ACADEMY

Flow Coaching Academy methodology developed at Sheffield Teaching Hospitals (UK)[12] incorporates many system thinking tools. It involves the setting up of "big rooms" to incorporate stakeholders from across clinical pathways. Team coaching is adopted so that perspectives and interrelationships are shared, and processes are mapped so that boundaries are understood. The process starts with cross pathway engagement and interrogation of the system employing the 5Vs process:

- Value—What is important for patients and families?
- Vision—What are the aims of working more collaboratively across a system?
- eVidence—What metrics will teams use to help them understand the system?
- inVolve—How will the team involve staff and patients from across the pathway?
- Visualization—How will the team make the evidence accessible to help others?

By collaboratively working at regular big room meetings, iterative PDSA cycles of improvement are measured to ensure that the impact of interventions on the system is understood. This approach has now been adopted at multiple sites across the UK to guide pathway improvement. For example, at Imperial College Hospital, by effective cross-system working, the length of stay for diabetic foot patients has been reduced by 25%.[13]

Why Now in Perioperative Medicine?

By appreciating the system components, stakeholders, and their perspectives and examining organizational boundaries, more holistic efficient care can be achieved. The aspiration of perioperative medicine clinicians to achieve the Institute for Healthcare Improvement (IHI)'s triple aim[14,15] of simultaneously improving patient outcomes and population health and reducing healthcare costs can only be achieved with cross-sector working and system appreciation.

One of the biggest challenges facing health care currently is sustaining the workforce. The COVID-19 pandemic has significantly stressed the human element of the healthcare system. Before the pandemic, high levels of burnout were already being reported across healthcare systems.[16] More recent iterations of the Triple Aim have included provider experience, generating a "Quadruple Aim" that includes the parallel scheme of work by the IHI: "joy at work."[15] We know staff engagement scores correlate with patient outcomes,[14] and thus working to improve practitioners' experience aligns with improving patient outcomes and demonstrates the interdependence of key components of healthcare systems on successful patient outcomes (Fig. 9.5).

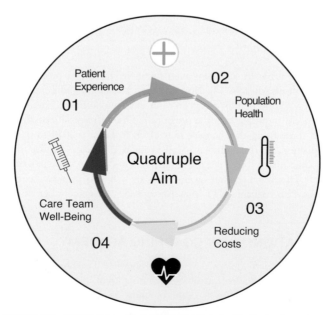

Fig. 9.5 The Quadruple Aim. (Adapted from Feeley D. The Institute for Healthcare Improvement. The triple aim or the quadruple aim? Four points to help set your strategy. http://www.ihi.org/communities/blogs/the-triple-aim-or-the-quadruple-aim-four-points-to-help-set-your-strategy.)

PERIOPERATIVE EXAMPLES

To be effective, prehabilitation programs must account for the structures of local funding and delivery systems to integrate and provide preoperative comprehensive cancer care. In the UK, Manchester's Prehab4Cancer program has successfully been integrated with existing "Greater Manchester Active" structures and fitness providers to integrate exercise into cancer pathways.[17]

In perioperative medicine, there is widespread evidence that preoperative psychological factors can influence a multitude of outcomes after surgery, from length of stay to functional recovery and quality of life scores.[17,18] The best methods for psychological preparation of a patient to ensure they are "mentally fit" for surgery are not yet established. In the design of future perioperative patient programs, it may be necessary to collaborate across the healthcare system with mental health services to deliver interventions to truly enhance postoperative recovery. To ensure that we are truly system thinking, the system must be viewed from the patients' perspective and patients must be involved in the design and delivery of perioperative programs.

Conclusion

In health care, we operate in increasingly complex systems. By adopting a system thinking mindset and understanding interconnections, boundaries, and different stakeholder perspectives, we can better diagnose system problems. By understanding the behaviors generated by the system structure and the mental models governing the system, we are best placed to plan iterative improvements. For better perioperative care to be realized, we need to think and work in systems.

References

1. Nelson E, Batalden P, Godfrey M. *Quality by Design: A Clinical Microsystem Approach.* California. Jossey-Bass; 2007.
2. Peden CJ, Campbell M, Aggarwal G. Quality, safety, and outcomes in anaesthesia; what's to be done? An international perspective. *Br J Anaesth.* 2017;119(S1):i5–i14.
3. Arnold RD, Wade JP. A definition of systems thinking: a systems approach. *Procedia Comput Sci.* 2015;44 (C):669–678.
4. Richmond B. System dynamics/systems thinking: let's just get on with it. *Syst Dyn Rev.* 1994;10 (2–3):135–157.
5. WHO. Systems Thinking for Health Systems Strengthening. In: WHO, 2017. http://www.who.int/alliance-hpsr/.
6. Williams B, Hummelbrunner R. Systems concepts in action: a practitioner's toolkit. *Vasa.* 2008;66:37–39.
7. The Systems Thinker. All methods are wrong. Some methods are useful. https://thesystemsthinker.com/%EF%BB%BFall-methods-are-wrong-some-methods-are-useful/.
8. Harari D, Hopper A, Dhesi J, et al. Proactive care of older people undergoing surgery (POPS): designing, embedding, evaluating and funding a comprehensive geriatric assessment service for older elective surgical patients. *Age Ageing.* 2007;36(2):190–196.
9. Spurgeon P, Flanagan H, Cooke M, et al. Creating safer health systems: lessons from other sectors and an account of an application in the Safer Clinical Systems programme. *Health Serv Manage Res.* 2017;30 (2):85–93.
10. Dixon-Woods M, Martin GP, Tarrant C, et al. *Safer Clinical Systems: evaluation findings Learning from the independent evaluation of the second phase of the Safer Clinical Systems programme.* London: Health Foundation; 2014. https://www.health.org.uk/publications/safer-clinical-systems-evaluation-findings.
11. Humphries A, Peden C, Jordan L, et al. Using the Safer Clinical Systems approach and Model for Improvement methodology to decrease venous thrombo-embolism in elective surgical patients. *BMJ Qual Improv Rep.* 2016;5. u210590.w4267.
12. Flow Coaching Academy. *Improving communication: the ladder of inference*; 2020. https://flowcoaching.academy/news/improvingcommunication-the-ladder-of-inference.
13. Putting feet first. *FCA Imperial The Diabetic Foot Big Room case study.* https://flowcoaching.academy/case-studies?page=2.

14. The Institute for Healthcare Improvement (IHI). The IHI triple aim. http://www.ihi.org/Engage/
Initiatives/TripleAim/Pages/default.aspx.
15. Sikka R, Morath JM, Leape L. The Quadruple Aim: care, health, cost and meaning in work. *BMJ Qual Saf.*
2015;24(10):608–610.
16. West M, Dawson J. *Employee engagement and NHS performance.* London: Kings Fund; 2012. https://www.
kingsfund.org.uk/sites/default/files/employee-engagement-nhs-performance-west-dawson-leadership-
review2012-paper.pdf.
17. Moore J, Merchant Z, Rowlinson K, et al. Implementing a system-wide cancer prehabilitation programme:
the journey of Greater Manchester's "Prehab4cancer". *Eur J Surg Oncol.* 2020;47(3):524–532.
18. Levett D, Grimmett C. Psychological factors, prehabilitation and surgical outcomes: evidence and future
directions. *Anaesthesia.* 2019;74(s1):36–42.

Further Reading and Resources

Thinking Tools Studio. Habits of a systems thinker courses. https://thinkingtoolsstudio.waterscenterst.org/
courses/habits.
Plack MM, Goldman EF, Scott AR, Brundage SB. *Systems Thinking in the Healthcare Professions: A Guide for
Educators and Clinicians.* Washington, DC: The George Washington University; 2019.
Richmond B. *The "Thinking" in Systems Thinking: Seven Essential Skills (Toolbox Reprint Series).* Waltham, MA:
Pegasus Communications; 2000.
Senge P. *The Fifth Discipline.* New York: Random House Business; 2006.

CHAPTER 10

Patient-Centered Care in Perioperative Outcomes

Angela M. Bader, MD, MPH

KEY POINTS

- Value in health care is defined as patient-centered outcomes (PCOs) relative to the cost of achieving those outcomes.
- PCOs must consider the health trajectory well past discharge.
- Patient outcomes include that there is concordance of the expectations of the planned procedure with patient preferences, goals, and values.

What Is Patient-Centered Care?

Patient-centered care requires that all disciplines involved in treating a specific surgical condition develop evidence-based collaborative care pathways with value-based metrics. The patient is at the center of the care, the patient's voice is an important part of the collaboration, and individual patient characteristics, both clinical and nonclinical, are accounted for. An effort is made to understand patient values and goals and to ensure that care aligns with these. Expectations and possible health trajectories are discussed realistically; evidence based collaborative pathways are used to achieve these goals. Metrics are patient centered and continue long past discharge. Equity is ensured by including the impact of disparities, culture, language, access issues, health literacy, and disabilities when planning care pathways. Enhanced patient engagement is key.

High-value health care should ensure patient-centered care as well. Specific elements include institutional buy-in, metric shift, condition-specific metrics leading to multidisciplinary care pathways, and patient-centered care aligned with individual values and goals.

INSTITUTIONAL BUY-IN

High-value, patient-centered care cannot be achieved without institutional alignment. The upper levels of the organization must value patient-centered outcomes (PCOs) and not just traditional metrics. Achieving buy-in from institutional leadership is often the most difficult step; however, clinicians without leadership support are unlikely to achieve desired goals. As payment models continue to transition from volume to value, the increasing focus on linking revenue to quality metrics may ease this transition. Unenlightened institutions may persist in old paradigms even in the setting of these transitions, which is likely to cause further disconnect between leadership and clinicians performing care.

METRIC SHIFT

Traditional metrics have focused on the absence of negative outcomes or process metrics rather than positive long-term PCOs. Arbitrary definitions of "in-hospital," "7-day," and "30-day" morbidity and mortality as definitions of success completely neglect the patient's goals in having the surgery; the patient has a procedure to achieve some positive impact on health trajectory and does not count success as merely being alive and uninjured on day 30. Why have these metrics become so ubiquitous? They are easy to measure and offer some overall information that can be used for benchmarking. Measuring PCOs that are condition specific and incorporate patient values and goals is hard. Process metrics such as "turnover time" or "operating room utilization" may be useful for operations planning and do play a role in the cost denominator of the value equation, but they do not relate to patient-centered care or PCOs. Judging clinicians by their ability to achieve these process metrics and not by their ability to achieve condition-specific PCOs can increase the institutional disconnect and impede patient-centered care.

CONDITION-SPECIFIC METRICS LEADING TO MULTIDISCIPLINARY CARE PATHWAYS

Some condition-specific metrics are provided by individual clinical organizations, but a more multidisciplinary framework is needed. Professor Michael Porter, who heads the Institute for Strategy and Competitiveness at Harvard Business School, founded the International Consortium for Health Outcomes Measurement (ICHOM), which is freely available via the Internet.[1] This work involves developing standard sets of outcomes that matter most to patients for specific conditions and driving international adoption and reporting of these measures to improve value of care provided (PCO/cost). The outcomes are divided into three tiers: tier one relates to acute surgical complications, tier two relates to self-reported health outcomes, and tier three relates to survival and disease control.

For example, using the ICHOM standard set for the condition "local prostate cancer":
Tier one outcomes: Acute major surgical and radiologic complications
Tier two outcomes: Urinary incontinence; urinary frequency, obstruction, or irritation; bowel irritation; sexual dysfunction
Tier three outcomes: Biochemical recurrence; metastases; cause-specific and overall survival

This type of analysis can used when developing PCOs using multidisciplinary collaboration, adding other outcomes as deemed necessary by the various disciplines involved. Based on the multidisciplinary outcomes desired, evidence-based collaborative care pathways can be developed. These should include attention to individual patient characteristics that can be addressed preoperatively using optimization and prehabilitation pathways and to postdischarge pathways and metrics obtained a sufficient amount of time after discharge to determine the overall impact of the perioperative care episode on health trajectory.

PATIENT-CENTERED CARE ALIGNED WITH INDIVIDUAL VALUES AND GOALS

Patient-centered care aligns treatment with individual preferences, values, and goals. Standard outcome sets are excellent for condition-specific measures. A comparison of probable outcomes with treatment options can enable patients to decide on a care plan most closely aligned with their goals. For example, balancing long-term survival and risk of recurrence after cancer surgery can be judged based on the impact of the procedure on self-reported health outcomes, acute surgical risks, and quality of life. Ensuring that treatment is aligned requires an investment on the part of clinicians, the patient, and often patient family members as well.

There are a number of barriers that must be overcome to ensure aligned care, such as insufficient patient engagement, inattention to patient factors, training deficiencies, time constraints, lack of emphasis on advanced care directives and proxies, and deficiencies in electronic medical record (EMR) documentation.

Insufficient Patient Engagement

We may not be asking all the right questions or really listening to the answers. Insufficient patient engagement is likely the most difficult barrier to overcome when attempting to achieve patient-centered care. Techniques outside the current EMR must be developed that allow easy access to patients from referral to long past discharge for engagement, education, and outcome measurement, so that information can continue to be collected and a conversation can be maintained. Current EMRs do not incorporate easily accessible systems that can record input based on time so that the continuum of perioperative care can be appropriately documented and mechanisms for patient education and engagement can be maintained.

Inattention to Patient Factors

We need to adapt our questions based on patient factors such as health literacy, culture, language, disparities, and access issues. These can all interfere with achieving the level of communication needed to ensure patient-centered care that is aligned with values and goals. Greater efforts must be placed on adapting patient engagement techniques to reflect these individual issues. Vulnerability screening for problems with issues such as hearing, vision, and cognitive dysfunction is of critical importance.

Training Deficiencies

We do not sufficiently train surgical and anesthesia residents to listen. We need to embed into residency programs sufficient training in communication to ensure that physicians have the skill sets needed to conduct appropriate conversations around patient-centered goals and alignment. Continuing education generally does not focus on the importance of acquiring these skills. Clinicians may feel uncomfortable conducting these conversations and may be unclear as to whether this is a part of their role as perioperative care providers.

Time Constraints

We do not sufficiently value time spent communicating with the patient. Time spent with the patient may not be considered "valuable" to operating room leadership because in most cases it does not translate directly into revenue. What is "valuable" often is translated into what is "billable," and significant effort is often placed on reducing any nonbillable time. The importance of time spent during preoperative assessment and optimization is disregarded in favor of reducing costs in the preoperative budget if the institution is using a siloed model of care. This is unfortunate because it does not give surgical providers sufficient financial "credit" for conducting conversations that will ensure alignment with patient values and goals, even though these conversations are critical for achieving PCOs. In addition, eliminating unwanted and potentially futile care has the potential not just to ensure alignment but also to eliminate waste of valuable healthcare resources, reducing overall healthcare costs.

Lack of Emphasis on Advanced Care Directives and Health Proxies

We do not pay enough attention to advanced care directives and healthcare proxies. This is of particular importance for patients who are undergoing high-risk treatment plans and who may become unable to speak for themselves because of the acuity of their care. These issues should be a standard part of preoperative care pathways. Advising patients to make sure their health proxy would know what their wishes are is also necessary to ensure patient-centered care and alignment with patient goals and values.

Deficiencies in Electronic Medical Record Documentation

EMRs are not built in a patient-centered format. EMRs were developed to record single patient encounters for ease of billing and are not well suited to document care along a continuum or to include significant patient engagement that continues well past discharge. We must demand that EMRs look at patients the way we do, rather than requiring us to put together a longitudinal picture of an episode of care from multiple disconnected encounters. Therefore to ensure patient-centered care, clinicians need to adapt their documentation systems so that important factors can be easily viewed by upstream and downstream providers. For example, easy identification of healthcare proxy and advanced directives, health literacy issues, and vulnerability screens are likely as important as allergies in terms of ensuring that appropriate treatment is given. Recording issues only in one clinician's assessment makes it difficult to ensure that downstream care is cognizant of the issues. Important issues should be displayed inside banners or similar techniques where these issues are easily visible when the chart is opened.

How Do We Measure Success?

There is no easy way to measure the success of collaborative care pathways with all of the various optimization, prehabilitation, and postdischarge care that may be incorporated. For example, reducing the incidence of postoperative delirium by implementing delirium prevention pathways can be measured, but the overall impact of all the perioperative elements on reducing postoperative cognitive decline is difficult to determine and likely the result of a bundle of care rather than one particular element. It is also difficult to measure whether we have successfully aligned patient preferences, values, and goals with treatment provided. For example, a palliative procedure may improve quality of life but have no impact on reducing mortality and should mortality occur, a causal attribution should not be made. Perhaps the best way to measure success is to determine as objectively as possible whether the care provided was consistent with patient values and goals. This may be done by surveys of patients and/or family members and comparing what is stated on advanced care planning documentation or do not resuscitate (DNR)/do not intubate (DNI) paperwork with what actually transpired. In summary, the best way to work toward achieving patient-centered care in perioperative outcomes is learning to incorporate the patient's voice, recognizing the skill and time that it will take to do this successfully. Empowering the patient in this way will yield great rewards in terms of achieving high-value health care that will impact individual patient outcomes and overall population health.

References

1. International Consortium for Health Outcomes Measurement. *https://www.ichom.org*. Accessed May 2, 2021.

CHAPTER 11

Shared Decision Making

Sally El-Ghazali, MBBS, MSc, FRCA, FFICM ■ Maria Khan, MBBS, FRCA ■
Ramai Santhirapala, MBBS, FRCA, FFICM, FHEA

KEY POINTS

- Shared decision making (SDM) is a patient-centered approach that encourages both healthcare professionals and patients to work collaboratively for the benefit of patients.
- Perioperative care is a collaborative multidisciplinary approach for patients contemplating surgery, and the patient's individual values and preferences should be at the center.
- One approach is the use and promotion of patient-facing resources, such as the "Benefits, Risks, Alternatives, and doing Nothing" (BRAN) model
- Another approach to use in conjunction with the BRAN model is the Best Case/Worst Case communication framework.
- SDM has been demonstrated to improve patients' engagement in health care, compliance with treatments, and, ultimately, satisfaction.
- Barriers to SDM include a lack of understanding about what SDM entails and how to implement it.

Introduction

Perioperative care is a collaborative multidisciplinary approach for patients contemplating surgery that centers individual values and preferences.[1] This personalized approach to perioperative care lends itself well to the shared decision making (SDM) model. The term SDM is defined as "… a process in which clinicians and patients work together to select tests, treatments, management or support packages, based on clinical evidence and the patient's informed preferences."[2] By using best practice evidence, clinicians can provide the information necessary to support and empower patients to make the best decisions for themselves.[2,3]

SDM is a patient-centered approach that moves away from traditional paternalism, recognizing both clinicians and patients as experts and partners in healthcare decisions.[4,5] Clinicians provide clinical expertise and knowledge about diagnosis and treatment, and patients act as the experts in their condition and have knowledge of their personal preferences. By sharing their respective knowledge, the patient and clinician can work collaboratively and choose the next best step in the patient's care and treatment.

Origins and Drivers

In 2012, the American Board of Internal Medicine launched a professionally led public-facing program called "Choosing Wisely."[6] Central to Choosing Wisely were aspirations of improving conversations between patients and healthcare professionals, which is a key underlying principle of SDM. The origins of Choosing Wisely are rooted in a collaborative effort between the American

Board of Internal Medicine, the American College of Physicians Foundation, and the European Federation of Internal Medicine termed "A Physician Charter."[7] This document highlights the importance of fair distribution of resources and encourages healthcare professionals to consider patient welfare, patient autonomy, and social justice. Since the launch of Choosing Wisely in the United States in 2012, more than 20 countries have joined this now international program. The Choosing Wisely UK program was launched in 2016 and has been led by the Academy of Medical Royal Colleges (AoMRC), which is the coordinating body of the 23 UK medical Royal Colleges and specialty societies.[8]

The drivers behind the promotion of SDM are multifactorial. As healthcare professionals in the UK, the Montgomery judgment alludes to a legal obligation to provide patients with the necessary information to make an informed decision as part of the consent process and therefore move from a paternalistic medicine model to a SDM one.[9] There is also the ethical considerations of SDM that support the principles of beneficence and nonmaleficence.[10] Additionally, there are political factors that encourage clinicians to endorse SDM in practice. SDM has been adopted in national policies after research revealed the benefits, particularly in high-risk surgical patients.[11]

Benefits of Shared Decision Making

Although some patients may choose not to make decisions with regards to their medical care, evidence suggests they still do want to be involved in the decision-making process.[12] SDM has been demonstrated to improve patients' engagement in health care, compliance with treatments, and, ultimately, satisfaction.[13,14] To facilitate SDM, it is imperative that the patient is fully informed of risks, benefits, alternatives, and the option of doing nothing. Patients should also be given the opportunity to ask further questions to support a conversation in ascertaining what matters to them. In the setting of perioperative care, this should ideally be performed in preoperative clinic to offer ample time and opportunity for informed consent.[4]

SDM can also help with the aspirations of the quadruple aim framework in transforming healthcare systems.[15] The quadruple aim encompasses improving patient experience, population health, cost-effectiveness, and healthcare team wellbeing.[16] Thus SDM allows for the appropriate resources to be allocated to each patient, which reduces duplication of work and resource waste, thus encouraging healthcare sustainability and reducing the environmental impact of health care.[17]

SDM may also have a positive impact on healthcare professionals. It may help alleviate the concerns of healthcare professionals who are worried about the impact of medical interventions on those patients who are not appropriately informed. This concept of "moral injury" is increasingly recognized as a contributor to burnout in health professionals. Collaborative working may help reduce the deleterious effects of this.[1]

Barriers to Shared Decision Making

Understanding the multifactorial barriers to SDM will enable us to overcome them. Commonly held views by clinicians are that they already practice SDM or that SDM is time consuming.[2] A lack of clinician understanding and no clear definition of SDM[10] may be the reason behind the belief that they already practice SDM. Patient surveys, however, have shown that at least half of patients would have liked more involvement in the decisions made about their care.[2]

Additionally, a clinician who may have developed preconceived ideas about the patient may be predisposed toward certain decisions before a consultation. Therefore some of the decision making may be influenced or have occurred before an in-depth discussion with the patient has taken place, thus impacting the ability to truly practice SDM. As a result, the clinician can shape the patient's "field of choice" in the consultation.[18]

Although SDM consultations may be perceived as more time consuming, taking time upfront to engage patients in decisions will reduce the overall time spent engaging those who are unsure or unhappy about the decisions made for them.[2] Another common belief is that patients do not want to be involved in the decision-making process.[19] Although this may be true for some, and in this scenario, clinicians have to make decisions in the best interest of the patient, this is not usually the case.[19]

Patients may have a great desire for more information about diseases and treatment options but not pursue it out of a desire to also be perceived as a "good patient."[2,19] This further perpetuates the belief that they do not want to be involved in the decision-making process. Social demographics appear to vary in the willingness to participate in the decision-making process, with young and highly educated patients more likely to actively seek involvement. Nevertheless, many older people and those from disadvantaged groups also want to actively participate but require adequate encouragement and the use of appropriate tools.[2]

The current lack of standardized tools for risk assessment and risk communication coupled with the current practice of risk discussions occurring after surgical consent has also proved to create barriers that need addressing for SDM to be implemented successfully.[10]

Practical Guidance

Strategies to promote uptake of SDM have predominately focused on patient interventions and the education of professionals.[20] SDM, however, is multidimensional and involves conversations between patient and the healthcare professional as well as multidisciplinary team working and systems that support the intervention. Therefore both professional-facing and patient-facing approaches are required to successfully implement SDM. Managers and leaders need to be actively involved in the process to enable productive engagement of relevant stakeholders. This is required to implement changes at both an individual and organizational level.[21]

Another imperative lever to implement SDM is education and training, not only highlighting the merits of SDM to healthcare professionals and patients but also showing how clinicians can effectively communicate to deliver an SDM standard. One particular approach is the use and promotion of patient-facing resources, such as the "Benefits, Risks, Alternatives and doing Nothing" (BRAN) model.[22] These are a set of questions that patients are encouraged to discuss with healthcare professionals to enable better decision making together. The questions are:

- What are the **B**enefits?
- What are the **R**isks?
- What are the **A**lternatives?
- What happens if I do **N**othing?

Another approach to use in conjunction with the BRAN model is the Best Case/Worst Case communication framework.[23] The Best Case/Worst Case combines a narrative description with handwritten graphics to describe how patients might experience a range of possible postoperative outcomes in the best case, worst case, and most likely scenarios. This helps to promote SDM by shifting the focus of decision-making conversations from an isolated problem to a discussion about treatment alternatives and outcomes.

Summary

SDM is a patient-centered approach that encourages both healthcare professionals and patients to work collaboratively for the benefit of patients. Healthcare professionals provide clinical expertise and knowledge about diagnosis and treatment, and patients are the experts in their condition and have knowledge of their personal preferences. SDM has demonstrated an improvement in patients' engagement in health care, compliance with treatments, and, ultimately, satisfaction. Nevertheless, barriers, including lack of understanding about what SDM entails and how to implement it, exist. Practical guidance involves both patient interventions and education and training of healthcare professionals to enable effective practice of SDM. The key to success in SDM is active involvement of all stakeholders. Understanding the benefits of SDM and how to mitigate barriers will lead to enhanced patient care.

References

1. Santhirapala R, Partridge J, MacEwen C. The older surgical patient—to operate or not? A state of the art review. *Anaesthesia.* 2020;75(Suppl. 1):e46–e53.
2. Coulter A., Collins A. Making Shared Decision-Making a Reality: No Decision About Me, Without Me. The Kings Fund; 2011. https://www.kingsfund.org.uk/sites/default/files/Making-shared-decision-making-a-reality-paper-Angela-Coulter-Alf-Collins-July-2011_0.pdf.
3. Barry M, Edgman-Levitan S. Shared decision making—the pinnacle of patient-centered care. *N Engl J Med.* 2012;366:780–781.
4. Simons M, Hetrick S, Jorm A. Shared decision making: benefits, barriers and current opportunities for application. *Australas Psychiatry.* 2010;18:394–397.
5. Santhirapala R, Mooneasinghe R. Primum Non Nocere: is shared decision-making the answer? *Perioper Med.* 2016;5:16.
6. Cassel C, Guest J. Choosing Wisely: helping physicians and patients make smart decisions about their care. *JAMA.* 2012;307:1801–1802.
7. ABIM Foundation, ACP-ASIM Foundation, European Federation of Internal Medicine. Medical professionalism in the new millennium: a physician charter. *Ann Intern Med.* 2002;136(3):243–246.
8. Academy of Medical Royal Colleges. https://www.aomrc.org.uk.
9. Chan S, Tulloch E, Cooper E, Smith A, Wojcik W, Norman J. Montgomery and informed consent: where are we now? *BMJ.* 2017;357:2224.
10. Santhirapala R, Pearse R. Shared decision making in perioperative care. In: Chereshneva M, Johnston C, Colvin J, Peden CJ, eds. *Raising the Standards: RCoA Quality Improvement Compendium [Internet].* 4th ed. Royal College of Anaesthetists; 2020:76–77. https://www.rcoa.ac.uk/sites/default/files/documents/2020-08/21075%20RCoA%20Audit%20Recipe%20Book_Combined_Final_25.08.2020_0.pdf.
11. National Institute for Health and Care Research. OSIRIS. *Optimising shared decision-making for high-risk major surgery.* https://www.fundingawards.nihr.ac.uk/award/RP-PG-0218-20001.
12. NatCen. British Social Attitudes survey; 2009. http://www.natcen.ac.uk/study/british-social-attitudes-25threport/findings.
13. Stiggelbout A, Van der Weijden T, De Wit M, et al. Shared decision making: really putting patients at the centre of healthcare. *BMJ.* 2012;344:256.
14. London: Health Foundation. Evidence: helping people share decision making; 2012. https://www.health.org.uk/sites/default/files/HelpingPeopleShareDecisionMaking.pdf.
15. Kunneman M, Montori VM. When patient-centred care is worth doing well: informed consent or shared decision-making. *BMJ Qual Saf.* 2017;26:522–524.
16. Sikka R, Morath JM, Leape L. The Quadruple Aim: care, health, cost and meaning in work. *BMJ Qual Saf.* 2015;24:608–610.
17. Naylor C, Appleby J. Sustainable health and social care: connecting environmental and financial performance. The King's Fund. http://www.kingsfund.org.uk/sites/files/kf/field/field_publication_file/sustainable-health-social-care-appleby-naylor-mar2012.pdf.
18. Clapp J, Arriaga A, Murthy S, et al. Surgical consultation as social process: implications for shared decision making. *Ann Surg.* 2019;269(3):446–452.
19. The National Institute for Health and Care Excellence. *Shared decision making.* 2019. https://www.nice.org.uk/advice/ktt23/resources/shared-decision-making-pdf-58758011521477.
20. Joseph-Williams N, Lloyd A, Edwards A, et al. Implementing shared decision making in the NHS: lessons from the MAGIC programme. *BMJ.* 2017;357, j1744.
21. Heifetz RA, Linksky M, Grashow A. *The Practice of Adaptive Leadership: Tools and Tactics for Changing Your Organisation and the World.* Harvard Business Press; 2009.

22. Santhirapala R, Fleisher L, Grocott M. Choosing Wisely: just because we can, does it mean we should? *Br J Anaesth. 2019*;122(3):306–310.
23. Taylor L, Nabozny M, Steffens N, et al. A framework to improve surgeon communication in high-stakes surgical decisions: best case/worst case. *JAMA Surg.* 2017;152(6):531–538.

CHAPTER 12

Clinical Outcomes and Measures in Perioperative Care

Elizabeth R. Berger, MD, MS ■ Chelsea P. Fischer, MD, MS ■
Clifford Y. Ko, MD, MS, MSHS

KEY POINTS

- To improve perioperative care and safety, relevant clinical outcomes and appropriate measures must be defined.
- The National Quality Forum (NQF) proposed that ideal clinical measures are:
  - Evidence-based and highlight a "performance gap."
  - Demonstrative of reliability and validity.
  - Feasible to collect without undue burden (routinely generated during care delivery; available in electronic medical record).
  - "Usable"—the measure should be able to be used for both accountability, such as for public reporting, and performance improvement.
- Despite many clinical outcome measures developed and used in the perioperative space, success has been variable regarding application, practical reliability, clinical meaningfulness, and overall sustained effectiveness in improving outcomes.
- Lessons learned include the need for consistent and appropriate risk adjustment and the importance of data source, case ascertainment, and collection methods.
- Coordination among experts, patient-centered goals, and thoughtful selection of clinical outcomes to measure will ultimately lead to improved patient care.

Importance of Clinical Outcome Measures

Clinical outcome measures serve as a way of understanding the results of healthcare delivery to patients, and monitoring of outcomes helps ensure safe and high-quality health care. Nearly a century ago, Massachusetts physician Ernest Codman recognized the importance of tracking patient "end results" to improve care for future patients. This practice did not become commonplace, however, until the Institute of Medicine (IOM) published *To Err Is to Human* in 1999, the landmark report outlining the substantial harm that medical errors inflict on patients, healthcare providers, and the healthcare system.[1] This report incited a national movement to design safer health systems and improve patient safety and quality. According to the IOM, healthcare quality is defined as "the degree to which health care services for individuals and populations increase the likelihood of desired health outcomes and are consistent with current professional knowledge."[2] Measurement of patient quality and safety is particularly relevant to surgical care because over 50 million in-patient procedures are performed annually, and an estimated 98,000 people die each year from hospital-related medical errors.[1] Additionally, perioperative complications are common and costly.[3–7]

Evaluation of healthcare quality can be understood through the conceptual framework of the Donabedian model, published in 1966 by Avedis Donabedian, which proposed a healthcare quality evaluation framework using a quality-of-care model and a triad of "Structure, Process, and Outcome."[8] Structure refers to the physical and organizational setting in which health care is delivered; process describes the actions of healthcare delivery; and outcome describes the end result of health care on patients and on population health status.[9] Data gathered using this model can create a better scientific understanding of health care as a system, inform healthcare quality, and, ultimately, improve patient outcomes. Because of this, the Donabedian model has remained a central pillar of contemporary evaluations of quality in perioperative care.

Before healthcare quality and safety can be improved, relevant clinical outcomes and appropriate measures must be defined. The National Quality Forum (NQF) has proposed a four-part process to evaluate the quality and appropriateness of collected measures.[10] First, the measure must be evidence-based and highlight a "performance gap," a variation in performance or substandard care that can be substantially improved. Second, the measure must demonstrate reliability and validity. The data elements should be replicable for consistent comparison across settings and should correctly represent the quality of care given. Third, the data must be feasible to collect without undue burden (routinely generated during care delivery; available in the electronic health record [EHR]). This allows for equitable implementation of data collection across hospital systems. Finally, the measure must be "usable"—it should be able to be used for both accountability, such as for public reporting, and performance improvement. Despite many clinical outcome measures having been developed and used in the perioperative space, success has been variable regarding their application, practical reliability, clinical meaningfulness, and overall sustained effectiveness. Lessons learned are many and include the need for consistent and appropriate risk adjustment and the importance of data source, case ascertainment, and collection methods.

Clinical Outcome Measures to Use in Perioperative Care

The first attempt to measure outcomes of surgical and perioperative care focused on inpatient mortality from administrative data sources. Since then, measures used have expanded to include other outcomes, process, structure, efficiency, and appropriateness measures to meet increasing demands for more information regarding quality of medical care. Because collecting limitless clinical outcome measures is not feasible, it is challenging but important to choose the most effective measures to improve care. The Centers for Medicare and Medicaid Services (CMS) had previously focused quality improvement (QI) efforts on collection of process measures, theorizing that by optimizing care processes, clinical outcomes would improve in turn. Process measures are advantageous in that they are actionable and can lead to increased adherence to the process. They are also helpful when an outcome measure is difficult to measure well (i.e., venous thromboembolism). Process of care measures have proved effective in improving clinical outcomes in areas such as surgical site infection (SSI), cardiac complications, and ventilator-associated pneumonia. Nevertheless, rigorous data and evidence proving causal linkage between processes and outcomes remains limited, and most outcomes have a multitude of plausible associated processes.

Clinical outcome measures such as mortality, complication rates (e.g., SSI, urinary tract infection, venous thromboembolism), length of stay (LOS), and readmission rates have been an area of focus for the last decade. Given that improving patient outcomes is a natural motivation for clinicians, these measures often have face validity with all perioperative team members. Other clinical outcome measures that have garnered recent attention are patient-reported outcomes (PROs) and value-based outcomes. PROs include aspects of patient function and quality of recovery; value-based outcomes include cost-effectiveness and resource use, as well as health-related quality of life.[11] A recent meta-analysis by Moonesinghe et al. states that patient-centered outcomes, such as PROs, are likely to become more commonplace given the increasing recognition that traditional outcomes of mortality or LOS incompletely evaluate the impact of clinical interventions on patients. Additionally, perioperative care advances have decreased the incidence of short-term outcomes (i.e., 30-day mortality), highlighting the need to focus on more prevalent outcomes such as complications, quality of life measures, or value-based care measures.[12]

Studies have shown that the action of measuring and reviewing outcomes, in and of itself, can improve outcomes, but to measure meaningful clinical outcomes requires high-quality, risk-adjusted data. This is often accomplished through clinical registries that provide nationally validated, risk-adjusted outcome data gathered by clinically trained personnel from medical records. In the United States, one example is the National Surgical Quality Improvement Project (NSQIP), which was borne out of a 1986 Congress mandate that the Departments of Veterans Affairs needed to report its surgical outcomes annually and compare them with the national average. In response, healthcare providers at the VA developed a statistically reliable database of patients' preoperative risk factors, intraoperative and in-hospital data, and postoperative outcomes and also employed methods for accurate risk adjustment.[13] Not only was benchmarking performed but also clinical outcomes improved, including mortality, complications, and LOS. Because of its success, a private sector NSQIP was developed by the American College of Surgeons (ACS) with currently over 800 hospitals participating in 12 countries. With over 15 years of experience of ACS NSQIP®, additional surgical specialties, procedures, and procedure-targeted variables have been identified, tested, and incorporated into ACS NSQIP®. Box 12.1 provides examples of some "core" clinical outcomes measured in all procedures in ACS NSQIP®, and Table 12.1 provides examples of "procedure-targeted" clinical outcomes in 10 specific

---

BOX 12.1 ■ ACS NSQIP® Core List of Clinical Outcome Examples

Postoperative Occurrences (Date of Occurrence Also Collected)

Superficial Incisional SSI
Date of Superficial Incisional SSI
Deep Incisional SSI
Organ/Space SSI
Wound Disruption
Pneumonia
Unplanned Intubation
Pulmonary Embolism
On Ventilator >48 Hours
Progressive Renal Insufficiency
Acute Renal Failure
Urinary Tract Infection
Stroke/CVA
Cardiac Arrest Requiring CPR
Myocardial Infarction
Blood Transfusion
Blood Units Transfused
Vein Thrombosis Requiring Therapy
C. diff
C. diff Diagnosis
C. diff Treatment Given
C. diff Tests Performed that Resulted Positive
Sepsis
Septic Shock
New Postoperative COVID–19 Diagnosis
Acute Hospital Discharge Date
Hospital Discharge Destination
Still in Hospital >30 Days
30-Day Mortality
End of Life/Withdrawal of Care

CPR, Cardiopulmonary resuscitation; *CVA*, cerebrovascular accident; *SSI*, surgical site infection.

TABLE 12.1 ■ Examples of ACS NSQIP® Procedure-Targeted Clinical Outcomes

Colectomy	Anastomotic Leak
	Prolonged Postoperative NPO or NGT Use
Appendectomy	Intraabdominal Abscess
Esophagectomy	Anastomotic Leak
Hepatectomy	Highest Drain Bilirubin POD#1
	Highest Drain Bilirubin POD#3 to POD#30
	Operative Drain Still Present at 30 Days
	Last Drain Removal Day
	Need for Invasive Intervention Postoperatively (excluding reoperation)
	Types of Required Invasive Intervention
	Peak Postoperative INR (on or after POD#5)
	Peak Postoperative Bilirubin (on or after POD#5)
	Peak Postoperative Serum Creatinine
	Bile Leakage
	Post Hepatectomy Liver Failure
	Post Hepatectomy Liver Failure Grade
Pancreatectomy	Highest Drain Amylase POD#1 (U/L)
	Highest Drain Amylase POD#2 to POD#30 (U/L)
	Date of Highest Amylase Level POD#2 to POD#30
	Drain Still Present at POD#30
	Last Pancreatic Drain Removal Day
	Postoperative Acute Pancreatitis (POAP)
	Pancreatic Fistula
	Postpancreatectomy Hemorrhage (PPH)
	Delayed Gastric Emptying
	Percutaneous Drain
	Percutaneous Drainage
	Intensive Care Unit LOS
Proctectomy	Anastomotic Leak
	Prolonged Postoperative NPO or NGT Use
Thyroidectomy	Postoperative Calcium Level Checked
	Postoperative Parathyroid Level Checked
	Postoperative Calcium and Vitamin D Replacement
	Significant Postoperative Hypocalcemia Before Discharge
	Significant Postoperative Hypocalcemia w/in 30 days
	Clinically Severe Hypocalcemia-Related Event
	Clinically Severe Hypocalcemia-Related Event, Type of Event
	Recurrent Laryngeal Nerve Injury or Dysfunction
	Neck Hematoma/Bleeding
Hysterectomy	Intestinal Obstruction
	Prolonged Postoperative NPO or NGT Use
	Anastomotic Leak
	Ureteral Obstruction
	Ureteral Fistula
	Bladder Fistula
Hip Fracture	Pathological Fracture
	New Postoperative Pressure Sore
	Postoperative Use of Mobility Aid
	Prescription of Postoperative Bone Protection Medication
	Place of Residence at 30 Days Postoperative
	Weight Bearing as Tolerated (WBAT) on POD#1
	Postoperative Delirium
Prostatectomy	Anastomotic Leak
	Rectal Injury
	Prolonged Postoperative NPO/NGT Use
	Ureteral Obstruction
	Urinary Leak/Fistula
	Lymphocele, Lymphatic Leak, or Other Fluid Collection

ACS, American College of Surgeons; *INR*, international normalized ratio; *LOS*, length of stay; *NGT*, nasogastric; *NPO*, nothing by mouth; *NSQIP*, National Surgical Quality Improvement Program; *POD*, postoperative day.

surgical procedures. In ACS NSQIP®, over 30 specific surgical procedures with procedure-targeted variables are available.

There are currently hundreds of clinical registries in health care and the volume of data collected in EHRs has enormous potential for further development of registries. Claims data are also acceptable alternatives to clinical data when collecting outcomes; however, they should be used with caution because their primary intention is to serve as financial records. Claims data have been shown to be inconsistent, subject to misinterpretation, and lacking clinical detail to appropriately evaluate and measure quality of care.[14,15] The future may additionally see data from patient-wearable technology and personal cellular phones incorporated into clinical outcome measurement.

Improving Perioperative Care With Clinical Outcome Measures

Collecting data on clinical outcome measures is a crucial first step to improve quality of care. Nevertheless, identifying poor outcomes alone does not inherently improve perioperative care. An essential component of improvement is understanding the data, frequent review, and feedback of outcomes to relevant stakeholders. Outcome risk-adjustment is important to making data interpretable and comparable to other institutions. Developing robust statistical methods to account for how patient factors (i.e., demographics and comorbidities) can influence clinical outcomes allows hospitals to benchmark their performance to peer groups. Without risk-adjustment, equitable comparison between hospitals is not possible given variation in the patient population served. Additionally, hospitals must engage in frequent review of outcomes, propose solutions, and provide feedback on both outcomes and progress to clinicians to ensure consensus and buy-in. Solutions must be tailored to the local environment to best accommodate local culture and resources and address identified poor outcomes in a continuous and reiterative process.[16]

Once a problem outcome is identified within the perioperative phases of care, the next step is to identify structures and/or processes to help with improvement. An excellent example of how structure and processes can improve outcomes is the demonstrable benefits of enhanced recovery programs for various surgical procedures.[17–19] Implementing evidence-based practices bundled within a structured care pathway delivered by multidisciplinary healthcare teams has shown faster recovery and fewer complications. Standardization across the entire perioperative care cycle (preoperative, intraoperative, and postoperative) creates more effective and efficient care. Nevertheless, standardized care should also consider the role of clinical expertise when rigorous, level 1 evidence is lacking. Patient values and goals are also important, and standardized care should be flexible enough to accommodate alignment with patient-centered goals.

Clinical outcomes within the perioperative care cycle have become, and will continue to be, important as healthcare reform brings greater focus to measurement and public reporting of outcomes. As healthcare systems grow increasingly more complex, QI efforts will only become more important and more complex. A multidisciplinary team approach and strong communication will be essential for improving the quality of care for patients. Coordination among experts, patient-centered goals, and thoughtful selection of clinical outcomes to measure will ultimately lead to improved patient care.

References

1. Kohn LT, Corrigan JM, Donaldson MS, eds. Institute of Medicine Committee on Quality of Health Care in America. In: *To Err Is Human: Building a Safer Health System.* National Academies Press; 2000.
2. Institute of Medicine Committee on Quality of Health Care in America. *Crossing the Quality Chasm: A New Health System for the 21st Century.* National Academies Press; 2001.
3. Centers for Disease Control and Prevention. Number of all-listed procedures for discharges from short-stay hospitals, by procedure category and age: United States, 2010. https://www.cdc.gov/nchs/data/nhds/4procedures/2010pro4_numberprocedureage.pdf. Accessed April 20, 2021.

4. Maggard-Gibbons M. The use of report cards and outcome measurements to improve the safety of surgical care: the American College of Surgeons National Surgical Quality Improvement Program. *BMJ Qual Saf.* 2014;23(7):589–599.
5. Vonlanthen R, et al. The impact of complications on costs of major surgical procedures: a cost analysis of 1200 patients. *Ann Surg.* 2011;254(6):907–913.
6. Birkmeyer JD, et al. Hospital quality and the cost of inpatient surgery in the United States. *Ann Surg.* 2012;255(1):1–5.
7. Dimick JB, et al. Hospital costs associated with surgical complications: a report from the private-sector National Surgical Quality Improvement Program. *J Am Coll Surg.* 2004;199(4):531–537.
8. Donabedian A. Evaluating the quality of medical care. *Milbank Mem Fund Q.* 1966;44(3). Suppl:166–206.
9. Donabedian A. The quality of care. How can it be assessed? *JAMA.* 1988;260(12):1743–1748.
10. National Quality Forum. Measure evaluation criteria. https://www.qualityforum.org/Measuring_ Performance/Submitting_Standards/Measure_Evaluation_Criteria.aspx. Accessed April 20, 2021.
11. Myles PS. Perioperative outcomes: are we asking the right questions? *Can J Anesth.* 2016;63(2):138–141.
12. Moonesinghe SR, et al. Systematic review and consensus definitions for the Standardised Endpoints in Perioperative Medicine initiative: patient-centred outcomes. *Br J Anaesth.* 2019;123(5):664–670.
13. Rowell KS, et al. Use of National Surgical Quality Improvement Program data as a catalyst for quality improvement. *J Am Coll Surg.* 2007;204(6):1293–1300.
14. Hall BL, et al. Comparison of mortality risk adjustment using a clinical data algorithm (American College of Surgeons National Surgical Quality Improvement Program) and an administrative data algorithm (Solucient) at the case level within a single institution. *J Am Coll Surg.* 2007;205(6):767–777.
15. Lawson EH, et al. A comparison of clinical registry versus administrative claims data for reporting of 30-day surgical complications. *Ann Surg.* 2012;256(6):973–981.
16. Main DS, et al. Relationship of processes and structures of care in general surgery to postoperative outcomes: a descriptive analysis. *J Am Coll Surg.* 2007;204(6):1157–1165.
17. Berian JR, et al. Association of an enhanced recovery pilot with length of stay in the National Surgical Quality Improvement Program. *JAMA Surg.* 2018;153(4):358–365.
18. Liu VX, et al. Enhanced recovery after surgery program implementation in 2 surgical populations in an integrated health care delivery system. *JAMA Surg.* 2017;152(7):e171032.
19. The Royal College of Anaesthetists. *Perioperative Medicine: The Pathway to Better Surgical Care.* 2015. https://www.rcoa.ac.uk/sites/default/files/documents/2019-08/Perioperative%20Medicine%20 %20The %20Pathway%20to%20Better%20Care.pdf.

CHAPTER 13

Equity and Perioperative Care

Ronald Wyatt, MD, MHA ■ Laura K. Botwinick, MS

KEY POINTS

- Closing gaps in care outcomes by race, ethnicity, and other measures of health inequity must be an integral part of quality improvement.
- Health disparities exist in every aspect of perioperative care and medicine.
- Addressing health equity involves understanding the roles race and racism play in health care.
- Racism must be understood on an individual level and a system level.
- There are many actions that perioperative care professionals can take to address equity in care.

Understanding Health Equity

Health disparities exist in every aspect of medicine[1] and perioperative care is no exception.[2,3] Disparities in care span every aspect of perioperative medicine, including, but not limited to, anesthesiology,[4,5] blood transfusions,[6] surgery type,[7] maternal health care,[8] and even treatment of pain.[9,10]

Health equity is one of the six domains of quality,[11] but until recently it has not received appropriate attention. Disparities in care for racial, ethnic, and other historically marginalized groups are not only unjust but also can be understood in quality improvement terminology as *variations* in care quality[12] and as *defects* in care.[13]

Health equity is when everyone has a fair opportunity to attain their full health potential, and no one is disadvantaged from achieving this potential.[14] Health disparity is the difference in health outcomes between groups within a population. Health disparities are prevalent internationally and exist in high, middle, and low income countries alike.[15–17]

Inequities in care are not an inherent part of the healthcare system. Many healthcare organizations and clinicians are working to address closing gaps in care by seeking to better understand race, ethnicity, language, sexual orientation and gender identity, insurance status, ability, and other measures of equity.[18,19] This is accomplished in part by stratifying quality data by race, ethnicity, and language (REaL) and other measures, then seeing the gaps in quality and committing to closing them. Addressing disparities in care requires applying an equity lens to all quality and safety improvement activities.[20]

Healthcare disparities stem from factors both within and beyond the direct control of clinicians; however, there is much that those working within the healthcare system can do to close gaps in care outcomes by race, ethnicity, and other measures of equity both within the healthcare system and in the community.

Dr. Camara Jones identifies three types of racism: personally mediated, internalized, and institutionalized racism.[21] Personally mediated racism is the racism expressed between individuals.

Internalized racism is when people of color internalize negative messages about their own race, or when White people internalize ideas about their superiority. Institutionalized/structural racism is when the policies, practices, norms, laws, regulations, and standards of the institution, profession, and broader society are causing racial inequities.

Racism in the form of implicit and explicit bias can have dire consequences for the safety and quality of care.[22] In addition, structural racism in the broader society affects health outcomes and public health. As we have seen from the recent experience of the COVID-19 pandemic, poor underlying health due to structural inequities and inequitable access to quality health care has contributed to proportionally higher death rates in historically marginalized communities.

An emerging issue in health equity is the use of race correction in clinical medicine.[23] This is becoming recognized as incorrect practice. Race is a social construct not a biological one.[24] Race correction occurs in commonly used guides for care, commercial algorithms for predicting health outcomes and risk assessment, and scales for assessing care needs.[25] Examples are the atherosclerotic cardiovascular disease (ASCVD) risk calculator, spirometry tests, and the breast cancer surveillance consortium risk calculator.

Addressing Implicit Bias

Implicit bias (also called *unconscious bias*) is a common occurrence in health care and the broader society. It is when people act on biases they have that may not even be known to them. Diminishing a Black person's experience of pain is one way this can manifest. Spending more time with White patients than patients of color is another. Implicit bias can impact the treatment options provided and have harmful effects on the quality of care and health outcomes.

Evidence-based actions that can be taken to prevent bias from harming patients include taking time to recognize the person in front of you as an individual and consciously thinking about the person as the opposite of a stereotype.[26] Implicit biases can be acted on when practitioners are rushed and stressed. Take a moment before a patient interaction to be ready to see and hear the person in front of you.

Designing for Health Equity

Equity and equality are not the same concepts. A focus on health equity means that different efforts may be required to address the needs of marginalized communities to achieve optimum health. Winston Wong and colleagues give examples of how equity of care can be achieved by applying tailored approaches for different needs.[27]

Fig. 13.1 illustrates the difference between equal care and equitable care. Equal means providing the same thing to all, but that does not always result in meeting the needs of every individual.

What Perioperative Care Professionals Can Do to Address Health Equity

There is much that perioperative care professionals can do to affect equity and the quality of care[28-31]:

- Implicit bias, explicit bias, and structural racism should be addressed in the full continuum of perioperative care, which includes initial scheduling and optimization of people preoperatively to include addressing social factors and possibly any impact of previous trauma (e.g., trauma-informed care).
- Listen to patients and families, understand and respond to their needs, build a trusting relationship, and in so doing build trust in the healthcare institution. Address patient experience and include patients as active participants in their own care, including in the perioperative process.

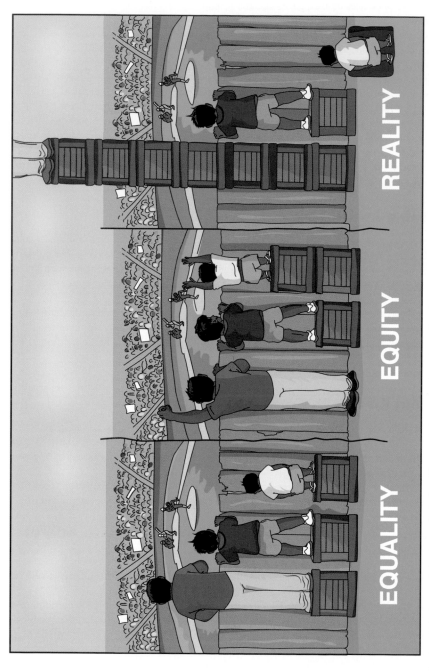

Fig. 13.1 A graphical example to demonstrate the difference between equity and equality. (Adapted from the Interaction Institute for Social Change.)

- Stratify outcomes data by REaL, by sexual orientation and gender identity (SOGI), and by other measures of disparity and work to close the gaps.
- Ensure people with limited English proficiency are offered interpretive services, especially in the consent process.
- Influence the healthcare system to change discriminatory policies in access to care, clinical care, human resources, and other business practices (i.e., eliminate institutional racism).[28]
- Build diverse and inclusive teams and support advancement of clinicians of color to leadership positions in the department and the organization.[29]
- Avoid race correction in clinical medicine.
- Expand care to incorporate social determinants of health. Examples in perioperative care would include social services and case management preoperatively to identify and address any postoperative needs such as housing, finances, and food insecurity.[30]
- Support community efforts to implement changes that impact health.[31]
- Advocate for public and private investments in public health and the social determinants of health to ensure a healthier population and improved outcomes in care.

References

1. Smedley BD, Stith AY, Nelson AR, eds. *Institute of Medicine, Unequal Treatment: Confronting Racial and Ethnic Disparities in Health Care.* Washington, DC: The National Academies Press; 2003.
2. Ravi P, Sood A, Schmid M, et al. Racial/Ethnic disparities in perioperative outcomes of major procedures: results from the national surgical quality improvement program. *Ann Surg.* 2015;262(6):955–964.
3. Elde S, Woo YJ. Racial and sex disparities persist in modern cardiac surgical outcomes. *Ann Surg.* 2020;272 (4):668.
4. Silber JH, Rosenbaum PR, Zhang X, et al. Influence of patient and hospital characteristics on anesthesia time in Medicare patients undergoing general and orthopedic surgery. *Anesthesiology.* 2007;106:356–364.
5. Estime SR, Lee HH, Jimenez N, et al. Diversity, equity, and inclusion in anesthesiology. *Int Anesthesiol Clin.* 2021;59(4):81–85.
6. Qian F, Eaton MP, Lustik SJ, et al. Racial disparities in the use of blood transfusion in major surgery. *BMC Health Serv Res.* 2014;14:121.
7. Muse IO, Joseph VA. Evidence of health care disparities in the perioperative setting. *ASA Monitor.* 2016;80:44–45.
8. Institute for Healthcare Improvement. Black maternal health: reducing inequities through community collaboration. http://www.ihi.org/resources/Pages/Publications/black-maternal-health-reducing-inequities-through-community-collaboration.aspx. Accessed 17 April 2022.
9. Wyatt R. Pain and ethnicity. *Am Med Assoc J Ethics.* 2013;15(5):449–454.
10. Hoffman KM, Trawalter S, Axt JR, Oliver MN. Racial bias in pain assessment and treatment recommendations, and false beliefs about biological differences between Blacks and Whites. *Proc Natl Acad Sci USA.* 2016;113(16):4296–4301.
11. Institute of Medicine. *Crossing the Quality Chasm: A New Health System for the 21st Century, Committee on Quality of Health Care in America.* National Academies Press; 2001.
12. Mate K. Why inequity should be treated as an unwanted variation in care. Institute for Healthcare Improvement; 2021. http://www.ihi.org/about/news/Pages/Why-inequity-should-be-treated-as-an-unwanted-variation-in-care.aspx. Accessed 17 April 2022.
13. Austin JM, Weeks K, Pronovost PJ. Health system leader's role in addressing racism: time to prioritize eliminating health care disparities. *Jt Comm J Qual Patient Saf.* 2021;47(4):265–267.
14. Whitehead M, Dahlgren G. *Concepts and Principles for Tackling Social Inequities in Health: Levelling up, Part 1.* World Health Organization, Regional Office for Europe; 2006.
15. Kruk ME, Gage AD, Arsenault C, et al. High-quality health systems in the Sustainable Development Goals era: time for a revolution. *Lancet Glob Health.* 2018;6(11). e1996–e1252.
16. National Academies of Sciences, Engineering, and Medicine. *Crossing the Global Quality: Chasm Improving Health Care Worldwide.* Washington, DC: The National Academies Press; 2018.

17. Durey A, Thompson SC. Reducing the health disparities of Indigenous Australians: time to change focus. *BMC Health Serv Res.* 2012;12:151.

18. Eberly LA, Richterman A, Beckett AG, et al. Identification of racial inequities in access to specialized inpatient heart failure care at an Academic Medical Center. *Circ Heart Fail.* 2019;12(11), e006214.

19. Institute for Healthcare Improvement. *Improving health equity: guidance for health care organizations, 7 guide*; 2019. http://www.ihi.org/resources/Pages/Publications/Improving-Health-Equity-Guidance-for-Health-Care-Organizations.aspx. Accessed 19 April 2022.

20. O'Kane M, Agrawal S, Binder L, et al. An equity agenda for the field of health care quality improvement. *National Academy of Medicine.* 2021. https://nam.edu/an-equity-agenda-for-the-field-of-health-care-quality-improvement/. Accessed 17 April 2022.

21. Jones CP. Levels of racism: a theoretic framework and a gardener's tale. *Am J Public Health.* 2000;90 (8):1212–1215.

22. Williams D, Lawrence J, Davis B, Vu C. Understanding how discrimination can affect health. *Health Serv Res.* 2019;54(S2):1374–1388.

23. Vyas DA, Eisenstein LG, Jones DS. Hidden in plain sight—reconsidering the use of race correction in clinical algorithms. *N Engl J Med.* 2020;383(9):874–882.

24. Boyd RW, Lindo EG, Weeks LD, McLemore MR. On racism: a new standard for publishing on racial health inequities. Health Affairs; 2020. https://www.healthaffairs.org/do/10.1377/hblog20200630.939347/full/. Accessed April 17, 2022.

25. Obermeyer Z, Powers B, Vogeliand C, Mullainathan M. Dissecting racial bias in an algorithm used to manage the health of populations. *Science.* 2019;366(6464):447–453.

26. Devine PG, Forscher PS, Austin AJ, Cox WTL. Long-term reduction in implicit race bias: a prejudice habit-breaking intervention. *J Exp Soc Psychol.* 2012;48(6):1267–1278.

27. Wong WF, LaVeist TA, Sharfstein JM. Achieving health equity by design. *JAMA.* 2015;313 (14):1417–1418.

28. Institute for Healthcare Improvement. *Improving health equity: eliminate racism and other forms of oppression. guidance for health care organizations*; 2019. http://www.ihi.org/resources/Pages/Publications/Improving-Health-Equity-Guidance-for-Health-Care-Organizations.aspx. Accessed 17 April 2022.

29. Salles A, Arora VM, Mitchell KA. Everyone must address anti-Black racism in health care, steps for non-Black health care professionals to take. *JAMA.* 2021;326(7):601–602.

30. Wyatt R, Laderman M, Botwinick L, Mate K, Whittington J. *Achieving health equity: a guide for health care organizations.* IHI White Paper: Institute for Healthcare Improvement; 2016.

31. Prevention Institute. *A practitioner's guide for advancing health equity*; 2013. https://www.preventioninstitute.org/publications/practitioners-guide-advancing-health-equity. Accessed 17 April 2022.

CHAPTER 14

Qualitative Research in Perioperative Medicine

Justin T. Clapp, PhD, MPH

KEY POINTS

- Uptake of qualitative methods in perioperative medical research has been relatively slow because of some misapprehensions about these methods.
- Qualitative methods are most appropriate for answering "how" questions about processes as they occur in their everyday contexts.
- Perioperative qualitative researchers should strive for greater flexibility in their interviews and for more observation-based data collection.
- During data analysis, perioperative qualitative researchers should focus less on intercoder reliability and more on robust discussion and debate about disagreements.
- Qualitative studies published in perioperative journals would benefit greatly from positing explanations for the thematic patterns they describe.

Qualitative Research in Perioperative Medicine

Qualitative methods are appearing with increasing frequency in high-impact journals in surgery, anesthesiology, and critical care. Nevertheless, their uptake remains relatively slow in the perioperative specialties. Misapprehensions about qualitative methods continue to keep many perioperative researchers from fully realizing their utility. In explaining the use of qualitative methods to address topics in perioperative medicine, this chapter attempts to clear up persistent confusions for perioperative researchers who are interested in or are already doing qualitative work, as well as those who do not do qualitative work themselves but are called on to evaluate qualitative studies (e.g., as journal reviewers) in their areas of content expertise. Readers are encouraged to explore the bibliography to see examples of high-quality qualitative studies in the perioperative space and to delve further into methodological issues.

What Is Qualitative Research, and What Kinds of Questions Can It Answer?

Qualitative and quantitative methods are less easily differentiable than might be presumed.[1] Both those methods labeled "qualitative" and those labeled "quantitative" deal with qualities *and* quantities. Analysis of interviews and fieldnotes must engage with the frequency with which certain types of utterances or events happen, whereas statistical analysis rests on qualitative assumptions about whatever attribute or event has been counted.

Perhaps the clearest difference between the two sets of methods is how they derive causal relationships. Quantitative researchers generally identify relationships by assessing covariance. Upon identifying a regularity in association between variables and controlling for other variables that might be responsible for this association, they infer a possible causal relationship. By contrast, qualitative researchers directly characterize causal processes in context.[2] Given this focus on process, qualitative methods are best suited for examining questions of "how." How do patients and surgeons arrive at decisions about whether to undergo elective surgery?[3] How does the pipeline of clinical research lead to the pursuit of more aggressive treatment in the critically ill?[4]

This process-oriented approach does not depend on preestablished comparisons in the way that quantitative methods do. Crucially, then, qualitative methods need not be hypothesis driven, and most often they are not. Qualitative researchers typically identify a process they are interested in characterizing and collect any data that they believe help explain this process.

Data Collection

Among qualitative studies published in perioperative journals and medical journals more broadly, interviewing has been by far the most common data collection approach. Interviewing—along with variant approaches such as focus groups—is invaluable for understanding how people experience the world, how they understand phenomena, and how they think through situations. In the perioperative space, interviewing can be productively used, such as to explore how patients experience surgery while under regional anesthesia[5] or to understand how patients process their decisions to undergo implantation of ventricular assist devices.[6]

A good interview is one that produces "thick" data—that is, the interviewee gives detailed, dense accounts of their thoughts and behaviors.[7] This requires interview questions that are adequately open-ended so that the descriptive onus is on the interviewee. Questions with discrete response options (e.g., yes/no), such as those that would be asked in a survey, should not make up the bulk of an interview guide. "Thick" interviews also require an interviewer who listens carefully during responses for opportunities to further probe into the factors that are causing interviewees to answer questions in certain ways. Although some of these follow-ups are predictable and can be prepared for, others are spontaneous.

Thus effective interviewing is a careful balance of structure and flexibility.[8] Some structure should be present, given that the researcher is interested in specific topics, but the objective of the interview is to follow the interviewee to the issues within a topical domain that *they* find most relevant. Researchers must be comfortable with the fact that interviews, although they might be similar in their broad structure, will spin out to some extent in their own individual directions. In the author's experience, many perioperative qualitative studies that are described as using "semistructured" interviewing do not actually allow for much flexibility, whether because of a concern that interviews should be standardized or because of an interviewer's reluctance to ask spontaneous probes.

A second prominent type of qualitative data collection is observation. Unfortunately, qualitative studies using observation are considerably less common in the medical literature than those using interviewing. Pioneered by anthropologists and sociologists—who often call observation "fieldwork"—the approach allows for direct characterization of activities in their everyday contexts.[9] In perioperative settings, it can be used to examine how clinical interactions lead to decisions about, for example, which type of anesthesia should be used for orthopedic surgery[10] or whether a high-risk operation is worth its possible postoperative complications.[11] Researchers can sometimes leverage audio and video recordings to help capture what they are observing. Data can also be collected via fieldnotes, in which the observer attempts to summarize relevant features of setting, activity, and discourse as comprehensively as possible.

Medical researchers are frequently concerned about the validity of the data produced by observation because of the notorious Hawthorne effect, which is when research subjects alter their behavior because of the presence of the observer. Anthropologists and sociologists, however, are considerably less concerned about this issue for two reasons.[12] First, observer effects tend to fade as subjects become accustomed to the presence of the observer. Second, if detected, these effects present an opportunity for discovery because behavioral alteration tells the researcher something about how a subject understands the topic of study—much in the way that changing the conditions in a laboratory experiment and examining the response tells us something about the entity being studied.

Data Analysis

Qualitative data analysis is pursued primarily through a coding process. Transcripts or fieldnotes are initially annotated to generate themes, which are formalized into a taxonomy that is then used to categorize the data. These themes can be imagined as occurring on a spectrum. On one end of the spectrum are descriptive themes that are clearly evident in the data. A snippet of an interview in which an intensivist discusses how she aims to involve patients in conversations about their care by eliciting their goals could be tabbed "patient communication." On the other end of the spectrum are more interpretive themes, which require more inference on the part of the researcher and often come from engagement with the literature. That same interview snippet could be tabbed "shared decision making." By having a mix of descriptive and interpretive codes, the analyst can be sure of capturing basic trends in the data while also pushing toward an assessment of the significance of these trends in relation to prior work.

There has been considerable contention and confusion in academic medicine about the issue of reliability in qualitative data analysis. When qualitative methods were first imported into medical research, discomfort with the "subjective" nature of the coding process led to a heavy emphasis on a team-based approach and the assessment of intercoder reliability. Qualitative methodologists, however, have argued that although it is desirable to attain a degree of consistency in basic descriptive coding, it is not reasonable to expect it when inferring the implications of the patterns identified by coding because there might be a number of valid explanations for these patterns.[13] Too much focus on reliability can actually inhibit explanation development[14] because the strength of an interdisciplinary, team-based qualitative approach is that each researcher will bring different expertise to a project. Disagreements that result based on these differing backgrounds are a boon for the rigor of a project, not an indicator of lack of validity. Accordingly, although team-based coding is still expected by most medical journals, the emphasis on rigid assessment of intercoder reliability is waning.

Explanation

The primary limitation of most qualitative work done in the medical sphere is that it stops short of developing explanations. Qualitative studies published in perioperative and other medical journals often collect data, sort them into codes, and then conclude the project and write it up. The result is a description of basic thematic patterns with little explanation of what processes might be responsible for these patterns.

This lack of explanation presents two problems for the overall enterprise of qualitative research in perioperative medicine. First, although remaining close to the data might seem like a good strategy for increasing the applied utility of qualitative work, it actually achieves the opposite.[15] Qualitative studies that do not take a shot at developing explanations give perioperative clinicians and researchers little idea of what to target when they are trying to improve their practice or design a new study. Second, this type of work harms the reputation of qualitative research in the perioperative space. When individuals unfamiliar with qualitative methods are exposed repeatedly to studies that stop at thematic trends, they begin to view these methods as "qualitative" in the way that natural and biomedical sciences use the term—as seeking to simply describe qualities. The explanatory power of qualitative methods goes unrealized, the generalizability of qualitative studies is diminished,[16] and the wider uptake of these methods is hindered.

Developing explanations for the trends made evident by coding requires additional engagement with the data and with prior literature on the research topic. How might the thematic patterns revealed relate to one another? What attributes of the people, settings, or behaviors studied might cause variation in these themes? How do these patterns compare to those discovered in prior work, and what might account for any differences? Do explanations offered in pertinent literature (including social scientific research) account sufficiently for these patterns, or do these patterns suggest that such explanations need revision?

Moving Forward

We are left with several aspirations for the future of qualitative methods in perioperative medicine. These methods should be used to address process-oriented questions in an open-ended approach that does not require a hypothesis. Perioperative qualitative researchers should cultivate flexibility in their interviewing and explore the benefits of using direct observation rather than relying almost totally on interviews. In analysis, they should cultivate an openness to disagreement and discussion rather than being preoccupied with intercoder reliability. And most important, qualitative studies in perioperative medicine should strive for deeper explanation rather than superficial reporting of themes.

Qualitative methods have made promising inroads in surgery, anesthesiology, and critical care. With attention to these goals, these approaches are set to flourish in the perioperative space.

References

1. Hammersley M. *What's Wrong With Ethnography?* Routledge; 1992.
2. Maxwell JA. Using qualitative methods for causal explanation. *Field Methods.* 2004;16(3):243–264.
3. Clapp JT, Arriaga AFM, Murthy SM, et al. Surgical consultation as social process: implications for shared decision making. *Ann Surg.* 2019;269(3):446–452.
4. Kaufman SR. *Ordinary Medicine: Extraordinary Treatments, Longer Lives, and Where to Draw the Line.* Duke University Press; 2015.
5. Karlsson A-C, Ekebergh M, Mauléon AL, Almerud Österberg S. "Is that my leg?" patients' experiences of being awake during regional anesthesia and surgery. *J Perianesth Nurs.* 2012;27(3):155–164.
6. Barg FK, Kellom K, Ziv T, Hull SC, Suhail-Sindhu S, Kirkpatrick JN. LVAD-DT: culture of rescue and liminal experience in the treatment of heart failure. *Am J Bioeth.* 2017;17(2):3–11.
7. Charmaz K. *Constructing Grounded Theory.* 2nd ed. SAGE Publications Ltd; 2014.
8. Yeo A, Legard R, Keegan J, Ward K, Nicholls CM, Lewis J. In-depth interviews. In: *Qualitative Research Practice: A Guide for Social Science Students & Researchers.* 2nd ed. SAGE Publications Ltd; 2014:177–210.
9. Jorgensen DL. Participant observation. In: *Emerging Trends in the Social and Behavioral Sciences.* American Cancer Society; 2015:1–15.
10. Graff V, Clapp JT, Heins SJ, et al. Patient involvement in anesthesia decision-making: a qualitative study of knee arthroplasty. *Anesthesiology.* 2021. https://doi.org/10.1097/ALN.0000000000003795.
11. Pecanac KE, Kehler JM, Brasel KJ, et al. It's big surgery: preoperative expressions of risk, responsibility, and commitment to treatment after high-risk operations. *Ann Surg.* 2014;259(3):458–463.

12. Monahan T, Fisher JA. Benefits of 'observer effects': lessons from the field. *Qual Res.* 2010;10(3):357–376.
13. Armstrong D, Gosling A, Weinman J, Marteau T. The place of inter-rater reliability in qualitative research: an empirical study. *Sociology.* 1997;31(3):597–606.
14. Morse JM. Critical analysis of strategies for determining rigor in qualitative inquiry. *Qual Health Res.* 2015;25(9):1212–1222.
15. Thorne S. Beyond theming: making qualitative studies matter. *Nurs Inq.* 2020;27(1):e12343.
16. Broom A. Conceptualizing qualitative data. *Qual Health Res.* 2021;31(10):1767–1770.

CHAPTER 15

Publication in Perioperative Medicine

Thomas R. Vetter, MD, MPH ▪ Angela M. Bader, MD, MPH

KEY POINTS

- Publication in perioperative medicine in a broad sense can be defined as work investigating the generation of value (quality ÷ cost) through the organization, operations, and metrics of care provided throughout the perioperative period.
- Publications in this area can include articles that are hypothesis driven with a scientific methodology ranging from randomized controlled trials to pre- and post-intervention work.
- Publications can also include work that has not always been strictly defined as research. Such publications would include descriptions of interventions at institutional levels, quality improvement efforts, and theoretical modeling for process improvement.
- To be successful in publishing in perioperative medicine, authors should diligently examine the type of research performed, the best fit category for the manuscript, and the journals most likely to accept such research and the manuscript.

Introduction

Perioperative medicine encompasses the interdisciplinary, collaborative, patient-centered, and integrated medical care of patients from initial consideration for surgery with a shared decision-making process through their entire postoperative course and postdischarge recovery.[1]

The practice of perioperative medicine identifies patients at increased risk for significant morbidity and mortality and proactively optimizes their care rather than simply rescuing them from complications. Providers with expertise in anesthesiology, surgery, and internal medicine have complementary expertise and thus ideally work together in delivering perioperative care.[2]

Although the various elements of perioperative care have historically been the topics of hypothesis-based research, perioperative medicine as a specialized area of investigation is relatively new. A well-accepted definition of perioperative medicine research does not exist. Few current journals consistently have content or a section devoted to this specialty. As previously noted, perioperative medicine is very broadly defined. Therefore research and publications in this field preferably include an interdisciplinary approach and patient-centered focus.

Perioperative Population Health Management: A Current Overarching Theme and Important Driver

Medical research typically focuses on a particular intervention in a very specific group of patients, looking at outcomes that may or may not be relevant from a larger perspective. For example, studying the effects of different anesthetic agents in geriatric surgery patients on a primary outcome occurring before hospital discharge, without considering overall geriatric vulnerability screening and delirium prevention, can lessen translational impact.

Unlike most medical research, perioperative medicine research is often translated to a population health management level. Therefore perioperative medicine research generally considers the impact of the intervention studied on a population level, with the goal being to improve value not only for an individual patient but also for a population, resulting in an overall improvement in population health management. Such research is thus expected to provide evidence that an intervention can be readily translated to improve perioperative care with appropriate implementation in the targeted population.[3]

The perioperative medicine and management literature has generally focused on the value of the care provided, initially defined as the ratio of quality (or outcomes) to the cost of achieving the desired outcomes. The numerator of this value ratio has subsequently been expanded:[4] Value = (Safe + Effective + Efficiency + Patient-Centeredness + Timely + Equitable) ÷ Cost.

The cost of an intervention is important in perioperative research findings, unlike other medical research that can examine technologies that would be prohibitively expensive on a population level. Nevertheless, direct and indirect perioperative costs remain underreported in the literature.

Three Key Perspectives That Warrant Further Research and Publication Emphasis

PATIENT-REPORTED OUTCOMES, INCLUDING HEALTH-RELATED QUALITY OF LIFE

Varied definitions and inconsistent reporting of outcomes across trials focused on similar clinical questions limit the value of this research. Such variability also undermines systematic reviews and meta-analyses aiming to synthesize relevant primary research about a particular question.[5]

The Standardised Endpoints in Perioperative Medicine (StEP) initiative defined which measures should be used in future research to facilitate a comparison between studies and to enable valid evidence synthesis through robust systematic reviews and meta-analyses.[5] Components of the StEP initiative have included clinical indicators[6] and patient-centered outcomes (PCOs),[6] also referred to as patient-reported outcomes. PCOs are increasingly measured in perioperative clinical trials and are receiving greater emphasis in perioperative publications.

LONGITUDINAL OUTCOMES BEYOND 30 DAYS POSTOPERATIVELY

A significant challenge in judging the quality of manuscripts submitted on perioperative interventions is that the metrics used as outcomes are traditional and not patient-centered. For example, judging success by the impact on morbidity and mortality whether in hospital, at discharge, or at 30 days is completely arbitrary and may not relate to more specific PCOs.

The absence of significant harm at 30 days does not imply that the surgery was not futile or in fact had any success at all. For example, if research on preoperative optimization strategies looks only at traditional morbidity and mortality metrics, there may be no perceived significant differences.

Looking at PCOs like decrease in non-home discharges, better functional recovery at 90 days, or less postoperative cognitive dysfunction at 90 days, however, may be much more relevant. Therefore valid publications in this area must be careful about choosing the appropriate metrics.

Furthermore, process measures such as "turnover time" are not PCOs. For example, an intervention that increases first case on time starts by 5% is a process metric, not a PCO. Manuscripts that focus only on process metrics as outcomes need to specify why these were chosen and discuss that this does not automatically improve PCOs or the health of the population. This research may have benefit if the manuscript delineates this as addressing the cost element of the value equation.

The healthcare strategy group at Harvard Business School has focused on this greater opportunity in defining appropriate outcomes. Their nonprofit organization, the International Consortium for Health Outcomes Measurement (ICHOM), is freely accessible on the Internet (https://www.ichom.org/). The mission of ICHOM is to define condition-specific standard outcomes that include morbidity and mortality as well as PCOs measured long after discharge. For example, prostate surgery and hip replacement have different PCO metrics. Authors should consider reviewing these standard sets and using a subset of these metrics when applicable.

PATIENT ENGAGEMENT AND EMPOWERMENT

The constructs of patient engagement and empowerment are of paramount importance in perioperative medicine research and publications. They are a distinguishing factor in this type of research. There is a continued clear need for publications addressing patient engagement and empowerment throughout the perioperative care period—including topics like high-quality shared decision making, futility of care, advanced care planning, health literacy, and goals of care conversations to ensure that the procedure planned is aligned with patient expectations, values, and goals.[7]

In addition, how to increase perioperative provider engagement and facility with these patient and family conversations is also important. Most surgeons and anesthesiologists have no formal training in conducting these discussions or ensuring that high-quality shared decision making has occurred. Manuscripts addressing educational methodologies, implementation of these conversations into workflows, and patient education in these areas would be of great interest.

Health Services Research and Quality Improvement Research

Health services research (HSR) should be conducted using the same scientific methodologies that would define a research manuscript in other areas of medicine. Journals may be interested in both HSR and quality improvement (QI) work, and authors should take some time to determine the best methodology for the type of work they are planning to do. A number of academic institutions have clearly defined checklists available from their institutional research review boards to help distinguish QI work from research in terms of the need for research board review, need for informed consent, and potential for publication. One example from Brigham and Women's Hospital, which is available on the web[8] (https://www.partners.org › Clinical-QI-Checklist), may help authors as they develop potentially publishable projects. Another example is a tool provided by the UK Medical Research Council, which has three questions to help distinguish research from QI.[9]

Simple (e.g., single institution) QI reports may be better suited to journals such as *BMJ Open Quality*, which provides templates for reporting based on the SQuIRE guidelines (see Chapter 16 on the SQuIRE guidelines). To achieve publication, more complex QI interventions should include a well-developed "theory of change," (see Chapter 21 on Programme Theory of Change) and adhere to standards of scientific rigor.[10,11] HSR can also include development and implementation of innovations, which may be perioperative pathways, healthcare economics, and large database studies.[11]

Increasing the Likelihood of Successful Publication

Representative journals that publish papers on perioperative medicine and on perioperative QI and HSR include *Anesthesia & Analgesia, Anesthesiology, British Journal of Anaesthesia, JAMA Surgery, Journal of Clinical Anesthesia, Journal of Perioperative Practice,* and *Perioperative Medicine*.

The major stakeholders in the publication of such medical literature include authors and readers, as well as the editors, peer reviewers, affiliated societies, owner, and publisher of the journal. All share the goal of publishing the best possible papers on a given topic. This process starts with a submitted manuscript that is written well.[12]

Key criteria that determine whether a submitted research manuscript will be accepted and published include:

- Novelty of study question or topic
- Impact of study question or topic
- Robust study design and valid data analysis
- Appropriate interpretation of study findings
- How likely is the paper to be viewed?
- How likely is the paper to be cited?

There is a significant risk for rejection when an article is framed as research but does not actually meet the requirements of true research methodology needed to assure validity and to define significance.[13] For example, lack of appropriate study population, unclear exclusion criteria, failure to adjust for possible cofounders, and the attribution of a causal relationship instead of simply association can all result in reviewers and editors requesting major revisions or rejecting the manuscript. It is very difficult in most cases to correct these major issues without redoing at least the analysis, and in some cases, new data would need to be collected to revalidate the findings. Authors should take great care when determining the methodology of their studies to prevent such issues from precluding successful peer review and publication. The "Statistical Analyses and Methods in the Published Literature" (SAMPL) guidelines are an excellent resource.[14]

"Writing a manuscript for a medical journal…is very akin to writing a newspaper article—albeit a scholarly one. Like any journalist, you have a story to tell. You need to tell your story in a way that is easy to follow and makes a compelling case to the reader."[15] The bottom line is that the authors' story must be interesting and written well.

References

1. Grocott MPW, Plumb JOM, Edwards M, Fecher-Jones I, Levett DZH. Re-designing the pathway to surgery: better care and added value. *Perioper Med (Lond)*. 2017;6:9.
2. Gooneratne M, Grailey K, Mythen M, Walker D. Perioperative medicine, interventions in surgical care: the role of replacing the late-night review with daytime leadership. *Future Hosp J*. 2016;3(1):58–61.
3. Aronson S, Westover J, Guinn N, et al. A perioperative medicine model for population health: an integrated approach for an evolving clinical science. *Anesth Analg*. 2018;126(2):682–690.
4. Mahajan A, Esper SA, Cole DJ, Fleisher LA. Anesthesiologists' role in value-based perioperative care and healthcare transformation. *Anesthesiology*. 2021;134(4):526–540.
5. Myles PS, Grocott MP, Boney O, Moonesinghe SR. Standardizing end points in perioperative trials: towards a core and extended outcome set. *Br J Anaesth*. 2016;116(5):586–589.
6. Haller G, Bampoe S, Cook T, et al. Systematic review and consensus definitions for the Standardised Endpoints in Perioperative Medicine initiative: clinical indicators. *Br J Anaesth*. 2019;123(2):228–237.
7. Goeddel LA, Porterfield JR, Jr., Hall JD, Vetter TR. Ethical opportunities with the perioperative surgical home: disruptive innovation, patient-centered care, shared decision making, health literacy, and futility of care. *Anesth Analg*. 2015;120(5):1158–1162.
8. Mass General Brigham. *Clinical quality improvement checklist from the Brigham and Women's HoSPITAL*. https://view.officeapps.live.com/op/view.aspx?src=https%3A%2F%2Fwww.massgeneralbrigham.org%2Fsites%2Fdefault%2Ffiles%2FClinical_QI_Checklist.doc. Accessed 7 November 2021.
9. Health Research Academy. Is my study research? http://www.hra-decisiontools.org.uk/research/question4.html. Accessed November 7, 2021.
10. Dixon-Woods M, Martin GP. Does quality improvement improve quality? *Future Hosp J*. 2016;3 (3):191–194.
11. Peden CJ, Ghaferi AA, Vetter TR, Kain ZN. Perioperative health services research: far better played as a team sport. *Anesth Analg*. 2021;133(2):553–557.
12. Sessler DI, Shafer S. Writing research reports. *Anesth Analg*. 2018;126(1):330–337.

13. Mascha EJ, Vetter TR. The statistical checklist and statistical review: two essential yet challenging deliverables. *Anesth Analg.* 2017;124(3):719–721.

14. Lang TA, Altman DG. Basic statistical reporting for articles published in biomedical journals: The "Statistical Analyses and Methods in the Published Literature" or the SAMPL Guidelines. *Int J Nurs Stud.* 2015;52(1):5–9.

15. Vetter TR, Mascha EJ. In the beginning-there is the introduction-and your study hypothesis. *Anesth Analg.* 2017;124(5):1709–1711.

The SQUIRE 2.0 (Standards for Quality Improvement Reporting Excellence) Guidelines: A Framework for Designing and Reporting Quality Improvement Studies, Application in Perioperative Care

Carol J. Peden, MB ChB, MD, FRCA, FFICM, MPH

KEY POINTS

- The SQUIRE 2.0 (Standards for Quality Improvement Reporting Excellence) guidelines provide a framework around which to construct and report an improvement project.
- The guidelines provide a format recognized by mainstream journals for the reporting of quality improvement studies.

Background

As quality improvement (QI) studies have become more widespread and researchers try to get studies published, the need for a structured method of formulating a QI study and reporting the findings has been recognized. The **S**tandards for **QU**ality **I**mprovement **R**eporting **E**xcellence (SQUIRE) guidelines were first published in 2008 and were revised to SQUIRE 2.0 in 2015 to reflect the increasing understanding of theories underpinning improvement work, the importance of the local context in which the study is undertaken, and the study of the actual improvement intervention.[1,2] The 2.0 version of the guidelines was evolved through expert opinion and feedback on the original version and was tested by expert authors who wrote sections of a manuscript using the guidelines. Feedback was provided by biomedical journal authors, resulting in further refinement.

Standardized guidelines and reporting for QI studies serve several purposes:

1. It helps the author/researcher to think about the structure of the study.
2. It aims to ensure that all relevant steps are reported so the reader can understand how the study was performed and in what context.
3. It increases the value of reported QI studies by ensuring reporting is done in a reliable and consistent way.
4. It provides a format that is recognized by major journals for QI studies.

Journals that use the SQUIRE guidelines include *BMJ Quality and Safety*, *the Journal of the American College of Surgeons*, *the Joint Commission Journal of Quality and Patient Safety*, and *BMJ Quality*

Open. The latter journal provides a good location to publish QI studies.[3] Although the SQUIRE guidelines have facilitated QI reporting and publication, QI studies can still be hard to get published in mainstream journals. Other relevant guidelines such as STROBE (**S**trengthening the **R**eporting of **OB**servational studies in **E**pidemiology) for observational studies can be used in addition, if appropriate. An overview of reporting tools including SQUIRE 2.0 and STROBE can be viewed on the EQUATOR (**E**nhancing the **QU**ality and **T**ransparency **O**f health **R**esearch) website.[4]

The sections of the SQUIRE 2.0 guidelines are divided into the familiar introduction, methods, results, and discussion sections but here are also framed as:

- Why did you start?
- What did you do?
- What did you find?
- What does it mean?

The SQUIRE 2.0 checklist contains 18 items (Box 16.1) and researchers should consider all items, but not all may apply and need not be reported.

BOX 16.1 ■ SQUIRE 2.0 Guidelines Checklist

Title/Abstract

1. Title Indicate that the manuscript concerns an initiative to improve health care (broadly defined to include the quality, safety, effectiveness, patient-centeredness, timeliness, cost, efficiency, and equity of health care).

2. Abstract
  a. Provide adequate information to aid in searching and indexing.
  b. Summarize all key information from various sections of the text using the abstract format of the intended publication or a structured summary, such as background, local problem, methods, interventions, results, and conclusions.

Introduction ***Why did you start?***

3. Problem Description Nature and significance of the local problem

4. Available Knowledge Summary of what is currently known about the problem, including relevant previous studies

5. Rationale Informal or formal frameworks, models, concepts, and/or theories used to explain the problem, any reasons or assumptions that were used to develop the intervention(s), and reasons why the intervention(s) was expected to work

6. Specific Aims Purpose of the project and of this report

Methods ***What did you do?***

7. Context Purpose of the project and of this report
Contextual elements considered important at the outset of introducing the intervention(s)

8. Intervention
  1. Description of the intervention(s) in sufficient detail that others could reproduce it
  2. Specifics of the team involved in the work

9. Study of the Intervention
  a. Approach chosen for assessing the impact of the intervention(s)
  b. Approach used to establish whether the observed outcomes were because of the intervention(s)

10. Measures
  1. Measures chosen for studying processes and outcomes of the intervention(s), including rationale for choosing them, their operational definitions, and their validity and reliability
  2. Description of the approach to the ongoing assessment of contextual elements that contributed to the success, failure, efficiency, and cost
  3. Methods employed for assessing completeness and accuracy of data

11. Analysis
  1. Qualitative and quantitative methods used to draw inferences from the data
  2. Methods for understanding variation within the data, including the effects of time as a variable

12. **Ethical Considerations**	Ethical aspects of implementing and studying the intervention(s) and how they were addressed, including, but not limited to, formal ethics review and potential conflict(s) of interest
Results	**What did you find?**
13. **Results**	**a.** Initial steps of the intervention(s) and their evolution over time (e.g., timeline diagram, flow chart, or table), including modifications made to the intervention during the project
	b. Details of the process measures and outcome
	c. Contextual elements that interacted with the intervention(s)
	d. Observed associations between outcomes, interventions, and relevant contextual elements
	e. Unintended consequences such as unexpected benefits, problems, failures, or costs associated with the intervention(s).
	f. Details about missing data
Discussion	**What does it mean?**
14. **Summary**	**1.** Key findings, including relevance to the rationale and specific aims
	2. Particular strengths of the project
15. **Interpretation**	**1.** Nature of the association between the intervention(s) and the outcomes
	2. Comparison of results with findings from other publications
	3. Impact of the project on people and systems
	4. Reasons for any differences between observed and anticipated outcomes, including the influence of context
	5. Costs and strategic trade-offs, including opportunity costs
16. **Limitations**	**a.** Limits to the generalizability of the work
	b. Factors that might have limited internal validity such as confounding, bias, or imprecision in the design, methods, measurement, or analysis
	c. Efforts made to minimize and adjust for limitations
17. **Conclusions**	**a.** Usefulness of the work
	b. Sustainability
	c. Potential for spread to other contexts
	d. Implications for practice and for further study in the field
	e. Suggested next steps
Other Information	
18. **Funding**	Sources of funding that supported this work. Role, if any, of the funding organization in the design, implementation, interpretation, and reporting

From Ogrinc G, Davies L, Goodman D, Batalden P, Davidoff F, Stevens D. SQUIRE 2.0 (Standards for QUality Improvement Reporting Excellence): revised publication guidelines from a detailed consensus process. *Am J Med Qual.* 2015;30(6):543–549.

Planning Your Study: Why Did You Start?

It is very useful to review the guidelines at the planning phase of any QI study. The guidelines provide a checklist to prompt consideration for your study and a framework around which to structure your project.

To answer the question "Why did you start?", define the problem you are trying/tried to solve and describe any background literature available. Can you explain why the problem is occurring? What is your proposed solution? Do you have a theory as to why this solution may work? For help with this, see Chapter 21 on developing a "Programme Theory" and a paper on demystifying theory.[5] Define the specific aims, and remember a good aim should be measurable and time defined. How will you measure your results?

Methods: What Did You Do?

The importance of context is now recognized in improvement work. What works in one context may not be reproducible in another. It is important that as part of the methods section, the reader of your paper has a clear description of the context in which this study was performed to understand adjustments that may have to be applied if they wish to replicate the study elsewhere. For example, in a paper describing implementation of a preoperative venous thromboembolism prophylaxis program before surgery, there is a clear description that this study took place in a UK National Health Service (NHS) preoperative surgical admissions area.[6] So, although the setting of a presurgical admissions unit may be replicable worldwide, the governing conditions of a national health system will differ elsewhere in the world, potentially rendering some aspects of the study harder to replicate.

The methods section (specifically SQUIRE item number nine) asks how the intervention will be studied. This is not the same as what will actually be done, but questions how the intervention will work to produce change, what helps to achieve success, and why the intervention may fail. For example, in the EPOCH (Enhanced PeriOperative Care for High Risk Patients) study, a QI intervention undertaken across many UK hospitals to improve high-risk surgery,[7] the intervention (an evidence-based clinical pathway supported by QI methodology) was studied with ethnography using formal observation in a subset of hospitals[8] and qualitative assessment through exit questionnaires to understand the barriers and facilitators for teams trying to implement the intervention.[9,10] Although the primary outcome of the intervention to reduce mortality from high-risk surgery at 180 days was not successful, the methods put in place to study the intervention provided a lot of useful information for future projects of this nature. For example, the more formal QI techniques teams used, the more successful they were, and teams who had good social connections within their organizations were more likely to be able to facilitate change.[9,10]

The SQUIRE guidelines emphasize the difference between "doing" an intervention and "studying" it, and improvement researchers should spend time considering both concepts as they plan and implement their project.

Results: What Did You Find?

It is helpful in the reporting of QI studies to include run charts (see Chapter 27) of progress against time. These should be annotated, if appropriate, to show interventions made through Plan Do Study Act (PDSA) cycles and iterative change during the project (Fig. 16.1). Although the SQUIRE guidelines do not specify detailing PDSA cycles as such, they do ask for the initial steps of the intervention and their evolution over time. Many projects reported in *BMJ Open Quality* list changes through descriptions of PDSA cycles as the project progressed.

Discussion: What Does It Mean?

In addition to the usual discussion of the study results and relevant other literature, the SQUIRE 2.0 guidelines suggest the need for discussion of the association between what was done and what happened, the impact on people and systems, the influence of context, and the costs and trade-offs. Importantly, the conclusion should include thoughts around the sustainability of any change achieved. These are all important additions to a normal academic discussion section and are highly relevant to achieving change in the real world.

Examples of Studies That Use SQUIRE 2.0 Guidelines

There are accompanying documents to the guidelines on the SQUIRE website that elaborate on them and give worked examples.[11] QI papers published in *BMJ Open Quality* use the SQUIRE approach. Some useful perioperative examples, in addition to those already given, include a study

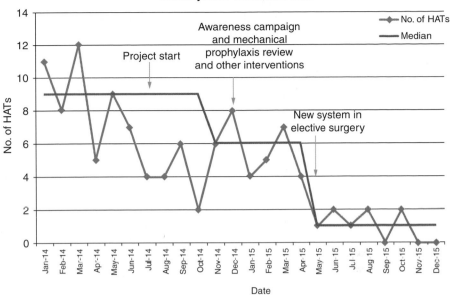

Fig. 16.1 Number of hospital-associated thromboses (*HATs*) over course of improvement project, annotated for iterative changes during the project. (Reproduced with permission from Humphries A, Jordan L, Crowe J, Peden C. Using the Safer Clinical Systems approach and Model for Improvement methodology to decrease venous thromboembolism in elective surgical patients. *BMJ Qual Improv Rep.* 2016;5[1].)

of increasing patient flow through a neurosurgical critical care unit[12] and one on improving hand-offs after cardiothoracic surgery.[13]

Conclusions

The SQUIRE 2.0 guidelines are an important resource for those involved in perioperative improvement. They provide a helpful checklist and framework to consider when planning a study and are a reporting structure accepted by leading journals.

References

1. Ogrinc G, Davies L, Goodman D, Batalden P, Davidoff F, Stevens D. SQUIRE 2.0 (Standards for QUality Improvement Reporting Excellence): revised publication guidelines from a detailed consensus process. *Am J Med Qual.* 2015;30(6):543–549.
2. Ogrinc G, Davies L, Goodman D, Batalden P, Davidoff F, Stevens D. SQUIRE 2.0—Standards for Quality Improvement Reporting Excellence—Revised Publication Guidelines from a Detailed Consensus Process. *J Am Coll Surg.* 2016;222(3):317–323.
3. BMJ Quality Open. *https://bmjopenquality.bmj.com.* Accessed May 27, 2021.
4. STROBE and the EQUATOR Network. *https://www.equator-network.org/reporting-guidelines/strobe/.* Accessed May 27, 2021.
5. Davidoff F, Dixon-Woods M, Leviton L, Michie S. Demystifying theory and its use in improvement. *BMJ Qual Saf.* 2015;24(3):228–238.
6. Humphries A, Jordan L, Crowe J, Peden C. Using the Safer Clinical Systems approach and Model for Improvement methodology to decrease venous thromboembolism in elective surgical patients. *BMJ Qual Improv Rep.* 2016;5(1).

7. Peden CJ, Stephens T, Martin G, et al. Effectiveness of a national quality improvement programme to improve survival after emergency abdominal surgery (EPOCH): a stepped-wedge cluster-randomised trial. *Lancet.* 2019;393(10187):2213–2221.
8. Martin GP, Kocman D, Stephens T, Peden CJ, Pearse RM. Pathways to professionalism? Quality improvement, care pathways, and the interplay of standardisation and clinical autonomy. *Sociol Health Illn.* 2017;39(8):1314–1329.
9. Stephens TJ, Peden CJ, Pearse RM, et al. Improving care at scale: process evaluation of a multi-component quality improvement intervention to reduce mortality after emergency abdominal surgery (EPOCH trial). *Implement Sci.* 2018;13(1):142.
10. Stephens TJ, Peden CJ, Haines R, et al. Hospital-level evaluation of the effect of a national quality improvement programme: time-series analysis of registry data. *BMJ Qual Saf.* 2020;29:623–625.
11. SQUIRE website. Explanation and elaboration. *http://squire-statement.org/index.cfm?fuseaction=page.viewpage&pageid=504.* Accessed May 27, 2021.
12. Meacock J, Mukherjee S, Sheikh A. Increasing patient flow through neurosurgical critical care: the Leeds Improvement Method. *BMJ Open Quality.* 2021;10: e001143.
13. Hamid S, Joyce F, Burza A, et al. OR and ICU teams 'running in parallel' at the end of cardiothoracic surgery improves perceptions of handoff safety. *BMJ Open Quality.* 2021;10(1):e001001.

CHAPTER 17

Leveraging the Perioperative Period to Address Population Health

Ryan Howard, MD ■ Michael Englesbe, MD

KEY POINTS

- Population health in the United States lags behind that of its peers.
- Undergoing major surgery serves as a teachable moment in which patients are especially motivated to adopt risk-reducing health behaviors.
- Perioperative interventions that screen for and intervene on modifiable health behaviors are feasible to implement and may significantly improve long-term outcomes.
- Health systems can take practical steps to integrate available resources into the perioperative pathway to help patients achieve lasting health improvements after surgery.

Introduction

Despite spending more on health care than any other country, population health in the United States (US) lags behind that of its peers. Compared with 10 other high-income countries, the US has the lowest life expectancy, highest chronic disease burden, and highest rate of preventable death.[1] The US also ranks 97th out of 163 countries in access to quality health care for its citizens.[2] On the Social Progress Index, the US is one of only three countries that is worse off in 2020 than it was when the Index began in 2011. The majority of these poor outcomes are driven by health behaviors and social determinants of health. These factors, such as smoking, physical inactivity, poor diet, alcohol use, and limited access to care, account for 70% of health outcomes and make up 9 of the top 10 risk factors for premature death in the US.[3]

Leveraging episodic care, such as undergoing major surgery, is a novel and potentially impactful way to address these problems. Over 50 million operations are performed each year in the US. Efforts to improve the value of surgical care have focused primarily on standardizing perioperative processes, reducing expenditure, and improving immediately measurable postoperative outcomes such as readmission or infection rates. Although these initiatives have been widely successful and become commonplace, surgical care has, at best, a marginal impact on the overall health of the population. This chapter reviews the evidence for addressing population health in the perioperative period and provides examples of quality improvement (QI) initiatives that have focused on these issues.

Surgery as a Teachable Moment and Missed Opportunity

A teachable moment is an event that motivates individuals to adopt risk-reducing health behaviors.[4] There is an abundance of evidence that major life events, such as a new diagnosis, a traumatic injury, and undergoing major surgery, serve as teachable moments. These events spontaneously prompt individuals to make health behavior changes they had previously not considered or had failed to make. For example, although less than 10% of smokers successfully quit each year, over 50% of smokers undergoing surgery for smoking-related diseases successfully quit after surgery.[5,6] In fact, even patients undergoing operations unrelated to tobacco use, such as elective joint replacement, are more likely to quit smoking.[7]

Not only are patients motivated to achieve health behavior change around the time of surgery, but there are also opportunities unique to the population of patients who undergo surgery. A recent study of more than 300,000 patients undergoing surgery in Michigan found that a quarter of patients smoked at the time of surgery, which is almost twice the national prevalence of tobacco use.[8] Moreover, patients with Medicaid or no insurance, for whom a surgical episode may represent one of their only interactions with the healthcare system, had a smoking prevalence of nearly 50%. Similarly, a 2020 study found that nearly a third of trauma patients had a new or unmanaged chronic medical or psychiatric condition at the time of presentation.[9] Although surgeons recognize the overriding importance of these health behaviors and chronic conditions, the majority do not engage patients in these domains, citing time constraints, lack of resources, or a belief that such efforts would simply be futile.[10]

Current Examples

Given the prevalence and effects of poor health behaviors and social strain among surgical patients, efforts to intervene around the time of surgery may be particularly effective. There are a number of initiatives that have attempted to leverage the teachable moment of a surgical episode to address these issues.

Perioperative smoking cessation interventions are an excellent example of achieving long-term health improvements after surgery. A randomized controlled trial of four simple intervention components before surgery (brief advice, brochures, telephone quit line referral, and nicotine replacement therapy [NRT]) found that patients randomized to the intervention arm were three times more likely to be tobacco free 1 year after surgery.[11] Multiple studies have corroborated the effectiveness of even simple interventions in the perioperative period. In Michigan, a statewide initiative that consisted of three simple components for vascular surgery patients (physician-delivered advice, quit line referral, and NRT) was independently associated with tobacco cessation 30 days after surgery.[12] Screening and referral for substance use disorder is also integrated into the trauma pathway in many health systems. As part of trauma center verification by the American College of Surgeons (ACS), centers are required to employ Screening, Brief Intervention, and Referral to Treatment (SBIRT) for all trauma patients who are intoxicated upon presentation.[13]

In the US, the Michigan Surgical and Health Optimization Program (MSHOP) and the ACS Strong for Surgery program are both initiatives that engage patients in health behavior improvement before surgery, also known as "prehabilitation." These programs engage patients in domains such as increased physical activity using a pedometer, medication management and glycemic control, smoking cessation, improved nutrition using healthy recipes, and other healthy lifestyle changes. These programs have been shown to reduce the incidence of postoperative complications, accelerate return to baseline functional status, and reduce hospital expenditures.[14] Although prehabilitation efforts are typically limited to health gains before surgery, their success reflects the impressive level of engagement that patients exhibit around the time of surgery. Moreover, these programs demonstrate that perioperative care can be coordinated in such a way as to bring inter-disciplinary teams together to address a wide range of patient needs.[15]

In 2018 Duke Health launched the Preoperative Anesthesia and Surgical Screening (PASS) clinic whose goal is "to more proactively and efficiently manage modifiable risks at the time a patient's surgical candidacy is first considered."[16] This centralized, highly interdisciplinary program screens surgical patients for a wide range of chronic health conditions, such as diabetes, malnutrition, obesity, smoking, exercise intolerance, frailty, stress, sleep apnea, and complex pain, and refers them to the appropriate providers and clinics to address these issues. As of April 2020, the PASS clinic has placed more than 5000 referrals to optimization programs. By centralizing the preoperative pathway, making it comprehensive in its scope, and taking a proactive approach to perioperative risk assessment and intervention, programs like the PASS Clinic have the potential to create value not only by optimizing immediate surgical outcomes, but by improving health outcomes long after the surgical episode has ended.[17]

In the UK, the National Health Service (NHS) program "Make Every Contact Count" also aims to leverage episodic care to impact population health.[18] Under this program, every interaction a patient has with the healthcare system is seen as an opportunity to screen for and address the health behaviors that have the biggest impact on an individual's life. A patient undergoing anything from a routine eye exam to an outpatient hernia repair to a major operation is asked about their diet, tobacco use, and physical activity and given resources or referrals to improve these behaviors.

At our own institution, we have recently integrated a screening and referral program for all surgical patients. As part of this program, all patients undergoing surgery are screened for active tobacco use (using the traditional social history) and food insecurity (using the two-question Hunger Vital Sign).[19] Patients who screen positive for smoking are referred to our institution's smoking cessation program, which offers multiple motivational interview sessions, NRT, and longitudinal follow-up to prevent recidivism. Patients who screen positive for food insecurity are referred to a nonmedical assistance program, where social workers identify resource needs, including food, housing, and transportation, and connect patients with local resources. The entire processes of screening and referral adds less than 30 seconds to the workflow of our preoperative clinic staff but has the potential to dramatically transform a patient's health trajectory after their surgical episode.

A Conceptual Model to Address Population Health Issues in the Perioperative Period

The aforementioned examples demonstrate that leveraging the perioperative period to improve population health is feasible and pragmatic. Many health systems already have existing resources dedicated to addressing patients' social needs or helping them quit smoking; however, they are not a part of the surgical pathway. Therefore we propose the following conceptual model as a way to integrate these resources into the surgical pathway (Fig. 17.1). According to this framework, a patient who undergoes surgery is screened for a number of intervenable conditions, such as smoking, alcohol use, physical inactivity, poor diet, obesity, mental health disorders, diabetes, and access to care. A positive screen in any of these areas would then translate into a referral to the appropriate resources. The goal is not to address every area before surgery but simply to use the surgical episode as an opportunity to connect patients with resources. This endeavor is overwhelming and thus would have to start small, as we have done by focusing only on smoking and food insecurity. The following simple, practical, and actionable steps can enable a surgical clinic or health system to begin a screening program for surgical patients:

- ▪ Integrate screening questions into the preoperative history and physical examination or through use of questionnaires to be filled out by patients while awaiting their appointment.

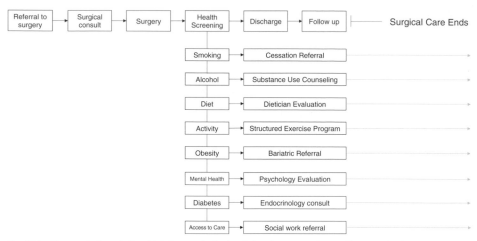

Fig. 17.1 Conceptual model in which the surgical episode involves screening and intervention for health behaviors and social determinants of health.

- Identify and partner with existing local resources. Many health systems already have programs in place to address tobacco use, healthy lifestyle changes, and access to care.
- Ensure that a positive screen for an unhealthy behavior or social need translates into a referral to the appropriate resources.
- Use departmental meetings to educate surgeons, anesthesiologists, physician assistants, and other perioperative staff on the importance of health behaviors and social needs.

We can envision how this perioperative pathway is different from traditional care using a hypothetical scenario. Consider a patient who is referred to a general surgery clinic with symptomatic cholelithiasis. She is a 54-year-old woman with a body mass index of 39 kg/m^2, active smoking, and poorly controlled diabetes. Unbeknownst to the surgeon, she also has a high-deductible health insurance plan, which has prevented her from regularly filling her insulin. Despite these medical issues, she has no contraindication for surgery and undergoes an uncomplicated, outpatient laparoscopic cholecystectomy. At her 2-week follow-up visit, her incisions are healed, she feels well, has returned to work, and therefore she is discharged from clinic. By every current quality metric, her episode of care was a success: She did not require hospital admission and she had an uncomplicated postoperative course. Nevertheless, her intervenable chronic conditions and lack of access to regular health care will shorten her life by more than a decade.[20]

Now envision a scenario in which this patient's surgical episode involves automatic screening that identifies intervenable issues such as obesity, tobacco use, uncontrolled diabetes, and poor healthcare access. This evaluation could result in a referral to the hospital's smoking cessation program, an endocrinology consultation with facilitated engagement, enrollment in a structured exercise program, and evaluation by a social worker with resources about more affordable insurance options. These simple steps could profoundly alter this patient's health trajectory long after her surgical care has ended. Success in even just one of these areas is likely to have a far bigger impact on this patient's longevity than her surgical care. The perioperative period is a time in which patients are highly engaged with the healthcare system and in some cases may represent their only engagement before they once again return to a living situation which limits their access to care. Capitalizing on this engagement as an opportunity to address fundamental health issues is a potentially powerful way to move the needle on some of our population's most urgent health needs.

References

1. Tikkanen R, Abrams MK. U.S. Health Care from a global perspective, 2019: higher spending, worse outcomes? Commonwealth Fund; 2020. https://doi.org/10.26099/7avy-fc29.
2. Social Progress Imperative. 2020 Social Progress Index. Washington, DC: Social Progress Imperative. www.socialprogress.org. Accessed February 24, 2021.
3. Institute for Health Metrics and Evaluation (IHME). United States of America. Seattle, WA: IHME, University of Washington; 2015. http://www.healthdata.org/united-states. Accessed August 17, 2020.
4. McBride CM, Emmons KM, Lipkus IM. Understanding the potential of teachable moments: the case of smoking cessation. *Health Educ Res.* 2003;18(2):156–170.
5. Warner DO. Surgery as a teachable moment: lost opportunities to improve public health. *Arch Surg.* 2009;144(12):1106–1107.
6. Mustoe MM, Clark JM, Huynh TT, et al. Engagement and effectiveness of a smoking cessation quitline intervention in a thoracic surgery clinic. *JAMA Surg.* 2020.
7. Shi Y, Warner DO. Surgery as a teachable moment for smoking cessation. *Anesthesiology.* 2010;112 (1):102–107.
8. Howard R, Singh K, Englesbe M. Prevalence and trends in smoking among surgical patients in Michigan, 2012–2019. *JAMA Netw Open.* 2021;4(3):e210553.
9. Spruce MW, Thomas DM, Anderson JE, Ortega JC, Mortazavi K, Galante JM. Trauma as an entry point to the health care system. *JAMA Surg.* 2020.
10. Barrett S, Begg S, Sloane A, Kingsley M. Surgeons and preventive health: a mixed methods study of current practice, beliefs and attitudes influencing health promotion activities amongst public hospital surgeons. *BMC Health Serv Res.* 2019;19(1):358.
11. Lee SM, Landry J, Jones PM, Buhrmann O, Morley-Forster P. Long-term quit rates after a perioperative smoking cessation randomized controlled trial. *Anesth Analg.* 2015;120(3):582–587.
12. Howard R, Albright J, Osborne N, Englesbe M, Goodney P, Henke P. Impact of a regional smoking cessation intervention for vascular surgery patients. *J Vasc Surg.* 2021.
13. Hays AM, Gilrain KL, Grunberg VA, Bullock A, Fizur P, Ross SE. Implementing and evaluating SBIRT for alcohol use at a level 1 trauma center: a behavioral medicine approach. *J Clin Psychol Med Settings.* 2020;27(2):376–384.
14. Howard R, Yin YS, McCandless L, Wang S, Englesbe M, Machado-Aranda D. Taking control of your surgery: impact of a prehabilitation program on major abdominal surgery. *J Am Coll Surg.* 2019;228 (1):72–80.
15. Peden CJ, Mythen MG, Vetter TR. Population health management and perioperative medicine: the expanding role of the anesthesiologist. *Anesth Analg.* 2018;126(2):397–399.
16. Aronson S, Murray S, Martin G, et al. Roadmap for transforming preoperative assessment to preoperative optimization. *Anesth Analg.* 2020;130(4):811–819.
17. Aronson S, Sangvai D, McClellan MB. Why a proactive perioperative medicine policy is crucial for a sustainable population health strategy. *Anesth Analg.* 2018;126(2):710–712.
18. Lawrence W, Black C, Tinati T, et al. 'Making every contact count': evaluation of the impact of an intervention to train health and social care practitioners in skills to support health behaviour change. *J Health Psychol.* 2016;21(2):138–151.
19. Cutts D, Cook J. Screening for food insecurity: short-term alleviation and long-term prevention. *Am J Public Health.* 2017;107(11):1699–1700.
20. Mokdad AH, Marks JS, Stroup DF, Gerberding JL. Actual causes of death in the United States, 2000. *JAMA.* 2004;291(10):1238–1245.

CHAPTER 18

Building for Sustainability

Lesley Jordan, MB ChB, FRCA

KEY POINTS

- Create passion for change and link to everyone's values.
- Team engagement, involvement, and ownership is essential to achieve and sustain change.
- Continuous transparent measurement must be established from the beginning.
- Maintain compliance measures and regular review, even after the aim is achieved to ensure success continues.
- Communicate and provide feedback on progress regularly.
- Ensure visible senior leadership and support.

Introduction

Improving patient care and experience is a fundamental aim for all healthcare systems but can be frustrating, demotivating, and a waste of valuable resources if improvement is short-lived. Unfortunately, only 30% of projects achieve and sustain their goal. Lack of resources are often assumed to be the cause of failure to sustain, but in 70% cases it is because of employee resistance or lack of management support.[1]

Right from the start, sustainability (i.e., "ensuring gains are maintained beyond the life of a project"[2]) needs be considered. Do not "dive straight in." Spend time planning, understanding the current system, considering who needs to be involved, and establishing measures to facilitate ongoing quality control and monitor improvement. With increasingly complex multidisciplinary pathways in perioperative medicine, these factors are particularly important.

Several models have been described to support achieving sustainability; all have similar components.[3,4] One of these, the National Health Service UK (NHS) change model, was created by NHS staff, who shared their experiences to produce an 8-point model (Fig. 18.1).[5] The factors included are: (1) shared purpose, (2) improvement methodology, (3) project management, (4) measurement, (5) system drivers, (6) mobilize and engage, (7) leadership, and (8) spread and adoption.

Shared Purpose

Describe and share the vision, linking to each other's values, to feel a connection and desire for it to succeed. Finding this "passion" for each individual requires time and active listening.

How can you demonstrate the existing problem and inspire feeling in others? Do you have patient stories to tell, or could you use a visual display?[6]

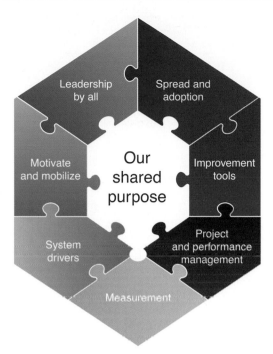

Fig. 18.1 NHS change model. The National Health Service UK (NHS) change model was created by NHS staff, who shared their experiences to produce this 8-point model. (Redrawn from Introduction to NHS change model. https://www.nhsggc.org.uk/media/235711/change-and-improvement-nhs_change_model_july20131. pdf. Accessed May 2021.)

Identify **all** staff who may be impacted or involved in the change or who have influence on it. There are stakeholder tools, which can help ensure no one is overlooked.[7]

Set up a multidisciplinary group of all involved, including physicians, nurses, front-line workers, and managers and administrators. This facilitates input and communication from the beginning.

Improvement Methodology and Project Management

Simple improvement tools such as the "Model for Improvement" provide structure and have been used successfully in many organizations (Fig. 18.2).[8]

- Allocate responsibilities and timelines.
- Do not forget the first two questions of the "Model for Improvement," which provide essential planning, ensuring a clear aim and measures. This will help clarify the "system" that must be changed.
- Create a process map with the team to identify issues with the current process and to support team engagement. Consider using a Fishbone diagram[9] to understand problems.
- Test ideas to see if they are effective. The key is to **LEARN** from what happened and "adapt, adopt, or abandon" the idea. Use the team to test and adapt ideas. This is crucial for success. It involves working with rather than imposing change on teams, ensures team ownership, and increases chance of sustaining improvements.
- Do not make the new process reliant on one individual because it will stop if they leave. This can occur when a project achieves its goals, but there is no ongoing feedback and those working on the project move on.[10]

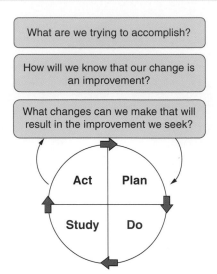

Fig. 18.2 The model for improvement. (Redrawn from Langley GL, Moen RD, Nolan KM, Nolan TW, Norman CL, Provost LP. *The Improvement Guide: A Practical Approach to Enhancing Organizational Performance*. 2nd ed. Jossey-Bass; 2009.)

Example: Staff moved on after implementation of an emergency laparotomy bundle and improvements decreased. Issues were knowledge decay and no team ownership of measures or feedback. The bundle was relaunched, considering sustainability from the outset. A multidisciplinary team (MDT) was established, compliance measures were collected by the team, with regular feedback and executive oversight, resulting in reliable processes and a sustained decrease in mortality.[11]

Measurement

Measurement is a key factor in sustainability.

Before starting:

- Establish baseline measures quantifying the problem
- Plan ongoing measurement to demonstrate impact of changes

In quality improvement the measurements required are different to those for research, which most healthcare staff are familiar with. Research is about finding new knowledge, so conditions need to be controlled and large numbers required to prove effectiveness. Improvement involves implementing proven changes in real life, or uncontrolled conditions, so measures do not need to be perfect. "Just enough" information is needed to understand what's happening. Using random sampling allows easy regular data collection[12] and enables the impact of changes to be demonstrated, so work can start while awaiting more permanent data.

For example, in a project to improve intraoperative and postoperative hypothermia, patient temperatures in the postanesthesia care unit after surgery were not available electronically and measurement and change took 2 years for implementation. Work started using weekly random patient sampling, monitoring the effect of varying interventions, and significant improvements were eventually achieved. Random sampling enabled improvement to be achieved, while awaiting more easily accessible data.[13]

Ensure measurements are collected and reviewed regularly. Even once goals are achieved, do not declare victory too early.[11] This ensures success is maintained.

For example, in the case study previously mentioned on temperature measurement, compliance improved to 90% within 6 months, but ongoing measurement showed a decrease immediately (Fig. 18.3). As compliance was reviewed regularly, investigation discovered shortage of fluid warming devices, which was a key improvement. This was then addressed promptly, and compliance improved. Without tracking the measures, practice could easily have reverted to the old norm

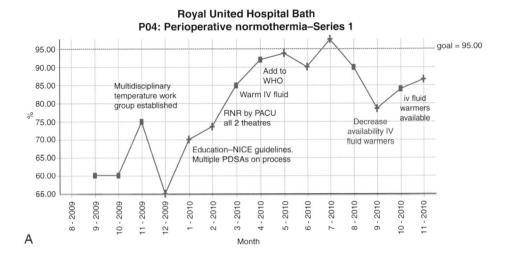

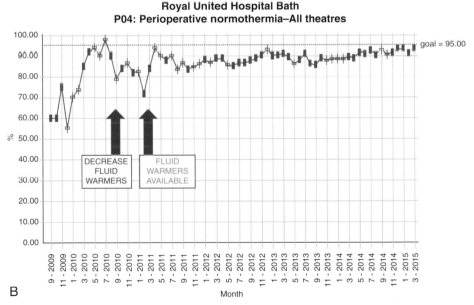

Fig. 18.3 (A, B) Annotated run charts demonstrating improvements in postoperative temperature, with reliable change enabled by random note reviews and monitoring compliance to identify issues early. (Redrawn from Jordan L. A quality improvement project: temperature on arrival in the post anaesthetic care unit (PACU). In: Colvin JR, Peden CJ, ed. *Raising the Standard: A Compendium of Audit Recipes*. 3rd ed. The Royal College of Anaesthetists; 2012, pp. 37–38.)

and all gains could have been lost. Tracking progress in this way also demonstrated the effectiveness of administering warmed intravenous fluids, persuading all team members to continue with the new process, resulting in a sustained change in practice.

Check that the change does not result in a negative impact elsewhere, which can hinder spread. Identify measures to collect for reassurance (balancing measures).

For example, when introducing a "briefing" before operating lists to improve communication, teamwork, and ensure availability of equipment, surgeons expressed concerns about delaying the list, resulting in overrunning or cancellation. Initial testing on one surgeon's lists, collecting balancing measures demonstrated the briefing took 5 minutes, no list overran, and staff were happy and engaged. The surgeons commented, 'They were the best lists for some time." Team engagement supported spread to other operating rooms, who were already requesting the intervention, having seen the positive effect on their colleagues. Collecting these balancing measures enabled concerns to be addressed from the beginning and the process became routine.

System Drivers

Align improvement to organizational strategies. Identify an executive sponsor to increase organizational support and improve sustainability. Consider this when planning the multidisciplinary stakeholder group. This will also be helpful in securing any funding required.

Are there are projects underway in the organization with similar goals to link with? (Remember the importance of understanding the system before starting.)

Mobilize and Engage

An essential aspect to implementing and sustaining successful change is engaging and involving all key personnel. Understanding the human dimensions of change is key.

Embed changes into routine practice so they become "how we do it around here." Nevertheless, human factors can make this difficult if the change is not easy, if multiple steps need to be remembered, or if the equipment required is not easily available. This can be exhausting, and the easiest response is to do what has always been done. This is important to realize: Staff are not usually resisting your change; it's just too difficult. Expecting staff to "work harder" or blaming them for resistance is not helpful.

Stop and pause, meet, and listen to staff and think about how to "make it easy to do the right thing."[14] Considering this at the beginning of the work helps prevent such problems.

There are a few possible ways to achieve this:

- Embed the change into existing processes:
  - For example, add temperature recording to the "sign in" of the World Health Organization (WHO) Surgical Safety Checklist.[13]
- Remove obstacles to doing the right thing.
  - Have equipment readily available (e.g., establish an "emergency laparotomy trolley" containing everything for goal-directed fluid therapy, specific endotracheal tubes for critical care, and promote delivery of essential bundle elements).[11]
  - Limit options (e.g., remove skin preparation and razors so only chlorhexidine and clippers are available in operating rooms and facilitate reliable processes to reduce surgical site infections)
- Ensure staff have received adequate training. If compliance with the process is low, check and make sure understanding is clear. Small clarifications may be needed to increase staff confidence. If they are busy and new processes are confusing, the easiest thing to do is what they have always done.

- Provide multiple "nudges" to help remind staff. Posters and checklists are useful. Place notices in prominent areas or immediately before a task is performed (e.g., "Stop before you block" notices on ultrasound machines screens that need to be moved before use may help decrease wrong side local anesthetic block).
- Communicating progress regularly supports continued staff engagement and helps drive further improvements.
- Celebrate success widely using your organizations communication teams. Recognizing achievements helps continued engagement. Consider describing the improvement in "patient terms" (e.g., number of lives saved, number of patients in whom a surgical site infection, or postoperative pneumonia was prevented). This can be extrapolated into costs saved. Business intelligence or finance teams can support this.
- Test the idea with enthusiastic teams/individuals. Do not start in the most difficult place because this will be more challenging. Make it easier by learning with supportive teams about what has not worked, refining the process to demonstrate success and making it easier to spread to any difficult areas or people.
- Include a patient or lay member in the team to give a different but exceptionally important perspective to the project, ensuring it remains patient centered. For example, in planning enhanced recovery pathways, patient expectations are a crucial element to success. Using patients to develop patient information ensures it is clear, understandable, and more likely to succeed.
- Have patients tell their own stories, which can be a powerful way to engage staff.

Leadership

Leadership is important to set the vision and shared purpose of the project and ensure the MDT is inclusive and well briefed with accurate facts and figures. Importantly, you do not need to be in a senior leadership position in your organization to lead change, but senior leaders play an important role in supporting anyone leading improvement. Ensure organizational leads are updated about the project so they can add valuable support.

Spread and Adoption

Using the quality improvement tools described to demonstrate the impact of the change, as well as any side effects and costs, is important in persuading others to adopt it. If the right people have been involved and influenced the change, spread and adoption to other areas is more successful. It is important not to spread until the change is working well in the initial group. Spread is then more successful because lessons learned can be implemented before spreading. When a change is spread, it is important to continue testing in the new area because different conditions may require further adaptation.

In summary, multiple factors need to be achieved to sustain improvements (Fig. 18.4). Key aspects are having supportive management, promoting a shared desire to improve, building an improvement culture, engaging and involving staff with robust feedback and communication, and evidencing improvement.[15] These factors must be considered at the beginning of any intervention. Sustainability requires considerable work after initial changes have been achieved,[10] and ongoing measurement and quality control must continue to be monitored through existing organization governance structures. Any decreases in performance must be investigated and managed early before gains are lost.

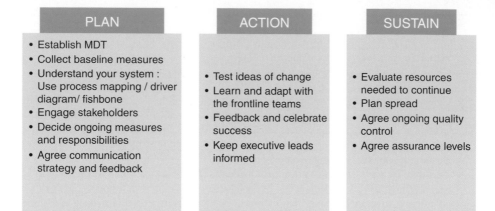

Fig. 18.4 Summary tool to aid in planning an improvement project and sustaining change.

References

1. Keller S, Schaninger B. *McKinsey and Company. Beyond Performance 2.0: A Proven Approach to Leading Large-Scale Change.* Wiley; 2019.
2. Clinical Excellence Commission (CEC). Enhancing project spread and sustainability. http://www.cec. health.nsw.gov,au_/data/assets/pdf_file/0007/258343/spread-and-sustainability.pdf. Accessed May 2021.
3. Harvard Business Review, Kotter JP. Leading change: why transformation efforts fail?; 1995. https://hbr. org/1995/05/leading-change-why-transformation-efforts-fail-2. Accessed May 2021.
4. Maher L, Gustafson D, Evan A. NHS sustainability model. https://www.england.nhs.uk/improvement-hub/wp-content/uploads/sites/44/2017/11/NHS-Sustainability-Model-2010.pdf. Accessed May 2021.
5. Introduction to NHS change model. https://www.nhsggc.org.uk/media/235711/change-and-improvement-nhs_change_model_july20131.pdf. Accessed May 2021.
6. Heath D, Heath C. Switch: How to Change Things When Change Is Hard. Cornerstone. ISBN: 9781847940322.
7. https://www.england.nhs.uk/wp-content/uploads/2021/03/qsir-stakeholder-analysis.pdf. Accessed May 2021.
8. Langley GL, Moen RD, Nolan KM, Nolan TW, Norman CL, Provost LP. *The Improvement Guide: A Practical Approach to Enhancing Organizational Performance.* 2nd ed. Jossey-Bass; 2009.
9. https://www.england.nhs.uk/wp-content/uploads/2021/03/qsir-cause-effect-fishbone.pdf.
10. Dixon-Woods M, McNicol S, Martin G. Ten challenges in improving quality in healthcare: lessons from the Health Foundation's programme evaluations and relevant literature. *BMJ Qual Safety.* 2012;21(10): 876–884.
11. Jordan LC, Cook TM, Cook SC, et al. Sustaining better care for patients undergoing emergency laparotomy. *Anaesthesia.* 2020;**75(10)**:1321–1330.
12. Perla RJ, Provost LP, Murray SK. Sampling considerations in health care improvement. *Qual Manag Health Care.* 2013;22(1):36–47.
13. Jordan L. A quality improvement project: temperature on arrival in the Post Anaesthetic Care Unit (PACU). In: Colvin JR, Peden CJ, eds. *Raising the Standard: A Compendium of Audit Recipes.* 3rd. The Royal College of Anaesthetists; 2012:37–38.
14. Reason J. 12 Principles of error management. http://aerossurance.com/helicopters/james-reasons-12-principles-error-management/. Accessed May 2021.
15. Scoville R, Little K, Rakover J, Luther K, Mate K. *Sustaining Improvement.* IHI White Paper, Institute for Healthcare Improvement; 2016. Available at ihi.org.

CHAPTER 19

Risk Management and Perioperative Quality

Steven E. Raper, MD, JD

KEY POINTS

- The medical malpractice system does a poor job of improving patient safety and quality.
- Targeted risk reduction initiatives are associated with lower malpractice costs.
- Initiatives can be tailored to individual departments or expanded entity-wide.
- Successful areas of focus include improving physician-patient communication, educating clinicians on the basics of medical malpractice, and developing procedure-specific electronic informed consent documents.

Healthcare risk management includes a number of diverse elements: claims and litigation, quality and patient safety, risk financing, regulatory compliance, emergency management, and occupational health and safety. Fundamentally, those responsible for risk management work to promote the healthcare organization's mission to keep people safe.[1] A comprehensive review of the many facets of healthcare risk management is beyond the scope of this chapter, but the intersection of medical malpractice and healthcare quality is a critical issue for which further analysis is needed. The relationship between perioperative preparation and postoperative care has improved perioperative outcomes. Developing useful cognitive aids, best practices in the use of checklists, and the concept of "failure to rescue" in surgical patients are all being explored with success.[2]

Nevertheless, medical errors leading to injury happen. Management of risks associated with medical malpractice is expensive. A random sample of 1452 closed malpractice claims were studied to determine whether a medical injury had occurred and, if so, whether it was because of medical error. Thirty-seven percent of the claims did not involve errors. Only 73% of the claims that involved medical errors were compensated. Claims in the study sample cost more than $449 million; total indemnity costs were more than $376 million and defense cost almost $73 million. The findings led the authors to conclude that most costs of the medical malpractice system are for litigation over medical injury errors and compensation, but the costs of medical malpractice litigation are "exorbitant."[3] In 2010 overall annual medical liability system costs, including estimates of defensive medicine, were stated as $55.6 billion in 2008 dollars, or 2.4% of total healthcare spending.[4]

Medical Malpractice as Deterrence: A Failed Approach to Quality and Patient Safety

Despite the high cost of the medical liability system, there are serious concerns about whether the medical malpractice system facilitates or hinders improvements in healthcare quality and patient safety. By providing access to the courts, the medical malpractice system has two aspirational goals: (1) to deter negligence and (2) to provide a remedy for patients injured by negligent medical care.[5] Neither goal appears to be adequately achieved. Improving healthcare quality would be expected to decrease negligence. One systematic review looked at the association between medical malpractice liability risk and healthcare quality and safety. Among 20 studies of patient mortality in nonobstetrical care settings, 16 found no evidence of an association with liability risk and 4 with only limited evidence. The authors concluded that greater tort liability—as currently practiced—was not associated with improved quality of care.[5]

In an observational study of short-term, acute-care general hospitals in the United States using publicly reported measures of state-specific malpractice environments, no consistent association between malpractice environment and hospital process-of-care measures was found. There was, however, evidence that defensive medicine was increased with malpractice risk. Specific examples included observations that hospitals in areas with a higher Medicare Malpractice Geographical Practice Cost Index (MGPCI) or a composite measure were associated with overutilization of cardiac stress testing and brain/sinus computed tomography (CT) scans, respectively. Also, the study found that acute myocardial infarction, heart failure, and pneumonia were more likely to have *higher* 30-day readmission rates in high malpractice risk environments.[6]

Therefore the goal of improving quality and patient safety is not achieved by increased malpractice risk. The goal of providing a remedy for patients injured by negligent care seems to also be unmet. Plaintiffs' attorneys work on a contingent basis, and generally take 30% to 40% of damage awards, plus expenses, but take nothing if the jury finds for the defendant.[7] Selecting the right client is critical to a personal injury attorney's professional survival. To be found worthy of representation, a variety of tests have been used, including: prior negligence by the defendant, how a jury would react, and the fact that the attorney may be involved in a case for years.[7]

The effort with which clients are selected for representation in medical malpractice litigation aside, many complaints are filed that do not support allegations of negligence. In a study of 98 claims, only 47 were confirmed as being the result of treatment in the given time period; of these, no negligence or even injury was found in more than half.[8] Of 98 claims, only 8 were considered to allege adverse events related to negligent treatment; 10 claims involved hospitalization that had produced injuries not thought to be because of physician negligence; and 3 cases exhibited some evidence of medical causation but not enough to pass the study's negligence criteria. Twenty-six of the reviewed claims—greater than half—provided neither evidence of medical injury nor negligence.[9]

The high bar set by malpractice attorneys for filing a claim on behalf of clients leads to a malpractice gap.[10] Again, the classic Harvard Medical Practice Study reviewed more than 31,000 medical records; 1100 medical injuries were noted. Of these, 280 were thought negligent but resulted in only 8 malpractice claims—less than 2%![9] As confirmation of the malpractice gap noted in the HMPS study, a review of claims filed in Utah and Colorado showed 18 malpractice claims in a sample of 14,700 hospital discharges. Fourteen of the 18 claims were not thought by reviewers to be because of negligence.[11] Another estimate of the litigation gap can be made by results of the statewide medical chart reviews, which estimated 27,179 negligent injuries and 3571 patient claims for 1984 treatment—one claim for every 7.6 estimated negligent injuries.[8] When calculating the claims data as a ratio based on sampling weight, the chances that a claim would be filed decreased to 1 in 50.[8]

Where, then, might attempts to decrease malpractice risk and improve patient safety and quality intersect? The University of Pennsylvania Health System (UPHS) has embarked on a years-long effort to reduce malpractice risk by focusing on certain quality metrics. A key component of this strategy is the Risk Reduction Initiative (RRI), which uses a "grassroots" or department-level approach to engage physicians and surgeons in risk mitigation activities to reduce malpractice costs. Clinical communities can be organized to achieve common quality improvement goals.[12,13] Using a faculty-driven approach, each clinical department proposes and executes one or more interventions in recognition of an area of high risk or prior malpractice claims data. To engage faculty and incentivize completion of the RRIs, a portion of the primary layer of malpractice premiums was offered for use in future quality and risk reduction activities. Since starting the RRI program, more than 250 proposals have been submitted by clinical departments (e.g., surgery, medicine, anesthesia) and $14 million have been awarded. Importantly, the number of malpractice claims and malpractice costs decreased.[14] Although it is difficult to assure cause and effect, the combined impact of these bottom-up department-initiated interventions and engaging faculty to become actively involved in risk mitigation as a means to patient safety and quality improvement is a positive strategy for reducing malpractice claims and costs.

Practical Strategies for Risk Reduction

Available evidence suggests improved communication between the patient and physician improves patient safety and quality while decreasing malpractice risk. Research has highlighted the importance of patient-provider communication in avoiding malpractice lawsuits.[15,16] The average MGPCI—and a separate developed composite measure—were negatively associated with Healthcare Consumer Assessment of Providers and Services (HCAHPS) doctor communication scores. Despite a hypothesis that providers would attempt to promote patient satisfaction through communication and other steps in high malpractice-risk environments, the data suggested that liability anxiety may impair communication between patients and physicians. An alternative interpretation was that poor communication (e.g., inadequate pain control and untimely delays in patient assistance) were the cause of patient dissatisfaction. Lower quality of care and higher malpractice claims therefore led to higher levels of MGPCI and composite risk.[6]

Improving Communication Skills

The UPHS Department of Surgery has focused a number of initiatives on improving surgeon-patient communication. There are a number of discrete circumstances in communicating with patients, each of which requires unique elements. Residents are expected to communicate effectively with patients across a broad range of socioeconomic and cultural backgrounds. We taught a course specifically on the disclosure of medical error. Residents viewed a web-based video didactic session and associated slide deck and then were filmed disclosing a wrong-site surgery to a standardized patient (SP). We quantitatively demonstrated competency across a wide range of domains of interpersonal and communication skills.[17]

This initial success led us to expand courses in communication skills to faculty. Current concepts of physician-patient communication were presented in a series of lectures; better patient care, fewer malpractice suits, and the move toward transparency of communication metrics were among the topics. Course attendees viewed and critiqued "Surgi-Drama" videos, with simulated patients in physician-patient communication scenarios done poorly and then well. Participation was robust and course content satisfaction was high. The percentage of "top box" Doctor Communication HCAHPS scores and the national percentile ranking showed a sustained increase out to 2 years from the dates of the courses.[18]

The courses on communication were so successful, we were asked to develop a similar course for advanced practitioners. The faculty course was adapted, and current concepts on provider-patient communication were discussed. Participants also asked to view and critique a video "provider-patient communication gone wrong" scenario. Lastly, participants were provided with techniques for improving provider-patient communication. The participants assessed the course. Provider communication scores were tracked from quarter 1, Fiscal Year 2014 to quarter 4 Fiscal Year 2017 and doctor communication scores showed sustained increases year over year, suggesting the various communication courses had a lasting impact on provider communication skills.[19]

We noted a dearth of literature educating surgeons in particular, and physicians in general, on techniques for improving the critical communication skill of listening. We developed a short course focusing on listening skills for academic surgical faculty. Surgical faculty were provided with a basic framework for communication specifically highlighting approaches to improve listening and a video identifying one resource should any faculty wish to sharpen their skills. The course was well attended. In particular, the benefits of good communication and materials on listening skills had the highest satisfaction scores. Although our course was focused on surgeons, the course could be readily adapted to any cohort of busy clinicians.[20]

Educating Surgeons on Medical Malpractice

Despite the fact that medical malpractice premiums are a major cost, surgeons often have little, if any, education in the basics of tort litigation or how to manage their risk. We developed one approach for educating academic faculty surgeons on current concepts of medical malpractice and provide some guidance on how to "tip the scales of justice" and hopefully mitigate the risks of being named in a medical malpractice lawsuit. A five-part course was developed, including a basic of the medical malpractice system, the high cost of malpractice insurance to the health system and surgeons individually, current departmental claims experience, strategies for decreasing the risk of being named in a claim, and an overview of state-level malpractice reforms. Eighty-four percent of faculty attended the course and, quantitatively, the course was reviewed very favorably by an anonymous satisfaction survey. Some unique facets of our approach included an emphasis on state law and department-specific data. Given the state-specific nature of malpractice claims and litigation and the specific circumstances of cohorts of faculty, individual departments must particularize similar presentations.[21]

Enhancing Informed Consent

A third major set of initiatives was the development of a procedure-specific, electronic consent process. This was a multiyear intradepartmental effort that has since reached a point where all clinical departments are moving to the electronic platform. The decision was made early on to develop the process in-house rather than subscribe to a commercial product. This allows for more flexibility in terms of surgeon-specific risk. This has major ramifications for perioperative medicine because an inefficient consent process leads to operating room (OR) delays, disruption of timed antibiotics, and potential discrepancies between procedures scheduled and actually performed, leading to an increased risk of wrong site surgery.[22] As with other communication strategies, an important part of the move to an electronic platform involved educating faculty on principles of consent, a constantly evolving but foundational part of the surgeon-patient relationship. A course was developed containing a concise, contemporary review of the principles of informed consent, which consisted of ethical imperatives, legal principles, the many stakeholders involved in creating current requirements, and new consent developments. An anonymous, voluntary evaluation tool was used to assess strengths and opportunities for improvement. Eighty-five percent of the surgery department faculty participated. Evaluations were overwhelmingly positive.[23]

In an attempt to confirm the UPHS data, previously cited, regarding the positive impact of the RRI program at the departmental level, the relative impact of the Department of Surgery initiatives was assessed compared with malpractice experience for the rest of the Clinical Practices of the University of Pennsylvania (CPUP). Malpractice claims, indemnity, malpractice premium data, and expenses were obtained from CPUP finance. Because actual dollars involved were considered too sensitive to present, cost data (yearly indemnity and expenses) and malpractice premiums (total and per physician) were expressed as a percentages of the 5-year mean value, preceding implementation of the initiative program. Department of Surgery claims were significantly lower than the rest of the health system. The data suggest that educating surgeons on better communication, malpractice, and other risk reduction initiatives may decrease malpractice costs. As part of a multiyear effort, emphasis on risk reduction strategies appears to be cumulative and should be part of an ongoing program.[24]

Conclusions and Summary

Although the work described here is confined to one university health system and to the initiatives of one department, the principles by which the risk reduction strategies were designed are universally applicable to other aspects of perioperative medicine. The data presented confirm the correctness of a multifaceted, comprehensive approach to reducing malpractice risk by focusing on select strategies designed to improve quality and patient safety.

References

1. Card AJ. The underlying narrative of risk management. *J Healthc Risk Manag.* 2017;37(2):6–7.
2. Staender S, Smith A. Enhancing the quality and safety of the perioperative patient. *Curr Opin Anaesthesiol.* 2017;30(6):730–735.
3. Studdert DM, Mello MM, Gawande AA, et al. Claims, errors, and compensation payments in medical malpractice litigation. *N Engl J Med.* 2006;354:2024–2033.
4. Mello MM, Chandra A, Gawande AA, Studdert DM. National costs of the medical liability system. *Health Aff.* 2010;29:1569–1577.
5. Mello MM, Frakes MD, Blumenkranz E, Studdert DM. Malpractice liability and health care quality: a review. *JAMA.* 2020;323(4):352–366.
6. Bilimoria KY, Chung JW, Minami CA, et al. Relationship between state malpractice environment and quality of health care in the United States. *Jt Comm J Qual Patient Saf.* 2017;43:241–250.
7. Werth B. *Damages. Berkeley Books*; 1998:44–45.
8. Weiler PC, Hiatt HH, Newhouse JP, Johnson WG, Brennan TA, Leape LL. *Chapter 4: Patient Injury and Malpractice Litigation in a Measure of Malpractice: Medical Injury, Malpractice Litigation, and Patient Compensation.* p70ff. Harvard University Press; 1993.
9. Localio AR, Lawthers AG, Brennan TA, et al. Relation between malpractice claims and adverse events due to negligence: results of the Harvard Medical Practice Study III. *New Eng J Med.* 1991;325:245–251.
10. Raper SE. Announcing remedies for medical injury: a proposal for medical liability reform based on the Patient Protection and Affordable Care Act. *J Health Care Law Policy.* 2013;16(2):309–352.
11. Studdert DM, Thomas EJ, Burstin HR, Zbar BIW, Orav EJ, Brennan TA. Negligent care and malpractice claiming behavior in Utah and Colorado. *Med Care.* 2000;38:250–260.
12. Aveling EL, Martin G, Armstrong N, Banerjee J, Dixon-Woods M. Quality improvement through clinical communities: eight lessons for practice. *J Health Organ Manag.* 2012;26:158–174.
13. Weiner BJ, Alexander JA, Shortell SM, Baker LC, Becker M, Geppert JJ. Quality improvement implementation and hospital performance on quality indicators. *Health Serv Res.* 2006;41:307–334.
14. Diraviam SP, Sullivan PG, Sestito JA, Nepps ME, Clapp JT, Fleisher LA. Physician engagement in malpractice risk reduction: a UPHS case study. *Jt Comm J Qual Patient Saf.* 2018;44:605–613.
15. Hickson GB, Federspiel CF, Pichert JW, Miller CS, Gauld-Jaeger J, Bost P. Patient complaints and malpractice risk. *JAMA.* 2002;287:2951–2957.

16. Levinson W, Roter DL, Mullooly JP, Dull VT, Frankel RM. Physician-patient communication: the relationship with malpractice claims among primary care physicians and surgeons. *JAMA*. 1997;277:553–559.
17. Raper SE, Resnick AS, Morris JB. Simulated disclosure of a medical error by residents: development of a course in specific communication skills. *J Surg Educ*. 2014;71(6):e116–e126.
18. Raper SE, Gupta M, Okusanya O, Morris JB. Improving communication skills: a course for Academic Medical Center Surgery Residents and Faculty. *J Surg Educ*. 2015;72(6):e202–e211.
19. Joseph J, Sicoutris C, Raper SE. Communication skills training for surgical inpatient advanced practice providers in an academic health-care system. *J Patient Exp*. 2020;7(1):42–48.
20. Raper SE, Joseph J, LaMarra D, Millstein JH. Educating surgeons on listening: a critical communication skill. *Ann Surg Edu*. 2020;1(2):27–34.
21. Raper SE, Joseph J, Seymour WG, Sullivan PG. Tipping the scales: educating surgeons about medical malpractice. *J Surg Res*. 2016;206(1):206–213.
22. Garonzik-Wang JM, Brat G, Salazar JH, et al. Missing consent forms in the preoperative area: a single-center assessment of the scope of the problem and its downstream effects. *JAMA Surg*. 2013;148 (9):886–889.
23. Raper SE, Joseph J. Informed consent for academic surgeons: a curriculum-based update. *MedEdPORTAL*. 2020;16:10985. https://doi.org/10.15766/mep_2374-8265.10985.
24. Raper SE, Rose D, Nepps ME, Drebin JA. Taking the initiative: risk-reduction strategies and decreased malpractice costs. *J Am Coll Surg*. 2017;225(5):612–621.

CHAPTER 20

Using Innovative Payment Models to Drive Improvement in Perioperative Care

Nicholas L. Berlin, MD, MPH, MS ■ Kevin Bozic, MD, MBA ■
Anaeze C. Offodile II, MD, MPH

KEY POINTS

- All payment models fundamentally seek to leverage financial incentives for healthcare organizations, providers, and patients to drive behavior changes that reduce spending on healthcare services and improve health outcomes.
- Understanding the basic design of payment models is necessary to take advantage of new opportunities to improve perioperative care.
- Episode-based bundled payment models are one of many innovative models that may impact perioperative care.
- Payment models often force providers or healthcare organizations to take on financial risk for the opportunity to gain additional revenue.
- Success in payment models depends on the ability of providers and healthcare organizations to deliver services efficiently, improve coordination of care across providers and treatment settings, improve health outcomes, and monitor use and costs of care.

Healthcare Spending in the United States

The United States (US) spent roughly $3.8 trillion dollars on health care in 2019, which represents approximately $11,582 per person and 17.7% of the gross domestic product (GDP).[1] Spending on surgical care is estimated to be nearly 30% of all US spending on health care.[2] There is a general perception that spending on health care in the US, inclusive of surgical services, is too high relative to health outcomes in other developed countries. The etiology for high spending includes an array of factors that fit into the existing fee-for-service model of care delivery, including wide unsubstantiated variations in price and intensity of services delivered, lack of price and outcomes transparency, aging population needs, higher unit prices of services relative to other industrialized nations, care fragmentation, malpractice concerns, and wasteful/unnecessary spending. Surgical care is a focus of policymakers given the episodic nature and documented variations in spending and clinical outcomes at the region, hospital, and provider level, suggestive of opportunities for care redesign to meaningful dampen spending and improve outcomes.

In the context of high spending on health care in the US, there has been a several decades-long effort by the Centers for Medicare and Medicaid Services (CMS) to control spending at the healthcare system level through a variety of payment models, some of which remain in existence today (Fig. 20.1). It is important to recognize that the intrinsic value of innovative payment models is largely anchored by the ability to modify financial incentives and drive behavior change that reduces spending. These models are often temporary and dynamic, but fit into the broader objective of improving delivery of efficient, high-quality care.

Why Is Payment Reform Important in Perioperative Medicine?

Payment reforms may significantly affect the quality and quantity of care across the five phases of the surgical continuum (i.e., preoperative, perioperative, intraoperative, postoperative, and functional recovery).[3] Providers should not only understand payment models as they are being discussed and implemented but should seek to provide input to limit unanticipated consequences, spillover effects, and ultimately improve the *value* of care delivered to patients.

Payment Models With Provider-Focused Incentives

EPISODE-BASED BUNDLED PAYMENTS

Bundled payments represent an arrangement wherein hospitals and providers are paid a predetermined lump sum in exchange for all services furnished to a patient during a time period or over the course of a defined clinical condition, across all appropriate care settings. Bundling, either at the procedure or condition-level, aims to indirectly increase financial accountability of providers and hospitals for spending on healthcare services. CMS sets a spending target for each episode for each hospital, and hospitals earn a financial reward when Medicare spends less than the target price. Conversely, hospitals pay a financial penalty when Medicare spends more than the target price. Evidence supporting bundling comes from the mandatory comprehensive care for joint replacement model and for patients undergoing orthopedic surgery in the voluntary bundled payment for care improvement (BPCI) program,[4,5] but the evidence supporting bundles for other surgical conditions is less certain.[5]

Optimistically, these programs have been shown to reduce spending by approximately 1% to 3% through decreased use of postacute care and other hospital resources, without affecting access or quality of care. These findings have led to further expansion of episode-based bundled payments to other surgical conditions with BPCI Advanced, which now features 13 surgical conditions. There is some evidence that private payers are now testing and implementing episode-based bundled payment models as well.[6,7] Expansion to surgical conditions with limited use of postacute care services is unclear, suggesting that a one-size-fits-all approach for bundling may not be appropriate.[8–11]

Practical Implications

Success in voluntary bundled payment programs requires first selecting surgical episodes that your organization feels will offer the greatest opportunities to reduce spending and improved health outcomes from the Medicare perspective. A granular understanding of your organization's historical performance relative to peer hospitals and practice-patterns associated with length of stay, 30-day readmissions, utilization, and discharge disposition (i.e., rehabilitation vs. skilled nursing facility) is requisite. These models also require the successful implementation of interdisciplinary care that optimizes value, reduces spending, and improves or maintains high-quality patient outcomes. Examples include enhanced recovery after surgery (ERAS) protocols, care pathways, checklists, and the de-escalation of low-value preoperative and postoperative laboratory and imaging (if the episode extends into the preoperative period). Regarding the former, routine preoperative testing before low-risk surgery has no known benefit and is an important target for de-implementation

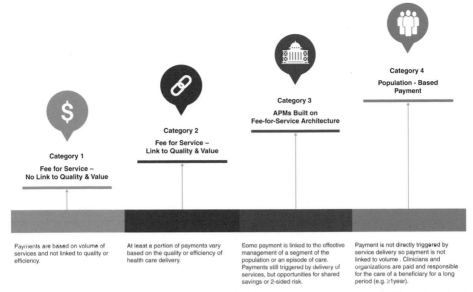

Fig. 20.1 Overview of Centers for Medicare and Medicaid Services payment models. (Reproduced with permission from The MITRE Corporation. In: Alternative Payment Model Framework. Health Care Payment Learning and Action Network. The MITRE Corporation; 2017. Figure 2, Page 11. https://hcp-lan.org/workproducts/apm-refresh-whitepaper-final.pdf. Accessed April 26, 2021.)

because it is overused, costly, and can lead to downstream care cascades involving invasive diagnostic testing.[12] Site-of-care optimization with respect to the setting of surgery receipt may also be helpful, in addition to a heightening cost awareness among providers. Reducing postoperative complications that require readmission or reoperation represents an opportunity to improve both quality of care delivered and reduce spending from the Medicare perspective. Additionally, the care standardization processes inherent to bundled payments represent an avenue for enhancing patient experience and reducing unnecessary care variation ("waste").

DIRECT PROVIDER CONTRACTING

Direct provider contracting (DPC) allows Medicare to contract directly with providers for a population of beneficiaries' entire healthcare spending via global capitated payments.[13] In this model, participants may be financially accountable for the costs of all care (not just primary care) delivered to patients within a population or region, respectively. Participation in these options is not limited to primary care physicians; clinicians from all specialties may engage in DPC. In general, the payment model options available under DPC seek to reduce program expenditures and improve quality of care and health outcomes for Medicare beneficiaries through alignment of financial incentives and an emphasis on beneficiary choice and care delivery while maintaining access to care for beneficiaries, including patients with complex, chronic conditions and seriously ill populations.

Practical Implications

Participants in the DPC programs must think more "globally" about expenditures for their patient population. Therefore surgeons, anesthesiologists, and others involved in the perioperative care process should think not only about how to reduce expenditures in ways that are successful for episode-based bundled payment programs (length of stay, readmissions, postacute care utilization, eliminating low-value routine preoperative testing) but also about how to best address more "upstream" factors, such as the appropriateness of a procedure and the comparative value of individual preference-sensitive surgical interventions. For providers engaged in DPC, eliminating routine preoperative testing, in the appropriate clinical scenario, might be an important source of spending reductions. Providers that are participating in DPC programs must also focus on appropriateness of discretionary surgical procedures that offer limited to no benefit over nonsurgical approaches yet remain commonly performed. The "global" perspective demanded by this payment model may result in improved and simpler care coordination and thus, improve patient experience and the quality of care delivered. Furthermore, a meaningful percentage of spending benchmarks are tied to performance metrics related to quality of care, thus preserving or perhaps incentivizing improvement in this aspect of care delivery for patients.

Payment Models With Patient-Focused Incentives

REFERENCE PRICING

With reference pricing models, the insurance provider places a limit on what it will contribute toward payment for a particular surgical procedure, assuring that the selected payment limit allows appropriate access for patients (typically, the payment is the median or some other midpoint in the distribution of prices in the local market).[14,15] Patients who select a provider that charges less than the purchaser's limit receive "full freight" coverage, with minimal cost sharing, and patients who select a provider charging above the contribution limit must pay the entire difference (termed a "reverse deductible"). When faced with paying the excessive rates charged by high-priced providers, most patients shift toward lower-priced providers. Reference pricing addresses the wide variation in the prices charged for similar services across the healthcare sector and has led to significant price reductions from hospitals where initial prices were above the California Public Employees' Retirement System (CalPERS) payment limit.[16] Similarly, reference pricing can result in an optimized site of care for elective, low-risk surgical procedures such as cataract removal, in addition to reduced spending.[17] Well-constructed reference pricing offers meaningful choices to consumers and savings to purchasers, with no sacrifice of quality and moves health care from a provider-dominated to a consumer-engaged system. Additionally, the upper limit of spending chosen by purchasers includes built-in quality metrics and many lower-priced providers may be delivering more efficient and higher quality care to patients, thus shifting patients toward providers that deliver higher quality care all together.

Practical Implications

Reference pricing models typically exist in markets with one or two dominant health insurance providers. For providers and healthcare organizations, reducing costs to bring prices near or below the limit will maintain patient referrals and volume while ensuring access to care. Reference pricing generally results in dramatic changes in spending at a health system level, primarily through the result of decreased revenue for hospitals and providers. If patients have limited understanding of their benefit structure and/or prices for healthcare services within a local healthcare market (i.e., health and financial literacy), they may experience high out of pocket costs if they unknowingly select a high-priced provider for a surgical procedure.

VALUE-BASED INSURANCE DESIGN

Value-based insurance design (V-BID) refers to mechanisms within insurance coverage that align patient out-of-pocket costs with the value of services delivered.[18] It is grounded in the principle that payers should remove or lower financial barriers for essential, high-value clinical services, thereby improving quality of care by encouraging, or discouraging, use of health services based on their potential benefit to patients' health relative to their costs. Conversely, in this model, patients pay more out-of-pocket for services of limited to no clinical benefit, thereby discouraging use of low-value services and reduced unnecessary spending. With regard to surgical procedures, V-BID has been conceptualized as a means to increase access and uptake of "high-value" surgical procedures such as bariatric surgery.[19] Although limited in use for perioperative care currently, V-BID leverages professional society recommendations from the Choosing Wisely campaign to create lists of "low-value" services, which typically include preoperative testing (e.g., cardiac tests, laboratory studies, chest radiography) before low-risk surgical procedures.[20]

Practical Implications

In V-BID models, patients and providers must be aware of when cost-sharing is reduced for high-value surgical and perioperative care and increased for low-value services. With awareness of different levels of cost-sharing, providers and patients can work together to optimize utilization of value-based care. Providers should actively engage in the design of tiers for cost-sharing with V-BID to ensure that access to surgical and perioperative care is maintained for services that may provide some clinical benefit, leaving the decision to pursue these types of services to the clinical decision-making of the providers and patients. Conversely, providers should actively seek to identify low-value and wasteful care in the perioperative period that provides limited to no clinical benefit.

References

1. Centers for Medicare and Medicaid Services. National health expenditures 2019 highlights. https://www.cms.gov/files/document/highlights.pdf. Accessed April 26, 2021.
2. Munoz E, Munoz W, 3rd, Wise L. National and surgical health care expenditures, 2005–2025. *Ann Surg.* 2010;251(2):195–200.
3. American College of Surgeons. New approach to surgical measurement: phases of surgical care. https://www.facs.org/advocacy/quality/phases. Accessed April 26, 2021.
4. Barnett ML, Wilcock A, McWilliams JM, et al. Two-year evaluation of mandatory bundled payments for joint replacement. *N Engl J Med.* 2019;380(3):252–262.
5. Agarwal R, Liao JM, Gupta A, et al. The impact of bundled payment on health care spending, utilization, and quality: a systematic review. *Health Aff (Millwood).* 2020;39(1):50–57.
6. Rastogi A, Mohr BA, Williams JO, et al. Prometheus payment model: application to hip and knee replacement surgery. *Clin Orthop Relat Res.* 2009;467(10):2587–2597.
7. Spinks T, Guzman A, Beadle BM, et al. Development and feasibility of bundled payments for the multidisciplinary treatment of head and neck cancer: a pilot program. *J Oncol Pract.* 2018;14(2):e103–e112.
8. Offodile AC, 2nd, Mehtsun W, Stimson CJ, et al. An overview of bundled payments for surgical oncologists: origins, progress to date, terminology, and future directions. Editorial. *Ann Surg Oncol.* 2019; 26(1):3–7.
9. Berlin NL, Chung KC, Matros E, et al. The costs of breast reconstruction and implications for episode-based bundled payment models. *Plast Reconstr Surg.* 2020;146(6):721e–730e.
10. Sheckter CC, Razdan SN, Disa JJ, et al. Conceptual considerations for payment bundling in breast reconstruction. *Plast Reconstr Surg.* 2018;141(2):294–300.
11. Liao JM, Wong SL, Chu D. Going beyond one size fits all in surgical bundled payments. *JAMA Surg.* 2020.
12. Berlin NL, Yost ML, Cheng B, et al. Patterns and determinants of low-value preoperative testing in Michigan. *JAMA Intern Med.* 2021.
13. Liao J, Navathe AS. *Medicare's direct provider contracting: to primary care and beyond."* *Health Affairs.* https://doi.org/10.1377/hblog20190626.900740.
14. Boynton A, Robinson JC. *Appropriate use of reference pricing can increase value.* *Health Affairs.* https://doi.org/10.1377/hblog20150707.049155.

15. Robinson JC, Brown TT, Whaley C. Reference pricing changes the 'choice architecture' of health care for consumers. *Health Aff (Millwood)*. 2017;36(3):524–530.
16. Robinson JC, Brown TT. Increases in consumer cost sharing redirect patient volumes and reduce hospital prices for orthopedic surgery. *Health Aff (Millwood)*. 2013;32(8):1392–1397.
17. Robinson JC, Brown T, Whaley C. Reference-based benefit design changes consumers' choices and employers' payments for ambulatory surgery. *Health Aff (Millwood)*. 2015;34(3):415–422.
18. Fendrick AM, Smith DG, Chernew ME. Applying value-based insurance design to low-value health services. *Health Aff (Millwood)*. 2010;29(11):2017–2021.
19. Gasoyan H, Tajeu G, Halpern MT, et al. Reasons for underutilization of bariatric surgery: the role of insurance benefit design. *Surg Obes Relat Dis*. 2019;15(1):146–151.
20. Kerr EA, Kullgren JT, Saini SD. Choosing wisely: how to fulfill the promise in the next 5 years. *Health Aff (Millwood)*. 2017;36(11):2012–2018.

Improvement Science Tools for Change

What is Program Theory and Why Is It Important to Perioperative Quality Improvement?

Clifford Y. Ko, MD, MS, MSHS ▪ Mary Dixon-Woods, BA, DipStat, MSc, DPhil

KEY POINTS

- The planning of quality improvement greatly benefits from articulating a program theory: It improves clarity around what the intervention is attempting to accomplish and the mechanisms of change.
- A program theory can also identify stakeholders and conditions for success.
- A program theory is based on the principle that the design and implementation of interventions are a reflection of underlying assumptions about a particular problem and how it can be addressed.
- A program theory can offer a theory-of-change that narratively explains the rationale and assumptions about mechanisms that are intended to link what is happening in the intervention to the intended outcomes.

Introduction: What Is Program Theory?

Those undertaking quality improvement (QI) in perioperative care are understandably concerned with knowing whether their interventions work. Increasingly, the importance of understanding *how* interventions work is recognized, too.[1] In this chapter, we outline the importance of program theory—which is principally concerned with the *how* question—for improving quality in perioperative care.

Theory is a word that attracts many definitions, many of them competing, contradictory, or even intimidating. In the context of QI, the concept of a *program theory* is a particularly useful one and is based on the principle that the design and implementation of interventions are always a reflection of underlying assumptions about a particular problem and how it can be addressed. Surfacing those assumptions and formalizing them into a program theory is an important responsibility of improvers because the assumptions are fundamental to understanding the goals of the intervention, the mechanisms through which it is intended to work, and the resources and activities needed to deliver it.

A program theory is a characteristically *small theory*[2]: It is specific to an intervention, rather than operating at a higher level of abstraction; it seeks to explain how the intervention is intended to lead to desired outcomes; and it is practical and accessible. A program theory may involve two things.[1] First, it can offer a theory-of-change that narratively explains the rationale and assumptions about mechanisms that are intended to link what is happening in the intervention to the intended outcomes, as well as identifying the stakeholders and identifying the conditions for success. For instance, an intervention to reduce mortality after emergency abdominal surgery was founded in an explicit program theory that identified the desired outcomes, the QI strategies to be used, the activities and resources, and the supporting evidence.[3]

To help in these tasks, the program team used *IF-THEN-SO THAT* statements such as the following:

- IF key professionals come together to form an improvement team and
- IF relevant data are reviewed and feedback is provided to teams regularly,
- THEN professionals can work as a team to define and achieve local improvement goals and
- THEN basic QI approaches can be employed to achieve the improvement goals
- SO THAT mortality after emergency laparotomy can be reduced.

Second, a program theory can use logic models, driver diagrams, or other visual methods to show the relationship between the intended outcomes and the components of the intervention. Depending on the approach chosen, these techniques may simply depict inputs, resources, activities, and outcomes and show the relationship between them, but they can also include other features of the program (e.g., relating to the contexts, the nature of the problem, assumptions, and rationale for change, and outputs and impacts). For instance, a QI initiative to involve families in patients' care after surgery developed a visual logic model showing the situation (including inadequate involvement of family caregivers), external factors (including ward cultures and family dynamics), the inputs needed, the intervention, the activities, and the immediate, intermediate, and ultimate outcomes.[4] Driver diagrams offer a more focused analysis of the outcomes sought (usually on the left of the diagram), the primary drivers (the broad areas requiring attention), and the secondary drivers (often relating to processes), as shown in the example in Fig. 21.1, aimed at improving surgery for older people.[5]

Why Use Program Theory in Perioperative Quality Improvement?

A key feature of improvement work, of course, is that those undertaking it are always, consciously or not, working with a set of assumptions and rationales about how their intervention is going to work, but using theory explicitly is helpful at every stage of a QI initiative.

Planning the intervention: Planning of QI greatly benefits from articulating a program theory. It improves clarity around what the intervention is attempting to accomplish, the mechanisms of change, who the stakeholders might be, and the relevant contexts. By encouraging improvers to be clear about the goals, inputs and resources, processes and activities, expected outputs and outcomes, relevant evidence, and what might facilitate or hinder the effort, program theory can support appropriate intervention development and anticipation of the resources needed, the actions to be taken, and the likely barriers.[6] Developing a logic model may be especially valuable in revealing elements that have not been thought through sufficiently or where there are differences of stakeholder opinion and where weaknesses or incoherence in the proposed intervention's causal logic might lie.[1]

Data: An explicit program theory helps to identify what data are needed and from whose perspective. For example, an initiative to reduce surgical site infections might begin by suggesting that data should be collected on variables such as 30-day occurrence, antibiotics used, timing of initial dose and re-dose, and operation type and length. Articulating the program theory, however, might reveal the importance of clinician behaviors and practices and thus reconfigure understanding of the types of data likely to be relevant. Articulating the program theory may also be important in identifying when patient-reported data is needed.

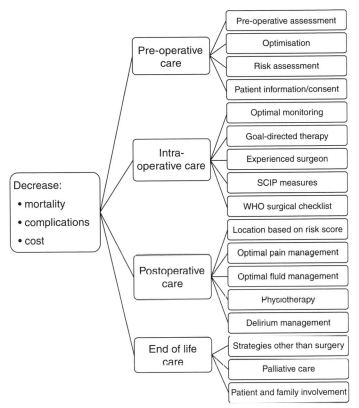

Fig. 21.1 Driver diagrams offer a more focused analysis of the outcomes sought (usually on the left of the diagram), the primary drivers (the broad areas requiring attention), and the secondary drivers (often relating to processes), as shown in this example, aimed at improving surgery for older people. *SCIP*, Surgical Care Improvement Project. (From Peden CJ. Emergency surgery in the elderly patient: a quality improvement approach. *Anaesthesia*. 2011;66[6]:440–445.)

Implementation: QI initiatives frequently experience challenges of implementation. Explicit articulation of a theory about how they will be introduced into practice, the influences on implementation, and the contextual influences is therefore helpful.[7] Further, QI initiatives may not be delivered exactly as planned.[8] Describing how the program was *supposed* to be carried out and subsequently recording how it *actually* was performed provides learning about to support future implementation.[9] Having a program theory can support assessment of whether the program was implemented with fidelity to the plan and can enable curation of evolution and mutation over time.

Evaluation: An explicit account of intervention components, processes, and assumptions underpinning an intervention provides a robust framework for both summative and process evaluation.[10,11] Process evaluation can allow assessment of whether the assumptions and rationales underpinning implementation actually play out in practice,[12] thus enabling analysis of whether any problems were because of failures of implementation or failures of theory, supporting replication of successful programs,[13] and highlighting what adaptations might need to be made to less successful efforts.

Developing a Program Theory

Developing a program theory for an improvement intervention in perioperative care may draw on a range of techniques and resources. Best practice requires a multistage, iterative approach and deep stakeholder engagement with a view to securing ownership and co-design, but a more pragmatic approach is often used, depending on available resources and program requirements. Recent high-quality examples of developing program theories in perioperative care are now available.[3,14] Whatever approach is chosen, the following steps are likely to be important.

UNDERSTAND THE PROBLEM AND THE RATIONALE FOR CHANGE

The rationale for change identifies why the program is needed, which may lie in a deficit in care (e.g., mortality after emergency surgery) or unwarranted variation (e.g., in start times for operations). The rationale can also include motivations for change, such as national policies, mandates, or local directives, as well as readiness and capacity for change of the practitioners, staff, and setting. Care is needed to ensure appropriate stakeholder involvement in formulating both the problem and the options for addressing it because the parties may not all share the same view.[15]

IDENTIFY WHAT NEEDS TO IMPROVE

Starting with the end in mind, outcomes are what needs to improve and should be informed by the rationale for change. The outcomes should be well defined, countable (measurable), and noticeable when improvement or change occurs, and matter to the stakeholders—both patients and staff.

IDENTIFY RELEVANT EVIDENCE

The forms of evidence likely to be useful include academic literature but also QI projects in similar areas, formal theories (e.g., about implementation or the role of audit and feedback), and informal theories.[1]

PRODUCE A PROTOTYPE IMPROVEMENT INTERVENTION AND CONSULT ON IT

The prototype should define the goals of the intervention, the program components and assumptions about how they will work, relevant features of context, and outcomes and how they will be measured. Consultation should involve those who will be involved in implementing and resourcing the intervention and those affected by it, including patients.

Identify What Is Needed to Support the Improvement Activity

The inputs are the resources that are necessary to perform the program and routinely include human resources, staff, time, and physical resources, taking into account available funding and other requirements. Activities are the processes performed to deliver the program. They might be grouped into different themes. For example, to decrease perioperative infections, program activities might include staff training, instituting clinical practices, data collection, and performance feedback.

FORMALIZE THE PROGRAM THEORY

Formalize the program theory using a theory of change and a logic model or other visual method and share it back with stakeholders, where appropriate incorporating any further revisions needed.

Conclusion

A good program theory can enable clarity about the components of a program, the mechanisms through which the program activities are thought to lead to the intended outcomes, and the key outcomes to be assessed. A well-formulated and clearly articulated program theory, ideally co-designed with stakeholders, including staff and patients, is fundamental to improvement in perioperative care.

References

1. Davidoff F, Dixon-Woods M, Leviton L, et al. Demystifying theory and its use in improvement. *BMJ Qual Safety*. 2015;24(3):228–238.
2. Lipsey MW. Theory as method: small theories of treatments. *New Dir Program Eval*. 1993;1993(57):5–38.
3. Stephens T, Peden CJ, Pearse R, et al. Improving care at scale: process evaluation of a multi-component quality improvement intervention to reduce mortality after emergency abdominal surgery (EPOCH trial). *Implement Sci*. 2018;13(1):142.
4. Eskes AM, Schreuder AM, Vermeulen H, et al. Developing an evidence-based and theory informed intervention to involve families in patients care after surgery: a quality improvement project. *Int J Nurs Sci*. 2019; 6(4):352 361.
5. Peden CJ. Emergency surgery in the elderly patient: a quality improvement approach. *Anaesthesia*. 2011; 66(6):440–445.
6. Balayah Z, Khadjesari Z, Keohane A, et al. National implementation of a pragmatic quality improvement skills curriculum for urology residents in the UK: application and results of 'theory-of-change' methodology. *Am J Surg*. 2021;221(2):401–409.
7. Dixon-Woods M. The problem of context in quality improvement. The Health Foundation; 2014. https://health.org.uk/sites/default/files/ PerspectivesOnContextDixonWoodsTheProblemOfContextInQualityImprovement.pdf.
8. Bion J, Richardson A, Hibbert P, et al. 'Matching Michigan': a 2-year stepped interventional programme to minimise central venous catheter blood stream infections in intensive care units in England. *BMJ Quality & Safety*. 2013;22(2):110–123.
9. Dixon-Woods M, Leslie M, Tarrant C, et al. Explaining Matching Michigan: an ethnographic study of a patient safety program. *Implement Sci*. 2013;8(1):70
10. Davidoff F, Dixon-Woods M, Leviton L, et al. Demystifying theory and its use in improvement. *BMJ Quality & Safety*. 2015;24(3):228 238.
11. Funnell SC, Rogers PJ. *Purposeful Program Theory: Effective Use of Theories of Change and Logic Models*. John Wiley & Sons; 2011.
12. Weiss CH, Connell JP. Nothing as practical as good theory: exploring theory-based evaluation for comprehensive community initiatives for children and families. In: *New Approaches to Evaluating Community Initiatives: Concepts, Methods, and Contexts*. The Aspen Institute; 1995:65–92.
13. Dixon-Woods M, Bosk CL, Aveling EL, et al. Explaining Michigan: developing an ex post theory of a quality improvement program. *Milbank Q*. 2011;89(2):167–205.
14. Jasper EV, Dhesi JK, Partridge JS, et al. Scaling up perioperative medicine for older people undergoing surgery (POPS) services; use of a logic model approach. *J Clin Med*. 2019;19(6):478–484.
15. Martin G, Ozieranski P, Leslie M, et al. How not to waste a crisis: a qualitative study of problem definition and its consequences in three hospitals. *J Health Serv Res Policy*. 2019;24(3):145–154.

CHAPTER 22

An Overview of Common Improvement Methodologies and Their Background

Caoimhe C. Duffy, MD, MSc, CPPS, FCAI ■ Meghan B. Lane-Fall, MD, MSHP, FCCM

KEY POINTS

- Description of the quality improvement (QI) methodology used is essential to ensuring the process can be replicated.
- The most common QI methodologies are Six Sigma, Lean Thinking, Model for Improvement, Statistical Process Control, and Theory of Constraints.
- It is important to recognize the key features of each QI methodology to differentiate between them.
- There is no superior QI methodology; success is rooted in implementation of the chosen QI method.

Quality improvement (QI) activities are used to support constructive change and are plentiful in the perioperative care space.[1] Nevertheless, inadequate reporting of the precise QI methodologies used impedes accurate replication of effective interventions in practice, increases duplication, and limits opportunities to accrue learning and benefit patients.[2] There is no consensus definition of QI interventions and techniques, and confusion can arise when a myriad of terms that refer to QI methodology, including "approaches," "interventions," or "techniques," are applied interchangeably.[2]

Process-improvement methodologies, such as Total Quality Management, Statistical Process Control, Theory of Constraints, and, more recently, Lean Thinking and Six Sigma, originated in mass manufacturing industries over the last 50 years and have been slowly adopted into healthcare QI.[3] Other chapters in this book will deal with individual methodologies in greater detail, but this chapter provides a summary of key approaches.

Six Sigma and Lean Thinking

Six Sigma (SS) and Lean Thinking are two prominent QI methodologies adapted to several areas of health care since 1998. SS is a process that was developed by the Motorola Corporation in 1986, with the aim of improving quality by identifying and correcting the causes of errors.[4] SS is most notably leveraged in the operating room (OR) to achieve reductions in time, costs, and errors.[5] Lean Thinking evolved from the Toyota Production System in 1990, which uses an ongoing cycle of improvement to focus on mapping out and adapting process pathways to preserve the steps that provide "value" and eliminate waste sources. A synergistic Lean Six Sigma (LSS) approach, using a 5-stage system known as DMAIC (Define, Measure, Analyze, Improve, Control), benefits from the statistical rigor of SS and the cyclical waste-reduction seen in Lean Thinking.[6]

Model for Improvement

The Model for Improvement (MFI), developed by "Associates in Improvement" in 1996 and popularized by the Institute for Healthcare Improvement (IHI), is widely used in health care, particularly as part of a collaborative approach to improving processes and outcomes.[7] MFI combines iterative measurements of small changes into a Plan-Do-Study-Act (PDSA) process, which starts by asking three simple questions: *What are we trying to accomplish? How will we know that a change is an improvement?* and *What changes can we make that will result in an improvement?*[8] After these questions have been addressed, changes can be introduced and tested using the PDSA model (Fig. 22.1).

The impact of MFI appears to depend on the focus of change, the participants and their host organization, and the style and method of implementing the change. PDSA cycles have been studied far more extensively than other approaches, although there is little evidence to suggest that their use is more cost-effective.[9] PDSA cycles may not always be used as intended and strategies for improving their application have been identified.[10,11] Within the perioperative environment, patient flow is imperative to efficiency, patient satisfaction, and quality. PDSA cycles can rapidly allow review of current patient flow, and teams can subsequently institute change and check to improve efficiencies.[12,13]

Statistical Process Control

Statistical Process Control (SPC), developed by Shewhart in the 1920s to improve industrial manufacturing, is used by The Joint Commission to analyze hospital performance metrics.[14] The SPC approach is based on learning through data and on the theory of variation (understanding

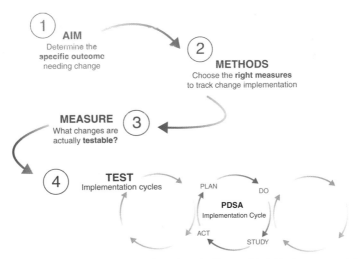

Fig. 22.1 A conceptual approach to using the Associates for Process Model for Improvement, the approach commonly used by the Institute for Health Improvement (IHI).

common and unique causes). The SPC strategy incorporates analytic study, process thinking, prevention, stratification, stability, capability, and prediction. SPC incorporates measurement, data collection methods, and planned experimentation. Graphical methods, such as Shewhart charts (more commonly called "control charts"), run charts, frequency plots, histograms, Pareto analysis, scatter diagrams, and flow diagrams are the primary tools used in SPC (Fig. 22.2).[15]

Clinical indicators can be plotted on a process control chart (e.g., postdural puncture headaches). The control chart can then reflect the number of indicators as a proportion of the variable sample size (e.g., the total number of neuraxial anesthetics performed). Control limits can be established based on the binomial distribution of the data. Data can be monitored for points that fall outside of the control limits or emerging trends. In a system without special causes for variation, a run or trend has approximately the same probability of occurring as a point outside of a control limit. Control charts allow a visual guide to discriminate between changes that yield improvement and those that do not (more details are given in the chapter on SPC).

SPC is a versatile tool that can be applied to perioperative QI.[12] Its application may be limited by having very large or very small data sets and the ability to measure a change in improvement as a proportion of the identified variable.[3]

Theory of Constraints

The Theory of Constraints (TOC) was developed from the Optimized Production Technology (OPT) system.[16] Systems can be held up at bottlenecks (constraints), which can be viewed as opportunities for improvement. TOC outlines a simple, logical approach to these problems. After identifying the constraint, there is a stepwise progression from making improvements, through the use of existing resources, to realigning the overall system to alleviate the constraint to considering entirely new actions that might be necessary to address the constraint. Importantly, the process should be repeatable to avoid inertia, and inherent to TOC methodology is the ability to address constraints as they arise. The complexity of the OR system makes TOC methodology very appealing. As part of Goldratt's theory, there are five focusing steps in the process of ongoing improvement: Identify, Exploit, Subordinate, Elevate, and Reassess (Table 22.1).[17]

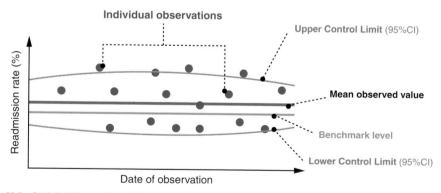

Fig. 22.2 Statistical Process Chart. In this example, readmission rates after surgery for a given time period (y-axis, %) were plotted against time as a run chart. The mean observed value, upper control limits, and lower control limits were highlighted, as was the benchmark performance level.

TABLE 22.1 ■ **Five Steps of Goldratt's Optimized Production Theory**

Step	Description	Clinical Example
Identify the constraint.	This can be a physical or policy constraint.	*Missing patient documentation in the preoperative area causing OR inefficiencies.*
Exploit the constraint.	Achieve the best possible output from the constraint, removing limitations to process flow and reducing nonproductive time.	*Create a checklist of documentation required before arriving in the preoperative area.*
Subordinate other activities to the constraint.	Link other operations to suit the constraint, smooth workflows, and avoid work in process inventory.	*Patients arrive to the preoperative area with all documentation completed.*
Elevate the constraint.	If the system constraint still does not have sufficient output, invest in new equipment or increase staff numbers to improve output.	*Increase the number of preoperative nursing staff reviewing patients.*
Return to Step 1 and reassess.	Assess to see if another operation or policy has become the constraint.	*Availability of surgeons to complete the surgical consent.*

OR, Operating room.

Summary

In general, common improvement methodologies are similar to each other with only subtle differences. It is important to recognize the key features of the main approaches. The differentiating factors between approaches pertain to where the emphasis is placed on the core concept of variation, flow, and user focus. There is no evidence that newer methods are superior to older methods, and the key to each methodology is implementation.

References

1. Jones EL, Dixon-Woods M, Martin GP. Why is reporting quality improvement so hard? A qualitative study in perioperative care. *BMJ Open.* 2019;9(7):e030269.
2. Jones EL, Lees N, Martin G, Dixon-Woods M. How well is quality improvement described in the perioperative care literature? A systematic review. *Jt Comm J Qual Patient Saf.* 2016;42(5):196–206.
3. Boaden R. Quality improvement: theory and practice. *Br J Health Care Manag.* 2009;15(1):12–16.
4. Mason SE, Nicolay CR, Darzi A. The use of Lean and Six Sigma methodologies in surgery: a systematic review. *Surgeon.* 2015;13(2):91–100.
5. Niñerola A, Sánchez-Rebull MV, Hernández-Lara AB. Quality improvement in healthcare: Six Sigma systematic review. *Health Policy.* 2020;124(4):438–445.
6. Schleelein LE, Vincent AM, Jawad AF, et al. Pediatric perioperative adverse events requiring rapid response: a retrospective case-control study. *Paediatr Anaesth.* 2016;26(7):734–741.
7. Agency for Healthcare Research and Quality. Module 4. Approaches to Quality Improvement. https://www.ahrq.gov/ncepcr/tools/pf-handbook/mod4.html.
8. Martin GP, Dixon-Woods M. After Mid Staffordshire: from acknowledgement, through learning, to improvement. *BMJ Qual Saf.* 2014;23(9):706–708.
9. ØVretveit J, Bate P, Cleary P, et al. Quality collaboratives: lessons from research. *Qual Saf Health Care.* 2002;11(4):345–351.

10. Knudsen SV, Laursen HVB, Johnsen SP, Bartels PD, Ehlers LH, Mainz J. Can quality improvement improve the quality of care? A systematic review of reported effects and methodological rigor in Plan-Do-Study-Act projects. *BMC Health Serv Res.* 2019;19(1):683.
11. McNicholas C, Lennox L, Woodcock T, Bell D, Reed JE. Evolving quality improvement support strategies to improve Plan-Do-Study-Act cycle fidelity: a retrospective mixed-methods study. *BMJ Qual Saf.* 2019; 28(5):356–365.
12. Brown B, Khemani E, Lin C, Armstrong K. Improving patient flow in a regional anaesthesia block room. *BMJ Open Quality.* 2019;8:e000346.
13. Valentine EA, Falk SA. Quality improvement in anesthesiology: leveraging data and analytics to optimize outcomes. *Anesthesiol Clin.* 2018;36:31–44.
14. Best M, Neuhauser D. Walter A Shewhart, 1924, and the Hawthorne factory. *Qual Saf Health Care.* 2006;15 (2):142–143.
15. Thor J, Lundberg J, Ask J, et al. Application of statistical process control in healthcare improvement: systematic review. *Qual Saf Health Care.* 2007;16:387–399.
16. Goldratt EM, Cox J. *The Goal: Excellence in Manufacturing.* Great Barrington, MA: North River Press; 1984.
17. Dettmer WH. *Goldratt's Theory of Constraints: A Systems Approach to Continuous Improvement.* ASQ Quality Press; 1997.

CHAPTER 23

The Model for Improvement: A Tool to Drive Perioperative Improvement

Madeleine Roper, MB ChB, FRCA ■ Kevin Rooney, MB ChB, FRCA, FFICM, FRCP Edin

KEY POINTS

- The Model for Improvement provides a template to test, implement and study change.
- To drive improvement, bold, specific, time-bound, aligned, ambitious, and numeric aims must be developed.
- Measurement is central to a team's ability to monitor and improve care.
- Not all changes will result in improvement.
- Diagnose what is wrong with the system that requires improvement and then develop a theory of change.
- Use the Plan Do Study Act (PDSA) cycle to test the theory of change under a variety of different conditions.

Background

Imagine you have just started working in a new department and have been asked to assist the Lead Clinician with a perioperative quality improvement (QI) project. The traditional audit review cycle of performance, followed by efforts to improve, has been completed twice now. It has become obvious that education, awareness, and telling people to do better has not worked. From past experience, you share that although information and training is needed and beneficial, it is not enough on its own to make improvement happen. To achieve meaningful change in a complex healthcare system, formal improvement methodology must be applied using, for example, the Model for Improvement (MFI).

"Every system is perfectly designed to get the results it gets" is a statement that has been widely popularized in the healthcare improvement world, originating from Paul Batalden of the Institute for Healthcare Improvement (IHI).[1] IHI's work also suggests that to achieve meaningful change in a system, the change agent requires "will, ideas, and execution."[1]

- The "will" to make the system better comes from creating emotion by demonstrating poor performance or less than optimal patient outcomes, as identified through patient experience and measurement of clinical outcomes. These findings provide the "*why*" we should do this.
- The change "ideas" come from those with a lived experience of the challenge who want to share their ideas and change things for the better. The ideas provide the "*what*" to do.
- The "execution" involves the skills required to make change happen. It is the "*how*" to do it.

The Model for Improvement: The Theory

The MFI (Fig. 23.1) is a foundational tool used in QI. The MFI was developed by the Associates in Process Improvement[2] and was derived from the work in industry of Walter Shewhart and W. Edwards Deming.[3] The simple Plan-Do-Study-Act (PDSA) cycle uses small, rapid cycle changes designed to test, measure impact, and test again, in a much more agile and proactive manner than a traditional clinical measurement and improvement cycle.[2] Other models of improvement based on Deming and Shewhart's work also use the PDSA cycle, which may also appear as a PDCA cycle (Plan-Do-*Check*-Act; although correctly the PDCA terminology refers to the quality control circle defined by Deming). Perioperative physicians who have participated in programs such as the UK-based Scottish Patient Safety Programme[4] or the IHI 5 Million Lives Campaign[5] will be well versed with the MFI and the PDSA tool.

There are three questions central to the application of the MFI[2]:
1. What are we trying to accomplish?
2. How will we know that a change is an improvement?
3. What change can we make that will result in an improvement?

The Model for Improvement: The Practice

WHAT ARE WE TRYING TO ACCOMPLISH?

The first question states our aim (e.g., we wish to improve outcomes for patients admitted with a fractured neck of femur). Our aim statement should be not only ambitious but also achievable. It is important that we consider and carefully define what we wish to measure and at what time point (see Chapter 26 on Measures). Do we wish to improve operative or nonoperative outcomes? Let's look at a different statement, such as: "Improve the percentage of patients discharged directly to home after operative fixation of a fractured neck of femur." This is better but still a little vague. By how much do we wish to improve discharge to home? Over what time frame do we wish to see this improvement

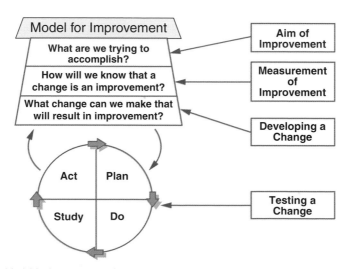

Fig. 23.1   The Model for Improvement. (Adapted from Langley GJ, Moen RD, Nolan KM, Nolan TW, Norman CL, Provost LP. *The Improvement Guide: A Practical Approach to Enhancing Organizational Performance.* San Francisco: Jossey-Bass, 2009.)

achieved? A clear aim statement should be specific, timebound, aligned with organizational goals, and numeric. As such, a good aim statement for this project would be:

"We aim to improve the number of patients who have undergone operative fixation of fractured neck of femur who are discharged directly to home by 10% by December 2022."

HOW WILL WE KNOW THAT A CHANGE IS AN IMPROVEMENT?

To answer the second question in the MFI, we will need to have measures. Measurement is central to a team's ability to monitor and improve care. It is an integral part of both clinical audit and QI. In our example, we have generated a clear outcome measure based on our theory of change (i.e., that if we better identify high-risk patients early, we can manage their care more proactively and improve outcomes). The measure we define is discharge to home of patients who have undergone operative fixation of fractured neck of femur. This lets us know how our system is performing and could be described as the voice of the patient.

To achieve our outcome we need process measures. In other words, are the steps in the system performing as planned? This could be described as the voice of the workings of the system and can be described as what we believe we can do that will improve the outcome, such as reduce the time from admission to theatre/operating room (OR) (process measure: time from admission to theatre) or reduce the time to first patient assessment by a geriatrician.

Finally, we need balancing measures. These are necessary to capture the unanticipated consequences of our actions. When we change a system, we must also consider how our changes affect other parts of the system. For example, if we prioritize time to the OR for fractured neck of femur patients, does this negatively impact waiting times for other urgent cases?

Now that we have our measures identified, we can develop our change ideas.[6] You will already have worked on developing the "will" for change by highlighting less than optimal management or poor outcomes for this group of patients, but how do you generate ideas for change, and where will you be able to make improvements? Much as we diagnose our patients, it is important that we diagnose our system and develop a theory for change. You could generate a process map of the patient journey (see Chapter 29 on Process Mapping) and then consider where you as a perioperative physician could make change happen. Are there other centers which have better outcomes for this group of patients—why is that and what do they do differently? Does your unit follow best practice? Have you asked the patients what could make their experience better? By generating ideas in this fashion, you can develop change concepts and a driver diagram (see Chapter 30 on Driver Diagrams). For example, if the audit showed that only 30% of patients had a nerve block and this appeared to be user-dependent, you could develop a change concept aimed at reducing variation in anesthesia and pain management for patients undergoing hip fixation. Reduction in unnecessary variation of care is a key factor in any successful QI initiative.

DEVELOPING AND TESTING A CHANGE

The third question in the MFI is: "What change can we make that will result in an improvement?" Our diagnosis of our system, namely the fractured neck of femur pathway, will have provided us with a theory of change to test. Although "all improvements require change, not all change will result in an improvement"[2]; as such, it is very important that measurement is a key part of the PDSA cycle (Fig. 23.2).[2]

In our example of the fractured neck of femur pathway, let us say that part of your theory of change is that you want every patient to have a Nottingham Hip Fracture Score calculated and documented preoperatively.[7] You believe that this will help you predict risk in terms of surgical morbidity and mortality and determine what level of care the patient will require postoperatively. To achieve this, you plan to inform the anesthesia team by email and place posters in key OR locations. You complete a PDSA cycle by doing the following:

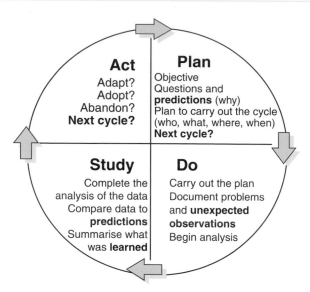

Fig. 23.2   The Plan-Do-Study-Act Cycle.

Plan to put a poster with a QR code for the risk calculator in the OR coffee rooms and inform the anesthesia and orthopedic teams through email. Do this and study what happens. Start to test on a small scale (e.g., with one team in one trauma OR on one day). Start with a team that is enthusiastic about the idea. If all the patients get a Nottingham Hip Fracture Score calculated and documented, start testing on different days. You may then find that the process becomes less reliable, so then you must study why it has become unreliable. The score may have been done but not documented and as a result it was not used to inform the postanesthetic care for the patient. Study: How do you get round that? What have you learned about your change idea? Act: Develop a new idea to deal with this challenge (e.g., use of a Nottingham Hip Fracture Score sticker) and test again. The cycle goes on, testing theories about what will work and learning from what does not work (see Fig. 23.2). If it works during a weekday night, does it work on a weekend night? Do not assume your process is reliable until you know it works with different teams and at different times of the day and night. It must work even if you are not there and cannot be seen as a person-dependent process.

Brown et al. demonstrated the effective use of the PDSA cycle in improving patient flow through the regional anesthesia block room in University Hospital in Ontario, Canada.[8] They set out clear aims: (1) Have 90% of patients arrive in the surgical preparation unit 60 minutes before scheduled surgery; (2) have 90% of patients arrive in the block room within 15 minutes of calling the surgical preparation unit; and (3) have 90% of patients arrive in the OR within 10 minutes of their scheduled start time. They ran three simultaneous PDSA cycles over a 6-month period. The first was focused around an audit and feedback loop of patient transit times, the second around patient movements through the surgical unit preoperatively, and the third around communication between the perioperative teams. Through frequent review of their data (i.e., the "study" component of the cycle), they were able to recognize the limitations of their aims and make changes throughout the process (e.g., by anticipating the days of the week with higher throughput and requesting support from other anesthetists). They were also able to use their data to demonstrate improvements in patient flow to advocate for improved information technology (IT) systems, allowing staff to enter and view patient data electronically during the patient's perioperative journey, which, in turn, enhanced communication between the teams involved. This ultimately resulted in statistically significant improvements in all areas set out in their initial aims. Remeasuring baseline data at 10 months also suggested that their improvements could be sustained in the long term.

Davies et al. also demonstrated effective use of the PDSA cycle in improving preoperative fasting times in their high throughput plastic surgery department.[9] They recognized an issue with prolonged preoperative fasting times and set an aim to reduce fasting time by 50% over 12 months. Collection of data through patient questionnaires and review of case notes allowed them to quantify the baseline average fasting times for both food and clear fluids. They then used two separate PDSA cycles. The first focused on communication and education of both staff and patients, with updated guidelines made available to staff and written information made available to inpatients. The second PDSA cycle was implemented after review of the first data set, which recognized a limitation in improvement because of availability of snacks and drinks outside normal catering times. Introduction of postoperative snacks and prescription of carbohydrate drinks for 6:00 AM on the morning of surgery allowed for a further improvement in fasting times, with a prediction of sustained improvement at the time of publication.

Although the PDSA cycle may initially appear unfamiliar to perioperative physicians, it is essentially similar to making a differential diagnosis and subsequent management plan, familiar in clinical practice. The "Plan" is the differential diagnosis and theory about what is wrong. The "Do" or "Doing" is the treatment plan or solution to be tested. The "Study" is to determine and observe whether the treatment plan or solution/test actually worked. The "Act" is to determine whether to continue with the treatment plan and solution, alter it slightly, or try something completely new. To try a new theory or solution, we start a new PDSA cycle.

Summary

In conclusion, the MFI consists of three questions and the PDSA cycle. The purpose of the PDSA cycle is to:

- Learn how to adapt a change to the unique conditions within a defined setting.
- Increase the belief, through testing, that the change will result in an improvement in the test area.
- Minimize resistance when spreading the change by demonstrating results.
- Evaluate the resources needed, and unanticipated side effects of the changes made.

Correctly used, the MFI and the PDSA cycle are valuable tools for perioperative improvement. To apply the MFI and PDSA cycles appropriately, clinicians should ensure that the small tests of change and the results are documented, and measurements of the impact of the iterative changes are made regularly.[10]

References

1. Institute for Healthcare Improvement. Science of improvement: how to improve. http://www.ihi.org/resources/Pages/HowtoImprove/ScienceofImprovementHowtoImprove.aspx. Accessed May 19, 2021.
2. Langley GJ, et al. *The Improvement Guide: A Practical Approach to Enhancing Organizational Performance.* San Francisco: Jossey-Bass; 2009.
3. Peden CJ, Rooney KD. The Science of Improvement as it relates to quality and safety in the ICU. *J Intens Care Soc.* 2009;10(4):260–265.
4. Scottish Patient Safety Programme. https://ihub.scot/improvement-programmes/scottish-patient-safety-programme-spsp/. Accessed March 25, 2022.
5. Institute of Healthcare Improvement. 5 Million Lives Campaign. http://www.ihi.org/Engage/Initiatives/Completed/5MillionLivesCampaign/Pages/default.aspx. Accessed March 25, 2022.
6. Lloyd RC. *Quality Health Care: A Guide to Developing and Using Indicators.* Sudbury, MA: Jones and Bartlett; 2004.

7. Moppett IK, Parker M, Griffiths R, Bowers T, White SM, Moran CG. Nottingham Hip Fracture Score: longitudinal and multi-assessment. *Br J Anaesth.* 2012;109(4):546–550.

8. Brown B, Khemani E, Lin C, et al. Improving patient flow in a regional anaesthesia block room. *BMJ Open Qual.* 2019;8, e000346.

9. Davies A, Pang WS, Fowler T, et al. Preoperative fasting in the department of plastic surgery. *BMJ Open Qual.* 2018;7, e000161.

10. Taylor MJ, McNicholas C, Nicolay C, Darzi A, Bell D, Reed JE. Systematic review of the application of the plan-do-study-act method to improve quality in healthcare. *BMJ Qual Saf.* 2014;23(4):290–298.

CHAPTER 24

Lean in Health Care

Scott Falk, MD

KEY POINTS

- Lean is a process improvement methodology developed by Toyota in 1930s Japan.
- In Lean, frontline workers such as nurses and physicians lead the improvement work.
- Lean application in health care begins by exploring the "voice of the customer," which has evolved to encompass patient-centered care models.
- The classic Lean technique to gain an in-depth understanding of the problem is to "walk the Gemba," or go out and actually see the problem.
- Lean work focuses on steps that add value to the patient and on the removal of wasted steps and processes, such as waiting or duplication.
- Techniques, such as development of a project charter, process mapping, and identification of value-added steps and waste, are commonly used.

Lean is a process improvement methodology that seeks to optimize the relationship between customer needs and a product.[1] The methodology focuses on a deep understanding of customer needs along with elimination of waste in the manufacturing process. For our purposes in this chapter, our customer is the patient and the manufacturing process is the provision of appropriate care to that patient. Ultimately our goal is to understand what our patients value and provide that to the patient in the most efficient way. One pitfall that occurs early in Lean journeys is that the expert group expresses that they know what the customer needs and wants more than the customer and that customers are too simplistic to know what they actually want or need. This inevitably leads to a mismatch, typically with an overproduced product that customers may not want to pay for. In auto manufacturing, this may lead to cars with unused features; in health care, patients may be subjected to tests or procedures with little intrinsic value to the goals important to them.

To really understand Lean, it is important to dissect the history of this methodology, which has its origins in 1930s Japan. Toyota was originally a textile company that evolved into auto and truck manufacturing in the 1930s. As they scaled up manufacturing, it became evident that there were many defects in the engine blocks being produced. To address this problem, "Kaizen" improvement teams were started.[2] These teams consisted of the personnel actually doing the manufacturing work. Involving those who are "doing" the work instead of those who are "supervising" the work is a key principle to successful improvements. Kaizen events continue today within Lean organizations, with the workers leading the improvement efforts rather than being instructed on how to improve. In health care, this translates into the frontline medical workers such as nurses, physicians, and providers driving improvement efforts. In the 1950s, there was a paucity of manufacturing resources in Japan. These limitations led to changes in production with "pull" systems and "just in time" production. These systems matched production to actual sales rather than market projections. By streamlining the delivery of not only the end product but also the supplies necessary to manufacture automobiles, economic efficiency was achieved while matching product specifically to customer demands. In essence, a car was manufactured to customer specifications quickly and efficiently after a sale.[3] Using "just in time" techniques for healthcare supplies and delivery of care has been an approach used to yield economic benefits with better matching of care and products to patients,[4] although some of the disadvantages of this approach surfaced during the COVID-19 epidemic, with, for example, inadequate personal protective equipment (PPE) being immediately available. The principles of Lean manufacturing were first adopted into health care in the early 2000s.[5] Since that time, the healthcare industry has embraced Lean techniques to deliver more efficient, higher value care.

The application of Lean into health care begins by exploring the "voice of the customer." The simplest way to do this for any aspect of care is to ask patients a series of three questions[6]:

1. What works well in the current process?

2. What does not work for you in the current process?

3. If you could change one thing to make this better, what would it be?

"Voice of the customer" has evolved to encompass patient-centered care models in which communication and care are tailored to patient and group needs.[7]

After conducting the first step of analysis to determine patient needs, an improvement group focuses on defining the opportunity. Formal definition should always occur because this will help the project group gain clarity and stay within the bounds of the project. Process Improvement methodology describes using a "charter" document to refine the exact work that will occur. A charter should include an opportunity statement, the scope of the project (both from a process step perspective and location perspective), goals and metrics for successful conclusion, and team members (Fig. 24.1). Goals for Lean improvements should always be SMART—**S**pecific, **M**easurable, **A**chievable, **R**elevant, and **T**ime-Bound (Fig. 24.2).

After defining the opportunity for improvement and goals, the team must then gain an in-depth understanding of the problem. The classic Lean technique used to do this is to "walk the Gemba," or go out and see. It is derived from the Japanese term *genba* (although the correct spelling is with an N, Gemba is an American adaption derived from the pronunciation), which means "the actual place."[8] The improvement team should use this time to develop a process map, which is a visualization of the work that is occurring. There are many different types of process maps that can be applied. It is

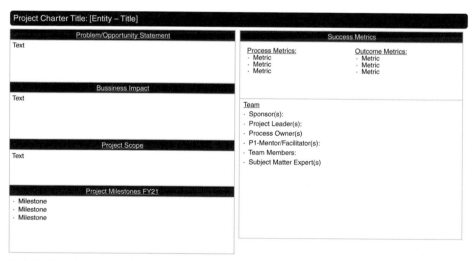

Fig. 24.1 "Charter" document used in process improvement to refine the exact work that will occur. A charter should include an opportunity statement, the scope of the project (both from a process step perspective and a location perspective), goals and metrics for successful conclusion, and team members.

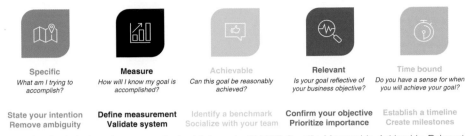

Specific	Measure	Achievable	Relevant	Time bound
What am I trying to accomplish?	How will I know my goal is accomplished?	Can this goal be reasonably achieved?	Is your goal reflective of your business objective?	Do you have a sense for when you will achieve your goal?
State your intention Remove ambiguity	Define measurement Validate system	Identify a benchmark Socialize with your team	Confirm your objective Prioritize importance	Establish a timeline Create milestones

Fig. 24.2 Goals for Lean improvements should always be SMART: Specific, Measurable, Achievable, Relevant, and Time-Bound.

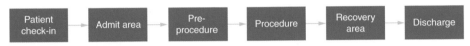

Fig. 24.3 A high-level process map. This process map is a six- to eight-step visualization of a process that provides an overview from which to work.

important to build the process map that will best allow teams to visualize the work and identify steps that may be considered wasteful. A common recommendation is to create a high-level process map as a first step. This process map is a six- to eight-step visualization of a process that provides an overview from which to work (Fig. 24.3). From this other process, maps can be built to suit project needs (Table 24.1) (see also Chapter 29 on Process Mapping). As process maps are created, the improvement team should be actively looking at which process steps and decisions add value and which are waste because waste elimination will be where improvements are focused.

For a process step or part of a product considered to be value added, it must meet one of the following criteria:

1. The customer/patient recognizes the value.
2. It changes the form, fit, or function of work toward something the customer/patient expects.
3. It is done right the first time.
4. The customer/patient would pay for it—more of it is better.

If a process step or part of a product does not meet any of those criteria, it would be considered nonvalue added. Nonvalue-added work can be broken up into **essential work** (necessary in the process because of regulatory or supporting value) and **waste** (defined as activity that is not value or enabling and should be completely eliminated).

In health care, process improvement elimination of the eight following wastes (Box 24.1)[6] is essential:

- defects
- overproduction
- waiting
- knowledge wasted/confusion
- transportation
- inventory
- motion and excess processing

Once the waste has been identified as a root cause of the defined problem, the improvement team can begin work to optimize the process for improved value to the patient. There are many classic Lean interventions that are popular in health care, including standard work (checklists), fail-safe inclusion, workspace optimization (5S: **S**ort, **S**et in order, **S**hine, **S**tandardize, **S**ustain), Kanban, Poka-Yoke (error proofing), and visual controls (Figs. 24.4 and 24.5 and Box 24.2).

TABLE 24.1 ■ Process Maps and Their Uses

Process Map	Description	When to Use
High-level process map	• View from 30,000 feet • Depicts major elements and their interactions • 5–8 steps total	Early in the project to identify boundaries and scope
Detailed process map	• A detailed version of the high-level process map • Fills in all of the steps within the high-level steps	• To see a detailed process in a simple view • Helps to identify and follow decision points
Supplier, input, process, output, customer (SIPOC)	Process snapshot that captures information that is critical to a project	• To come to an agreement on project boundaries and scope • To verify that process inputs match the outputs of the process • Quality issue
Visual stream map (VSM)	• Captures all key flows (of work, information, materials) in a process and important process metrics • Requires a current and future state to be done	• To identify and quantify waste • Helps visualize the improvement opportunities • Flow or time issue
Swim lane flowchart	Emphasizes the "who" in "who does what"	• To study handoffs between people and/or work groups in a process • Especially useful with administrative (service) processes
Spaghetti map	Depicts the physical flow of work or material in a process	To improve the physical layout of a workspace (unit, office, floor)

BOX 24.1 ■ The Eight Wastes Essential to Eliminate in Healthcare Process Improvement

Defects	Errors, duplicate work, checking, inspection, incomplete/incorrect information ■ Lab tests are performed twice because of errors.
Overproduction	Preparing more than necessary or preparing too much, large deliveries, more information than can be processed ■ There are too many unnecessary paper reports.
Waiting	People (patients or workers) waiting, waiting for something to arrive ■ Operating room (OR) tech waits "N" minutes to begin and is not free to do other tasks.
N (k) knowledge underutilization	Not using staff efficiently ■ Numerous ideas are "lost" only to be rediscovered later.
Transportation	Moving materials and/or moving people ■ Patient gets wheeled back and forth between the floor and radiology because of a scheduling mix-up.

BOX 24.1 ■ The Eight Wastes Essential to Eliminate in Healthcare Process Improvement (continued)	
Inventory	Work waiting, patients waiting, batching (waiting to be worked)
	■ Medicines held over the shelf-life because of excess ordering
Motion	Unnecessary human movement
	■ Pharmacy tech spends X minutes looking in multiple places for a particular medicine.
Excessive processing	Things we are doing that do not add value to the process; unnecessary information
	■ Nurse records respiratory rate on X different forms in the chart.

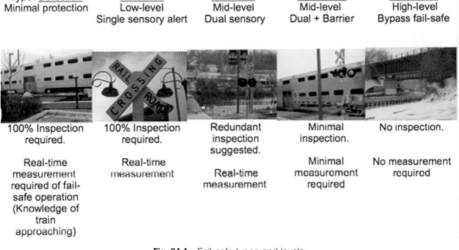

Level 1	Level 2	Level 3	Level 4	Level 5
Type: Detection	Detection	Detection	Prevention	Prevention
Minimal protection	Low-level	Mid-level	Mid-level	High-level
	Single sensory alert	Dual sensory	Dual + Barrier	Bypass fail-safe
100% Inspection required.	100% Inspection required.	Redundant inspection suggested.	Minimal inspection.	No inspection.
Real-time measurement required of fail-safe operation (Knowledge of train approaching)	Real-time measurement	Real-time measurement	Minimal measurement required	No measurement required

Fig. 24.4   Fail-safe types and levels.

As always, it is important to keep in mind that no matter what we are changing, we must be able to measure relevant metrics from before and after the intervention.

Lean methodology has been successfully applied to improve operating room (OR) efficiency and quality. In a 2019 study, Lean methodology was used to reduce OR turnover times from a mean of 37 minutes to a mean of 14 minutes; 10% of process steps were deemed nonvalue added and eliminated, and an additional 25% of steps were changed from sequential to synchronous.[9] Another published improvement project using Lean methodology to improve inventory and function in a neurosurgical OR suite demonstrated a reduction in surgical site infections and a reduction in supply costs.1 Another study used Lean methodology to improve first case starts. By eliminating nonvalue steps in the admission and preoperative process, first case on time starts went from 23.5% to 73%.[11]

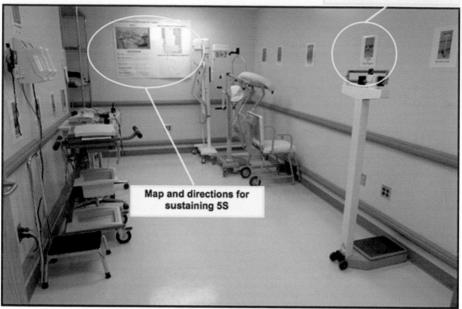

Fig. 24.5 5S with visual controls.

BOX 24.2 ■ Poka-Yoke: Real-World Examples

- Overflow drains on a sink (the holes high up on the side) prevent making a mess when filling the basin up with water.
- Most computer manufacturers poka-yoke their cables so their plugs only fit in one way. This prevents damage to the system.
- Printers stop printing when the paper runs out. This keeps them from spreading ink all over the internal mechanisms of the machine.
- A sensor in a gas nozzle knows when your tank is full. This is a poka-yoke that prevents dangerous messes by shutting off the pump.
- The ice maker in your freezer shuts off when the bucket is full.
- Your washing machine ends the spin cycle when it is out of balance.

Sustaining positive change is another key to success for Lean improvement projects. The most common tools to achieve this are run charts and control charts (see also Chapter 27 on run charts and Chapter 28 on control/SPC charts). Run charts look at your metric over time (Fig. 24.6), and control charts do the same and use statistical bounds to ensure a process remains in control, accounting for normal variation and special cause variation (Fig. 24.7).[6] If sustainment tools are in use, it will be readily noticed when the improvement change reverts to baseline. Further, these tools can be

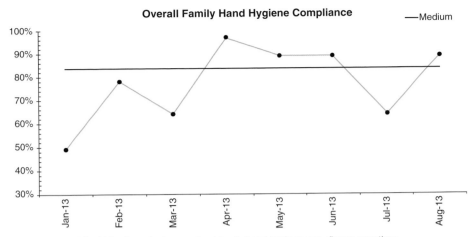

Fig. 24.6 Run chart example of family hand hygiene compliance over time.

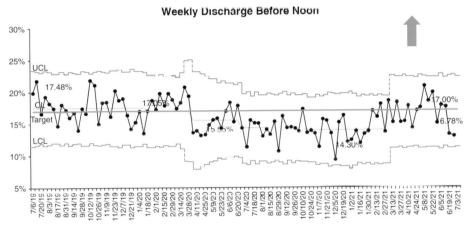

Fig. 24.7 Control chart of weekly discharge before noon with a median and upper control limit (*UCL*) and lower control limit (*LCL*) .

used as baseline metrics for continued improvements; after all, Lean improvement is a journey, not a destination.

References

1. Womack JP, Jones DT. *Lean Thinking: Banish Waste and Create Wealth in Your Corporation.* Simon and Schuster; 2003:10.
2. Sugimori Y, Kusunoki K, Cho F, Uchikawa S. Toyota production system and Kanban system: materialization of just-in-time and respect-for-human system. *Int J Prod Res.* 1977;15(6):553–564.
3. Goddard Walter E. *Just-in-Time: Surviving by Breaking Tradition.* Essex Junction, VT: Oliver Wight Ltd; 1986.
4. Jarrett PG. An analysis of international health care logistics: the benefits and implications of implementing just-in-time systems in the health care industry. *Int J Health Care Qual Assur Inc Leadersh Health Serv.* 2006;19(1):i–x.

5. Young T, Brailsford S, Connell C, Davies R, Harper P, Klein JH. Using industrial processes to improve patient care. *BMJ.* 2004;328(7432):162–164.

6. Falk, SA, n.d. Penn Medicine Academy—Performance Improvement in Action Course.

7. Newell S, Jordan Z. The patient experience of patient-centered communication with nurses in the hospital setting: a qualitative systematic review protocol. *JBI Database System Rev Implement Rep.* 2015;13(1):76–87.

8. Womack J. *Gemba Walks.* Lean Enterprise Institute, Inc.; 2011:348.

9. Cerfolio RJ, Ferrari-Light D, et al. Improving operating room turnover time in a New York City Academic Hospital via Lean. *Ann Thorac Surg.* 2019;107(4):1011–1016.

10. Leming-Lee T', Polancich S, Pilon B. T, Polancich S, Pilon B. The application of the Toyota production system LEAN 5S methodology in the operating room setting. *Nurs Clin North Am.* 2019;54(1):53–79.

11. Coffey C Jr, Cho ES, Wei E, et al. Lean methods to improve operating room elective first case on-time starts in a large, urban, safety net medical center. *Am J Surg.* 2018;216(2):194–201.

Other Reading

Smith I, Hicks C, McGovern T. Adapting Lean methods to facilitate stakeholder engagement and co-design in healthcare. *BMJ.* 2020;368:m35.

Scoville R, Little K. *Comparing Lean and Quality Improvement.* IHI White Paper, Cambridge, MA: Institute for Healthcare Improvement; 2014. ihi.org.

CHAPTER 25

Other Performance Improvement Tools: From Compliance to Excellence

Kaveh Houshmand Azad, MSc

KEY POINTS

- Improving healthcare processes and outcomes and maintaining these achievements within the healthcare system is a multifaceted journey.
- Different services, systems, and processes each present their own unique set of "Opportunities for Improvement" (OFI).
- Depending on the complexity of the OFI—and, equally important, the level of organizational maturity—the approach used is different.

Improving healthcare processes and outcomes and maintaining these achievements within the healthcare system is a multifaceted journey. The continuum in Fig. 25.1 depicts a model of different improvement methodologies and approaches to address a wide range of organizational needs. Although this model does not claim to include all existing improvement methodologies, it represents a spectrum of the most common approaches used by healthcare institutions in the United States (US) and across the globe.

In general, we can group these methods into three main *zones*, based on their primary focus and application:

1. **Compliance Zone**: Methodologies in this zone primarily focus on organizational processes and compliance with regulatory, healthcare, or internally defined requirements. Compliance with ISO 9001 requirements[1] (e.g., policies, procedures, records) and with The Joint Commission requirements[2] are two common examples of this category. Later in this chapter, we will review ISO 9001 in more detail.

2. **Improvement Zone:** Although not entirely separate from the concept of compliance, the methodologies in this zone assume that the basic compliance measures are already in place and direct their attention to continuous improvement. These methodologies are best known for their "project" approach. Lean and Six Sigma are two of the best-known models in this zone that are often used by healthcare institutions. An earlier chapter (see Chapter 24) deals with Lean and we will discuss Six Sigma in more detail in this chapter.

3. **Performance Excellence Zone**: Performance excellence frameworks provide a model to integrate the culture, vision, tools, and measurements for improvement across different functions and areas of the organization. These models are the embodiment of Dr. Deming's "Total Quality Management,"[3] often structured around specific criteria element. The High Reliability Organization Maturity Model,[4] Baldrige Criteria for Performance Excellence,[5] and European Foundation for Quality Management (EFQM)[6] model are some examples for these frameworks, and we will review the Baldrige model in more detail later in this chapter.

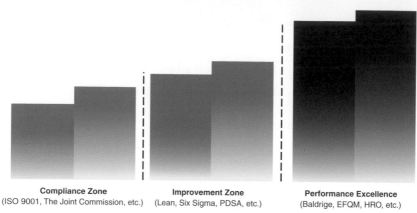

Compliance Zone	Improvement Zone	Performance Excellence
(ISO 9001, The Joint Commission, etc.)	(Lean, Six Sigma, PDSA, etc.)	(Baldrige, EFQM, HRO, etc.)

Fig. 25.1   Different zones and methodologies of healthcare performance improvement. A wide range of performance improvement methods can support healthcare organizations in their journey to excellence.

ISO 9001 Quality Management System

ISO 9001[1] refers to a family of quality management system standards that allow the organization to define, document, implement, measure, and improve its performance through cycles of continuous improvement. Rooted in established national standards for quality management (such as UK standard BS 5750 and US Defense Standards), the first edition of ISO 9001 standard was introduced in 1987 by the International Organization for Standardization (ISO). Although the early adoption was mainly embraced by engineering and manufacturing companies, by year 2000 more than 3700 healthcare organizations had pursued the standard. This number has significantly grown since, and health care is among the leading industries to apply ISO 9001 principles to their systems and processes.

The most recent version of ISO 9001 standards (BS EN ISO 9001:2015) requires organizations to "…to establish, implement, maintain and continually improve a quality management system, including the processes needed and their interactions, in accordance with the requirements of this International Standard" and is built based on the following overall framework (Fig. 25.2):

- Leadership: Securing leadership commitment (administrative and physicians), establishing clear policies and quality and performance objectives, and communicating these policies across different levels and areas of the organization
- Planning: Assessment, identification, and action planning for risks; quality objectives and planning to achieve them; and change management
- Provision of support: Resources, such as people, infrastructure, environment for the operations of processes, education, and training.
- Monitoring and measuring resources: Organizational knowledge, competencies, communication, and awareness.
- Documentation of information: A reliable documentation structure, which involves its creation, updates, and revision control
- Operational (and clinical) planning and control: Core and supporting processes
- Customer (and patient) communications
- Determining the requirements for products and services: Care delivery and its outcomes and ongoing review and updates as needed
- Controlling externally provided processes, products, and services
- Performance evaluation: Monitoring, measuring, analyzing, and evaluating systems

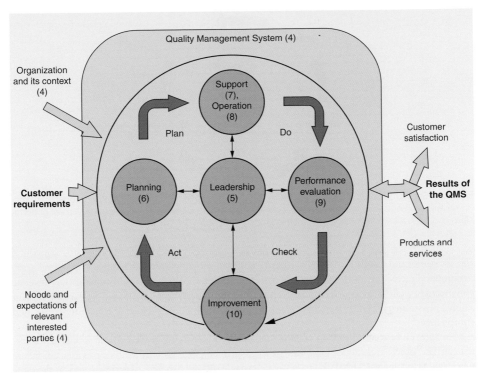

Fig. 25.2   The ISO 9001 process approach requires the organization to identify, plan for, and improve its processes and their interrelations using PDCA/PDSA cycles. (From ISO 9001:2015. Quality management systems—requirements. British Standards Institution. https://www.iso.org/standard/62085.html. Accessed December 1, 2021.)

- Review and improvement of customer (patient) satisfaction
- Leadership/management review: Ensure that organizational goals and strategies are achieved
One of the most important aspects of ISO 9001 Standards is a platform for accreditation and recognition. Although most healthcare organizations (hospitals and outpatient clinics alike) make a strategic decision to implement ISO 9001 on a voluntarily basis, in recent years ISO-based approaches have allowed hospitals to demonstrate necessary compliance with the Centers for Medicare and Medicaid Services (CMS) Conditions of Participation through means other than The Joint Commission Standards and Survey. This approach provides the opportunity to apply quality management principles, using a Plan-Do-Check/Study-Act (PDC/SA) approach.

Six Sigma

Six Sigma is both a methodology and a management philosophy and emphasizes continuous identification and elimination of defects (process and outcomes) by combining quality and project management tools. Although several versions of the methodology have been used since its inception in 1978, the Define, Measure, Analyze, Improvement, and Control (DMAIC) method has been universally adopted by many industries, including health care (Fig. 25.3).

The concept of Six Sigma in health care was first implemented by the Commonwealth Health Corporation (CHC) in partnership with General Electric (GE), resulting in an improved radiology throughout by 33% and decreased cost per radiology procedure by 21.5%.[7] Since then, numerous

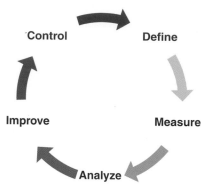

Fig. 25.3   Six Sigma DMAIC (Define, Measure, Analyze, Improve, and Control) methodology. This data-driven approach is used to identify, quantify, optimize, and sustain system and process improvement opportunities and plays a key role in Six Sigma methodology.

success stories and research articles have been published showing a favorable impact on several organizational dimensions, most importantly patient satisfaction, financial improvement (i.e., revenue enhancement, cost saving), operational excellence (i.e., speed and timeliness of services, patient safety, physician efficiency, resource planning, defect reduction such as medication error), and compliance.[8]

Six Sigma is beyond a problem-solving toolbox. This methodology uses several sophisticated statistical (and other) techniques (e.g., design to experiment, regressions, analysis of variance, failure mode and effect analysis [FMEA]) to better investigate different sources of variation and, at the same time, places equal emphasis on change management and empowering project stakeholders to customize the project for their environment. This is especially important in health care, considering the importance of adoption of developed solutions among different clinicians and patient populations.

The Joint Commission has also included Six Sigma as one of its key components for the High Reliability Organization Model.[9] Table 25.1 presents a summary of Six Sigma phases and the aspects of each phase.

Baldrige Criteria for Performance Excellence

As a public-private partnership, the Malcolm Baldrige National Performance Excellence Award (and criteria)[5] was introduced in 1987 to recognize organizations who have exemplified system-based, outstanding and sustained results across different industries and organization sizes and models. Award winners are required to share information on their successful performance strategies with other US organizations (excluding proprietary information).

The Baldrige framework (Fig. 25.4) takes a holistic approach to organizational outcomes by defining the key outcomes in five key categories:

1. Healthcare and Process Outcomes: Being the most important type of outcome, these refer to results that are related to key patient (and other stakeholder) requirements, such as quality, safety, and efficacy of care (e.g., clinical outcomes, harm indices), as well as effectiveness and efficiency of care delivery processes (e.g., turnaround time, patient/procedure wait time)

2. Customer-Focused Outcomes: These are results related to the satisfaction and dissatisfaction of different customer groups (most importantly, patients and their families), as directly collected by the organization (e.g., rounding, real-time surveys) or by external organizations, such as the Hospital Consumer Assessment of Healthcare Providers and Systems (HCAHPS) or Clinician and Group Consumer Assessment of Healthcare Providers and Systems (CGCAHPS)

TABLE 25.1 ■ **Six Sigma Phases and the Aspects of Each Phase**

Six Sigma Phase	Objective	Key Common Tools and Techniques Used
Define	Identification and documentation of the project scope, and its stakeholders	• Voice of customer • SIPOC (supplier, input, process, output, customer) • Project charter
Measure	Establishment of a reliable measurable system and quantification of gaps in the process and its outcomes	• Initial process capability • Operational definition of key metrics • Validation of measurement system
Analyze	Identification (and quantification) of the factors contributing to the process	• Value stream mapping • Root cause analysis • Failure mode and effect analysis (FMEA) • Analysis of variance (ANOVA) • Design of experiment (DoE)
Improve	Implication of developed solution and deployment of the appropriate change management approach to ensure optimal results	• Implementation plan (action items, ownership, and timeline) • Optimization of solution and adjustments
Control	The ensuring of the sustainability of solutions in the long term	• Control plan • Process ownership transition plan

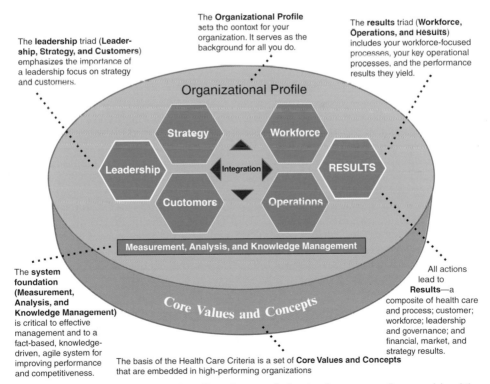

The **Organizational Profile** sets the context for your organization. It serves as the background for all you do.

The **leadership** triad (**Leadership, Strategy, and Customers**) emphasizes the importance of a leadership focus on strategy and customers.

The **results** triad (**Workforce, Operations, and Results**) includes your workforce-focused processes, your key operational processes, and the performance results they yield.

The **system foundation** (**Measurement, Analysis, and Knowledge Management**) is critical to effective management and to a fact-based, knowledge-driven, agile system for improving performance and competitiveness.

All actions lead to **Results**—a composite of health care and process; customer; workforce; leadership and governance; and financial, market, and strategy results.

The basis of the Health Care Criteria is a set of **Core Values and Concepts** that are embedded in high-performing organizations

Fig. 25.4 This framework depicts the key pillars of an organizational performance excellence model and the interconnectivity between different elements of the system. (From Baldrige Healthcare Excellence Framework 2021–2022, National Institute of Standard and Technology. https://www.nist.gov/baldrige/publications/baldrige-excellence-framework/health-care. Accessed December 1, 2021.)

3. Workforce-Focused Outcomes: These are results related to the environment for the key workforce segments (physicians, executive level, staff, and volunteers), on parameters such as capability and capacity, diversity, overall work climate (safety, security, benefits), and development opportunities

4. Leadership and Governance Outcomes: This summarizes the key senior leadership and governance, including those in charge of fiscal responsibility, legal compliance, ethical behaviors, and societal responsibility

5. Financial and Market Outcomes: This summarizes the financial measures of the organization, including financial return, viability, growth rate, and new markets

Using the data provided by the organization, each of these categories are independently reviewed and scored. The maturity of organizational data is assessed and based not only on the performance measures but also on historical trends and comparison with other performance metrics demonstrated by other healthcare organizations. The assessment also takes into the account the accuracy, integrity, reliability, timeliness, and security of the data.

It is important to note that the Baldrige model is not a methodology but rather a comprehensive set of key questions for organizational consideration and a road map for the organization's continuous improvement journey.

In general, both the Baldrige criteria and the assessment process encourage a more proactive, innovative, and integrated approach toward organizational opportunities, with common goals and collaboration, to share organizational knowledge across different organizational units.

There have been several studies done comparing other organizational excellence frameworks, such as The Joint Commission Standards[2] and the American Nurses Credentialing Center's Magnet Recognition Program Model,[10] with the Baldrige Framework.[5] Although there are several parallels within these models, the Baldrige framework provides the most comprehensive approach for different organizational processes and measures.

In addition to its comprehensive approach to performance excellence, the Baldrige program is also known for its annual recognition of the best performing organizations. Established in 1987, the Baldrige award is the most prestigious quality award in the nation, and it recognizes the best performing organizations based on their "Approach," "Deployment," "Learning," and "Integration" (ADLI) in performance excellence.

Although the implementation of Baldrige framework has a positive impact on all aspects of the healthcare organization and its operations, an economic evaluation of the Baldrige Performance Excellence Program[11] highlighted the particular importance of the benefit-cost assessment of 45 award recipients of the program. Using a counterfactual evaluation method, the implementation of the program shows a 3.0-to-1.0 cost saving, and the gains from consumer satisfaction could be as high as 107.0-to-1.0.

The comprehensive approach for the Baldrige program allows for sustained improvement over a variety of different healthcare measures. GBMC HealthCare System (Baltimore, MD) has achieved a 5-star rating (the highest) from the CMS, with a rating for communication with doctors that has consistently been in the top 10% of national hospitals. Sutter Davis Hospital (Davis, CA) has leveraged the Baldrige framework to exceed the 93rd percentile of California acute care hospitals in financial excellence in its earnings.

European Foundation for Quality Management

Another internationally recognized framework for performance excellence is the EFQM (Fig. 25.5).[6] Established in 1989, the impetus for the model was the work of Dr. Deming in total quality management. EFQM provides an overarching framework to enhance processes and their results. The model addresses several organization stakeholders, functions, and performance measures. Several studies, including a 10-year experience within the Trento Healthcare Trust, a large Italian

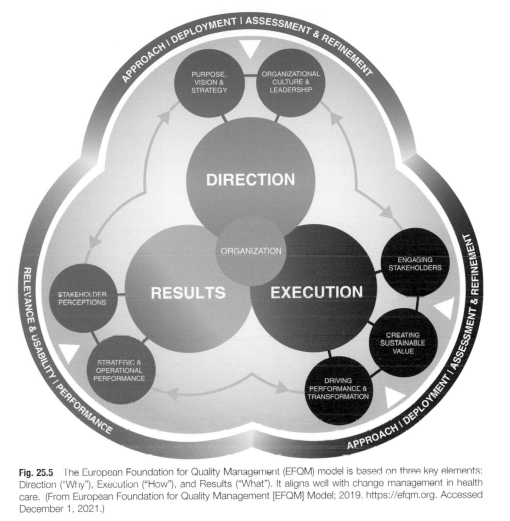

Fig. 25.5 The European Foundation for Quality Management (EFQM) model is based on three key elements: Direction ("Why"), Execution ("How"), and Results ("What"). It aligns well with change management in health care. (From European Foundation for Quality Management [EFQM] Model; 2019. https://efqm.org. Accessed December 1, 2021.)

healthcare system,[1,2] show significant improvement on customer satisfaction, people results, and key service delivery and outcomes.

In conclusion, it is imperative for healthcare organizations to assess and understand their current maturity level of systems and processes before selecting their improvement journey framework. Each methodology has its areas of strength and applicability, and it is important to choose the best fit for the organization and its environment to optimally address challenges and opportunities.

References

1. ISO 9001:2015. Quality management systems—requirements. British Standards Institution. https://www.iso.org/standard/62085.html. Accessed December 1, 2021.
2. The Joint Commission. Accreditation and Certification. https://www.jointcommission.org/accreditation-and-certification/. Accessed December 1, 2021.
3. Dr. Deming's Total Quality Management. Dr. Deming's 14 points for management. https://deming.org/explore/fourteen-points/. Accessed December 1, 2021.

4. Sullivan JL, Rivard PE, Shin MH, Rosen AK. Applying the high reliability health care maturity model to assess hospital performance: a VA case study. *Jt Comm J Qual Patient Saf.* 2016;42(9):389–411.

5. Baldrige Healthcare Excellence Framework 2021-2022, National Institute of Standard and Technology. https://www.nist.gov/baldrige/publications/baldrige-excellence-framework/health-care. Accessed December 1, 2021.

6. European Foundation for Quality Management (EFQM) Model; 2019. https://efqm.org. Accessed December 1, 2021.

7. Thomerson LD. Journey for excellence: Kentucky's Commonwealth Health Corporation adopts Six Sigma approach. *Ann Qual Congr Proc.* 2001;55:152–158.

8. Antony J, Snee R, Hoerl R. Lean Six Sigma: yesterday, today and tomorrow. *Int J Qual Rel Manag.* 2017;34(7):1073–1093.

9. The Joint Commission Center for Transforming Healthcare. https://www.centerfortransforminghealthcare.org/?_ga=2.66050535.851401032.1638322289-793861161.1638322289. Accessed December 1, 2021.

10. American Nurse Credentialing Center Magnet Recognition Program. https://www.nursingworld.org/organizational-programs/magnet/. Accessed December 1, 2021.

11. Link AN, Scott JT. Economic Evaluation of the Baldrige Performance Excellence Program. https://www.nist.gov/system/files/documents/2017/05/09/report11-2.pdf. Accessed December 1, 2021.

12. Favaretti C, De Pieri P, Torri E, et al. An EFQM excellence model for integrated healthcare governance. *Int J Health Care Qual Assur.* 2015;28(2):156–172.

CHAPTER 26

Building a Measurement System That Works: Milestones, Measure Development, and Sampling

Robert Lloyd, PhD

KEY POINTS

- Without data, you are merely a person with another opinion!
- Living in concept-land will never produce results!
- The milestones in the quality measurement journey provide the roadmap for successful results.

Every successful journey starts with a map and a plan. As the milestones along the journey are approached and passed, the traveler has an opportunity to assess progress made toward the journey's destination. Quality improvement (QI) is a journey, but it is a continuous journey that benefits from having milestones that help improvement team members evaluate progress and learn if the initial plan for the journey is leading in the desired direction, toward the expressed results. This chapter addresses a specific segment of the overall QI journey, namely the milestones in the quality measurement journey (QMJ). In this chapter, the first six milestones are discussed: concept, aim, related measures, operational definitions, data collection plan, and data collection (Fig. 26.1). In the next chapter, the analysis and action milestones are covered.

Moving From Concept-Land to Measurement-Land

All journeys start out as a concept and with thoughts such as, "Let's go and see the Grand Canyon." This is good, but it is just an aim, a desired outcome. The aim needs to be more concrete. So, the next version is "Let's take a road trip and travel Route 66 to get there!" This is a little more specific, but it is still in the concept phase. What is needed is to move out of concept-land and onto the road. It is only then that this trip can be laid out and evaluated. Measurement strategies and tactics for achieving the aim are required to move out of "concept-land" and into "measurement-land."

Many healthcare professionals live in concept-land with phrases such as, "We need to...":

- Reduce wait times
- Improve patient satisfaction
- Reduce waste and inefficiencies

There is nothing inherently wrong with concepts; they provide direction and a vision for what could be. If the concepts are to be realized, however, the measures that these vague notions reflect must be selected and defined to determine the direction implied by the concept. For example, if reducing harm is the concept, how can this be made more specific? Harm is a very broad concept,

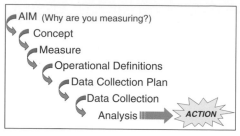

Fig. 26.1   Milestones in the Quality Measurement Journey. (From Lloyd R. *Quality Health Care: A Guide to Developing and Using Indicators*. 2nd ed. Jones & Bartlett Learning; 2019:100. Used with permission.)

but if we said that we will reduce harm by reducing the inpatient fall rate (i.e., the number of falls per 1000 inpatient days), then we have moved out of concept-land and into measurement-land.

IDENTIFY POTENTIAL MEASURES RELATED TO THE AIM

Once members of an improvement team establish a clear and defined aim with a time frame and an idea of the size of the problem (e.g., reduce patient complaints at the surgical clinic by 37% within 3 months; currently the clinic receives about 30 complaints each month), they then must identify potential measures related to this aim. Ideally, the process of identifying potential measures should begin by listening to those who come to the clinic. What does the concept of "complaint" mean to a patient? Are complaints, for example, about scheduling an appointment, lack of friendliness of the front desk staff, time spent in the waiting room, or the communication skills of the doctor? Many factors may be related to reducing complaints and enhancing patient satisfaction.

Once the improvement team has identified several potential measures related to the aim, the number of measures should be reduced into a more manageable set. These are referred to as the *vital few* measures. One way to do this is to create a family of measures, which consists of three types: **outcome, process,** and **balancing measures** (Box 26.1).

BOX 26.1 ■ Three Types of Measures

Outcome Measures (Select 1–2)

- Should be the qualities that the voice of the customer has indicated are most important
- Should reflect if the system and its processes are meeting the needs of the customer
- Should answer the question: Are our improvement efforts making a meaningful impact on what matters to those we serve?

Process Measures (Select 3–5)

- Should capture the voice of the process (i.e., factors that cause changes in the outcomes)
- Should reflect the parts/steps in the processes that the customers experience: Are the processes performing as planned? Are the processes reliable? Efficient? Patient-centered?
- Have you selected measures that are the causal factors that drive the outcome measures?

Balancing Measures (Select 1–2)

- Address the fundamental question: Are we producing unintended consequences in our efforts to improve?
- What other factors may be affecting results we have not thought about?
- Help us look at the system from different directions and perspectives
- Allow us to determine what happened to the system as we improved the outcome and process measures

DEVELOP OPERATIONAL DEFINITIONS

Having selected outcome, process, and balancing measures, the next milestone is to develop operational definitions for the selected measures. An operational definition:

- Gives communicable meaning to a measure
- Must be clear and unambiguous
- Must specify the measurement method, equipment, and, if appropriate, the criteria by which measurement decisions will be made

It is always possible to debate whether one operational definition will work better than another. Plus, there are no right, wrong, or universally accepted operational definitions. The key is that the operational definition must be acceptable to the members of the improvement team because this will guide data collection efforts.

For example, if the measurement concept is "wait time to see the doctor," the team must agree on how they will operationally define "time." Are they going to measure it in whole minutes, or minutes and seconds? When do they start tracking the time of this process and when does it end? Does time start when the patient signs in at the registration desk or when a receptionist checks the patient into the computer system? How do they record time? Is it measured by the clock on the wall or the time stamp on the computer registration screen? When does the time waiting to see the doctor end? Who records this time? The doctor? The nurse? If the improvement team develops a clear and unambiguous operational definition of the concept of time, they can measure it in a valid and reliable manner. If they do not have an agreed-on operational definition, then the data collected will be inconsistent and confusing.

Ask yourself, for example, what operational definitions you might give to the following concepts:

- Medication error
- Courtesy in answering the telephone
- Cleanliness of a patient room

After developing what you think is a clear, unambiguous, and communicable definition for each of your measures, you should be in a good position to move on to the next milestone: developing a data collection plan.

DEVELOP A DATA COLLECTION PLAN AND COLLECT DATA

At the data collection milestone, three key tactics should be considered:

- Stratification
- Sampling methods
- Frequency and duration of data collection

Stratification

Stratification is a practical rather than technical issue, which requires subject matter expertise rather than deep statistical knowledge. If you ask people who work in a process how or why things differ, they can tell you. People unfamiliar with the way a process works, and the variation in the process, can take a guess at stratification levels but it will be just that: a guess. Stratification basically consists of separating or classifying data into categories or homogeneous buckets that reflect common characteristics. The objective of stratification is to create mutually exclusive categories that allow the improvement team to discover patterns that would otherwise be confounded or masked if the data were aggregated. The goal of stratification is to minimize within group variation to maximize the learning that can come by comparing dissimilar groups. Frequently used stratification levels include:

- Age and gender
- Severity levels of patients
- Socioeconomic status

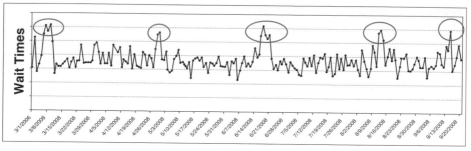

Fig. 26.2   Wait times by week.

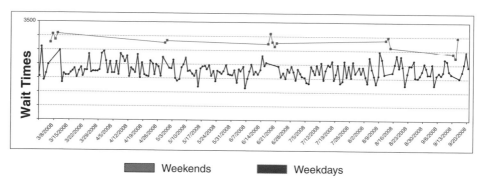

Fig. 26.3   Wait times by week stratified by weekends and weekdays.

The key to using stratification successfully is to decide on stratification categories *before* data collection. If the data is stratified after collection, it will have to be manually teased apart, which leads to rework and potential improper classification. Fig. 26.2 shows the classic stratification problem. Notice the repeating spikes in the data pattern. Are these inherent to the process or do they reflect a special condition? Fig. 26.3 provides additional insight. There are two separate and distinct processes here for wait time, weekends, and weekdays. In this case, two separate charts should be made: one for weekend wait times and the other for weekday wait times. If they are combined, the data are confounded and summary statistics, such as mean and standard deviation, will be misleading. More importantly, the improvement team may make decisions that overreact to the weekend wait times, not realizing that they represent a completely different process than the weekday wait time process.

Sampling Methods

There are two primary reasons why sampling methods are used:

1. Not all the resources needed are available, including time, money, and people, to complete a total enumeration of all the data.
2. There are more data than is needed to understand the performance of the process.

The first reason is self-evident. The second reason requires comment. First, we are doing QI research, not academic research structured around experimental and quasi-experimental designs.[1] In experimental and quasi-experimental research, large databases may be assembled containing thousands or tens of thousands of observations. With QI research, we take a different approach and are interested in understanding the variation in a process as it lays itself out over time. This requires collecting small data sets by hour, day, week, or month and gathering sufficient data (typically 20 data points or more) to analyze variation in the data using a run chart or a Shewhart chart.[2–8] The goal of sampling is to represent the characteristics of a population or a process by directly observing a smaller subset of the population's data. The challenge is to obtain a sample that is representative of the population but not biased either positively or negatively from what would be discovered if all the data for the population under consideration was reviewed.

A variety of sampling methods have been developed over the years to help researchers enhance representativeness and reduce bias. Unfortunately, many healthcare professionals have never taken formal courses in sampling methods and their applications. As a result, samples are frequently taken that are not representative and lead to biased conclusions. Understanding sampling methods and approaches is straightforward and practical but does require discipline and training. Ishikawa[2] offers four conditions for developing a successful sampling strategy: accuracy, reliability, speed, and economy. Not every sampling plan will maximize these four conditions, but they provide excellent guidance for sampling efforts.

Sampling methods are grouped into two basic categories: **probability** and **nonprobability**. Although there are many techniques in each of these categories, as shown in Table 26.1, most people have a general sense of what a random sample is. A random number table or a random number–generating software program is used to provide observations selected "randomly" out of the total population. For example, a random number generator could be used to create a random sample of 5 patient wait times out of the 63 total patient wait times from the surgical clinic on Monday. If a second request is made, the next five randomly selected wait times will be different. All other probability sampling methods are merely variations on this simple random sampling approach.

With **nonprobability** sampling methods, there is more variation. *Convenience* and *quota sampling* frequently go together and are the least reliable of all sampling methods. For example, a TV station reporter might be told to go out and get comments from four people about a new tax proposal. The four people are not randomly picked but chosen to give good sound bites. The results are that the four sound bites are not representative of the population viewpoint, resulting in a biased sample. The other nonprobability sampling method, *judgment sampling,* may or may not involve random sampling but is different from the convenience-quota approach. Judgment sampling was advocated by Dr. Walter Shewhart and Dr. W. Edwards Deming as efficient approaches to sampling based on the judgment or knowledge of the workers. The workers know when there is variation in the process or system, so ask them about the variation and then develop a sampling strategy that captures that variation. For example, at the clinic where we are interested in patient wait times, talk to the workers about how the wait time process varies by day or during the week. One worker says, "It is nuts here between 9:30 and 11:00 AM." The next worker says, "Things are very busy on Mondays and Fridays but not as busy on Tuesdays." The third worker says, "I only work on Tuesdays and Thursdays and things are not too hectic on these days." Now we have judgment (knowledge) from those who work in the process; based on these insights we can develop a sampling strategy that may or may not involve probability sampling.

Developing appropriate sampling strategies is not a difficult task. It does, however, require knowledge of the various sampling approaches, the advantages and disadvantages of each approach, and when to apply a particular approach. The major sampling approaches are described in Table 26.1.

With knowledge of the advantages, disadvantages, and when to use each of these methods, you will be well on your way to collecting samples that are most likely to meet Ishikawa's four conditions. Any reputable statistics book, regardless of its age,[3] will provide an excellent review of these various sampling methods. There are also many good online resources to explore (e.g., the American Society for Quality [https://asq.org] is a credible source for obtaining knowledge about sampling methods and other QI tools). Practical guidance can also be found in Lloyd[4] and in Provost and Murray.[5]

TABLE 26.1 ■ Advantages and Disadvantages of Various Sampling Methods

Sampling Method	Description	Advantages	Disadvantages
Probability Sampling Methods			
Simple random sample	A random sample that is drawn in such a way that every member of a population has an equal chance of being included. A random number table or a random number generator is typically used to actually pull the sample.	• Requires minimum knowledge of the population in advance • Free of possible classification errors • Easy to analyze the data and compute errors • Fairly inexpensive	• Does not take advantage of the knowledge the researcher might have about the population • There could be overrepresentation or underrepresentation of subgroups within the population • Typically produces larger sampling errors than a stratified sample for the same sample
Stratified random sample	The population is divided into relevant strata before random sampling is applied to each stratum.	• Helps to reduce the chances of overrepresenting/underrepresenting subgroups within the population • Allows you to segment the data into "buckets" during the analysis phase • Creates more efficient samples • Reduces sampling error	• Requires knowledge of the presence of various characteristics within the population • Sampling costs can increase if knowledge of the population is shallow • If the strata are not highly homogeneous, then sampling error goes up and efficiency goes down
Proportional stratified random sample	The proportion (or percentage) of a particular stratum is determined in the population and then applied to the random sample.	• Adds even more precision than the stratified random sample • Increases sample representativeness • Creates very efficient samples • Reduces sampling error	• Requires more human and financial resources than other methods • Requires even more information about the population than stratified random methods
Systematic sample	Select every kth observation from the population after a random starting point has been selected.	• Very easy to conduct • Has "intuitive" appeal • Inexpensive to conduct	• Can produce bias because of periodic ordering of observation, which produces exclusion of segments of the population • Increased probability of sampling bias
Cluster sample	Clusters or "bunches" of the population are identified, and then random sampling is applied to each cluster.	• Can be low cost, especially if geographical clusters are used • If properly done, each cluster is a small model of the population • High level of practicality	• Clusters need to be as heterogeneous as possible • Typically has lower statistical efficiency • Large samples are often needed to ensure precision

Nonprobability Sampling Methods

Convenience sample	Observations are selected based on availability and convenience. Also known as "accidental" samples.	• Ease of obtaining a sample • Relatively low cost	• Extremely low generalizability • No way to determine sampling bias or sampling error
Quota sample	A population is divided into relevant strata. The desired proportion of samples to be obtained from each stratum is determined, and then a fixed quota within each stratum is set.	• Stratification effect is achieved if the strata are appropriately structured • In theory, it should be reasonably representative of the population • Human and financial costs can be kept to a minimum if the strata from which the quotas are to be drawn are grouped close together (to reduce the amount of travel the data collectors have to perform to gather the data)	• The people assigned to collect the quotas need to be scrupulous, free from selection bias, and able to follow the prescribed sampling design (otherwise this method becomes a convenience sample) • It is difficult to guarantee that the quotas were filled accurately • In-depth knowledge of the population is required • Nonrandom selection of the quotas can also introduce bias
Judgment sample	Subgroups are drawn from a process over time based on expert knowledge. The subgroup samples can be drawn either by random or nonrandom procedures.	• Samples in a subgroup can be small (3–5) because many subgroups will be selected • Data collection costs can be reduced • Provides a dynamic picture of the data and serves as the basis for process improvement • Minimum stratification effect is achieved	• Sampling bias and sampling error cannot be calculated • Expert knowledge of the process or population is required • Generalization of the judgment sample to larger populations cannot be done • Personal bias enters into the selection of the sample

From Lloyd R. *Quality Health Care: A Guide to Developing and Using Indicators.* 2nd ed. Jones & Bartlett Learning; 2019. Replication and/or distribution of this table without expressed written permission form Dr. Lloyd and Jones & Bartlett Learning is strictly prohibited.

Frequency and Duration of Data Collection

The final decisions needed about your data collection plan are centered around two basic questions:

- *How often* will you dip into a stream of data to obtain observations on the process? Will you collect data every hour? Every day? Once a week? Once a month?
- *How long* do you plan to continue collecting data? Will you collect data on an ongoing basis and not end until the measure of interest is always at the specified target or goal? Will you conduct periodic audits? Will you just collect data at a single point in time to "check the pulse of the process?"

The answers to these questions will demonstrate if you are genuinely on a QI journey for learning, or if you are using the "Q" word in name only. Remember that for QI, the standard is to collect data over time to understand the variation that lives in the process you are trying to improve. You cannot understand variation by collecting pre-post data or by conducting point prevalence audits (e.g., gathering data on Tuesday at 2:30 PM and using it to make assumptions about how the entire process operates). QI requires collecting data as close to the production of work as possible, which leads to development of data collection plans preferably by hour, day, week, or possibly month, but realize that monthly data, particularly monthly averages, can be very misleading. Finally, avoid quarterly data for any QI initiative. There is just too much variation that gets aggregated away in quarterly data. Quarterly data leads to judgment, not improvement.

In this chapter, the first six milestones in the QMJ have been discussed. The final two milestones, analysis and action, are discussed in the next chapter.

References

1. Campbell D, Stanley J. *Experimental and Quasi-Experimental Designs for Research.* Houghton-Mifflin; 1963.
2. Ishikawa K. *Guide to Quality Control.* Asian Productivity Organization/Quality Resources; 1982.
3. Selltiz C, Jahoda M, Deutsch M, Cook S. *Research Methods in Social Relations.* Revised One-Volume edition. Holt, Rinehart and Winston; 1959.
4. Lloyd R. *Quality Health Care: A Guide to Developing and Using Indicators.* 2nd ed. Jones & Bartlett Learning; 2019.
5. Provost L, Murray S. *The Health Care Data Guide.* Jossey-Bass; 2011.
6. Wheeler D, Chambers D. *Understanding Statistical Process Control.* SPC Press; 1992.
7. Mohammed MA, Worthington P, Woodall WH. Plotting basic control charts: tutorial notes for healthcare practitioners. *Qual Saf Health Care.* 2008;17(2):137–145.
8. Western Electric Company. Handbook Committee. In: *Statistical Quality Control Handbook.* 11th ed. AT&T Technologies Inc.; 1985.

CHAPTER 27

Analyzing Variation With Run Charts

Robert Lloyd, PhD

KEY POINTS

- Variation exists in all that we do.
- Variation needs to be understood as it lays itself out over time.
- Static displays of data using summary and descriptive statistics will not allow you to understand variation.
- The Run Chart provides a starting point to understand variation in a process.

In the previous chapter, six of the milestones in the quality measurement journey (QMJ) were discussed. Particular attention was given to identifying measures, classifying them as outcome, process and balancing measures, the need for operational definitions, and, finally, data collection strategies. In this chapter, the next question is addressed: Now that you have data, what do you do with it? If you are genuinely committed to quality as a clinical and business strategy, then there is only one option: to understand the variation that lives in the data. This is best achieved by using statistical process control (SPC) methods and, in particular, the run chart and Shewhart control charts. In this chapter, the focus will be on the run chart. Chapter 28 (SPC charts chapter) addresses the Shewhart control charts.

What Is a Run Chart?

A run chart is a graphic display of data that:
- Makes the variation in a process visible in a way that static or descriptive statistics cannot do
- Confirms whether a change has led to improvement
- Verifies if the process improvement has been sustained over time

A run chart provides a running record of a process over time. Clinically it is like monitoring an intensive care unit (ICU) patient's vital signs moment by moment as they occur over time. The run chart, therefore, offers a dynamic display of the data and can be used on virtually any type of data (e.g., counts of events, percentages, volume, time, or money). Because run charts require no statistical calculations, which are required with Shewhart control charts, they can be made by hand or with software. A major aspect of using the run chart is that it can be easily understood by everyone on the team. Skill with making and interpreting run charts can be developed in less than an hour. The major drawback in using run charts, however, is that they can detect some but not all types of special causes. This last point will become more apparent in the following sections.

Elements of a Run Chart

The elements of a run chart are shown in Fig. 27.1.
- The measure of interest (i.e., the observation) is always plotted on the vertical or Y axis. This could be time, a percent, a count of the number of patients seen each day, money, or a rate (e.g., an inpatient fall rate).

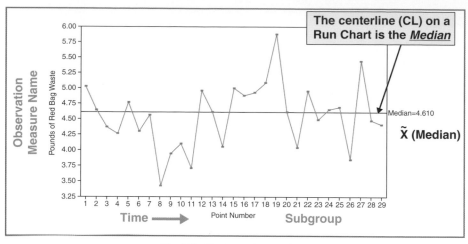

Fig. 27.1   Elements of a run chart.

■ The horizontal or X axis is used to display the data as it appears in chronological order. This is also referred to as the subgroup. An individual patient can be a subgroup of one. In this case, we would be plotting the wait time of each patient before seeing the doctor and the patients would be in chronological order (i.e., patient 1 came in at 9:35 AM, then patient 2 came at 9:51 AM, patient 3 at 10:09 AM, and so on). Day, week, or month could also be the subgroup. In any of these cases, we would need to decide if we are going to record the wait times of all the patients each day, week, or month or draw a sample of the patients from the day, week, or month and record their individual wait times (see the previous Chapter 26 for more details on sampling approaches). The key point is that the data must always be organized and presented in chronological order. Finally, note that you can start a run chart with the first data point. As a rule, however, you should have a minimum of 8 to 10 data points before placing the median on the chart and at least 10 data points before applying the run chart rules, which are explained in the next section.

■ The data values are plotted in chronological order and the data points (i.e., dots or some other symbol on the chart) are typically connected by a solid line. The connecting line should not be so thick that it obscures the dots. The dots provide the foundation for understanding the variation that lives in the process and should be easily discernable.

■ The centerline (CL) on the run chart is the median. The median is one of the three measures of central tendency (the others being the mean and the mode). The median is also the point in a rank ordered data set (highest to lowest data values) that divides the data set into an equal number of data points above and below the median (i.e., the 50th percentile). If you have an odd number of data points, then the median will be a discrete number. If you have an even number of data points, the median will be the average of the two middle values. If you make the run chart using statistical software, the median may be identified as the CL or symbolically as X (you will need to insert the $\sim$ above the X) (i.e., "X-tilde").

Analyzing a Run Chart

When you have sufficient data points (i.e., 10 or more), you can start to analyze the run chart. This is best accomplished by building skills in:

■ Determining the number of runs on the chart, and then
■ Applying the run chart rules to decide if your chart exhibits random or nonrandom variation.

DETERMINING THE NUMBER OF RUNS

A run is one or more consecutive data points *on the same side of the median*. Data points that fall exactly on the median should not be counted as part of a run. A run can consist of multiple consecutive data points, or a run can be only a single data point. It is important to remember that a run ends when the line connecting the dots crosses the median. When this happens, the run ends and you then begin counting the number of data points in the next run.

You have two options when counting the number of runs:

- Option 1: You can draw a circle around each run and count the number of circles you have drawn.
- Option 2: You can count the number of times the sequence of data points (the line on the chart) crosses the median and then add 1 to this count.

If you count the number of circles drawn around the runs (option 1) and compare it with the number of runs you get when you count the number of crossing and add 1 (option 2), you should arrive at the same number. If the number of runs using the two options does not match, then you have not applied one of the options correctly. The two counts should be the same! Fig. 27.2 shows option 1 for counting the number of runs. The chart has 7 runs. Note that two of the data points marked with blue boxes fall exactly on the median and are not part of any run.

Fig. 27.3 shows the same run chart as in Fig. 27.2 but using option 2 to count the number of runs. In this case there are 6 crossings of the median plus 1, which equals 7 runs, and this is what we discovered in Fig. 27.2 by circling the runs.

APPLYING THE RUN CHART RULES

Now that you have determined the median and the number of runs on the chart, some might ask, "So what? What do I do with this chart now?" The answer is simple: You need to analyze the chart to determine whether the measure of interest exhibits random or nonrandom variation and then make the appropriate decision on how to respond to the identified type of variation. The best place to start is by making sure you know the difference between random and nonrandom variation. Box 27.1 summarizes the two types of variation and their characteristics.

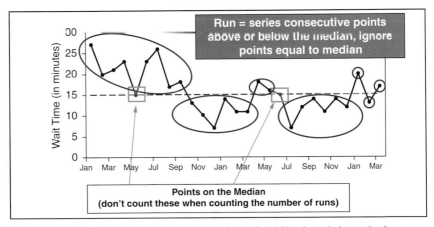

Fig. 27.2   Counting the number of runs using option 1 (the draw circles method).

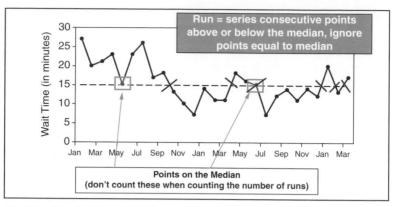

Fig. 27.3   Counting the number of runs using option 2 (the count the crossings method).

BOX 27.1 ■ Characteristics of Random and Nonrandom Variation

Random Variation

- Is inherent in the design of the process
- Is because of regular, natural, or ordinary causes
- Affects all the outcomes of a process
- Results in a "stable" process that is predictable
- Also known as random or unassignable variation

Nonrandom Variation

- Is because of irregular or unnatural causes that are not inherent in the design of the process
- Affect some, but not necessarily all, aspects of the process
- Results in an "unstable" process that is not predictable
- Also known as nonrandom or assignable variation

When analyzing run charts, the proper reference to the two types of variation is random and nonrandom variation. When you move to using Shewhart (control) charts, the two types of variation are referred to as common cause variation and special cause variation. This is because the Shewhart charts are more precise than run charts. There is a chance of missing a special cause on a run chart mainly because of using the median as the centerline rather than the mean as on a Shewhart chart and not having the upper and lower control limits. (See Chapter 28 for more details on this point.)

It is important to understand these two types of variation because you should only try to improve a process that reflects random variation. This is because a process demonstrating random variation is stable and therefore predictable. Being stable and predictable, however, does not mean that the performance of the measure and the process it represents is acceptable or capable of achieving the defined target or goal. You can have a stable process that is predictably bad, but because it is stable and predictable, you can take steps to run tests of change and see if the performance of the process can be improved. If, on the other hand, the run chart exhibits nonrandom variation, the measure and its related process are unstable and therefore not predicable. Trying to improve a process that is unstable and not predictable will only make performance worse.

It is easy to make a run chart. The real skill comes in properly interpreting the chart and making the correct decision about the performance of the process. There is a rich body of literature on understanding random and nonrandom variation.[1–4] Take time to read and study these concepts before starting to make and interpret run charts.

With knowledge of the types of variation, it is now time to apply the run chart rules for detecting nonrandom variation. There are many statistical rules that have been developed over the years to identify patterns of nonrandom variation. You will need to decide which set of rules is most appropriate for your organization. Consistency of rules and organization uses is critical. If everyone in the organization is not using the same rules to interpret the charts, some will see random variation, whereas others will see nonrandom variation.

The rules generally address a shift in the process, a trend, too much or too little variation in the data display, or an extreme (astronomical) data point. At the Institute for Healthcare Improvement (IHI), we have explored the various rules and settled on four that have been found to work well in health and social service settings when analyzing run charts. The four rules are:

- **Rule #1: A shift** in the process is defined by observing 6 or more *consecutive data points* above or below the median.
- **Rule #2: A trend** in the data is defined as 5 or more *consecutive data points constantly* increasing or decreasing. You do not count data points that repeat a value.
- **Rule #3: Too many or too few runs** reflect nonrandom patterns in the data. A random process should not be exhibiting patterns that are cyclical or display too much bunching of the data on one side or the other of the median. Table 27.1 should be used to determine whether the chart has too many or too few runs.[5] To use this table, you:
  - First calculate the number of "useful observations" in your data set. This is done by subtracting the number of data points on the median from the total number of data points. This number will be found in the left column of Table 27.1.
  - The lower number of runs is found in the second column.
  - The upper number of runs can be found in the third column.

TABLE 27.1 ■ **Table to Use With Rule #3: Too Many or Too Few Runs**

No. of Useful Observations	Lower No. of Runs	Upper No. of Runs
10	3	9
11	3	10
12	3	11
13	4	11
14	4	12
15	5	12
16	5	13
17	5	13
18	6	14
19	6	15
20	6	16
21	7	16
22	7	17
23	7	17
24	8	17
25	8	18
26	9	18
27	10	19
28	10	19
29	10	20
30	11	21
31	11	22

Reprinted with the permission of the Institute of Mathematical Statistics.

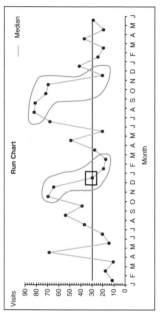

Rule 1: A Shift (6 or more consecutive
data points above or below the median)

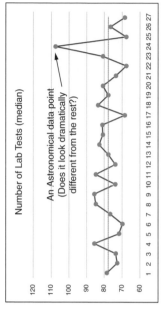

Rule 2: A Trend (5 or more consecutive
data points constantly going up or down)

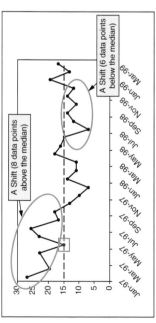

Rule 3: Too many or two few runs (based
on a statistical table)

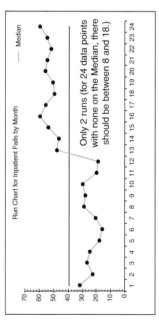

Rule 4: An Astronomical data point

Fig. 27.4　The four run chart rules for nonrandom variation.

- If the number of runs on the run chart falls below the lower limit or above the upper limit, then this is a signal of a nonrandom pattern in the data.
- **Rule #4: An "astronomical" data point.** This is not a statistical test but rather a visual inspection or filtering test. Remember that in any data set, you will find a high data point and a low data point. A high and low balance each other out. If a single data point, *and it is only one data point*, looks dramatically different from the rest then it is reasonable to conclude that this is an astronomical data point. The best way to confirm if the data point is astronomical is to place the data on a Shewhart (control) chart and see if the assumed astronomical data point exceeds either the upper or lower control limit on the Shewhart chart. (See Chapter 28 for more detail on Shewhart charts.)

The four run chart rules for detecting nonrandom patterns in the data are shown in Fig. 27.4. Additional detail on the rules and how to apply them in healthcare and social settings can be found in Lloyd[1] and Provost and Murry.[2]

In summary, the run chart is a fundamental tool for quality improvement teams. It is simple to make either by hand or with software, easy to analyze, and, most importantly, helps you determine the action(s) you need to follow. If you do not detect any nonrandom patterns in the data and the process is not capable of achieving the defined target or goal, then you can proceed to develop change ideas and run Plan-Do-Study-Act (PDSA) tests to see if the new ideas move the process in the desired direction. If, on the other hand, the run chart reveals the presence of nonrandom variation, then the correct decision is to investigate why the nonrandom variation exists and take steps to extricate the causes of this nonrandom variation from the process. If you ignore nonrandom variation, I cannot tell you exactly when it will reoccur, but it will. Why? Because the causes of nonrandom variation are inherent in the process or system and although they may be dormant at various times, they are essentially what Reason[6] calls "latent errors" that are merely waiting for the conditions to be right to reoccur. So, get some data, make a run chart, and start your quality journey!

References

1. Lloyd R. *Quality Health Care: A Guide to Developing and Using Indicators.* 2nd ed. Jones & Bartlett Learning; 2019.
2. Provost L, Murray S. *The Health Care Data Guide.* Jossey-Bass Publishers; 2011.
3. Wheeler D, Chambers D. *Understanding Statistical Process Control.* SPC Press; 1992.
4. Western Electric Company. *Statistical Process Control Handbook.* AT&T Technologies Inc.; 1985.
5. Swed F, Eisenhart C. Tables for testing randomness of grouping in a sequence of alternatives. *Ann Math Stat.* 1943;14:66–87.
6. Reason J. *Human Error.* Cambridge University Press; 1990.

Further Reading

Berman L, Raval MV, Goldin A. Process improvement strategies: designing and implementing quality improvement research. *Semin Pediatr Surg.* 2018;27(6):379–385.
Hamid S, Gallo Marin B, Smith L, et al. Improving sequential compression device (SCD) compliance in trauma patients at Kings County Hospital Center: a quality improvement report. *BMJ Open Quality.* 2021;10: e001171.
Peden CJ, Moonesinghe SR. Measurement for improvement in anaesthesia and intensive care. *Br J Anaesth.* 2016;117(2):145–148.
Perla RJ, Provost LP, Murray SK. The run chart: a simple analytical tool for learning from variation in healthcare processes. *BMJ Qual Saf.* 2011;20(1):46–51.

CHAPTER 28

Statistical Process Control Charts for Clinical Users

Gareth Parry, BSc, MSc, PhD ■ Joseph Incorvia, MS

KEY POINTS

- Quality improvement teams need a rigorous method to learn whether the changes they make lead to improvement.
- Statistical process control (SPC) charts visualize data over time, signaling whether a process is stable or whether a nonrandom special cause, suggesting improvement or deterioration, has occurred.
- A variety of SPC charts are available depending on the attributes of the measure.
- Quality assurance teams can use SPC charts to monitor performance over time, providing clear signals when an unusual event occurs.
- SPC charts are simple to operationalize by busy clinical teams.

Quality improvement in perioperative care focuses on teams, close to the point of care, iteratively testing changes to a process within a local setting.[1] To learn whether they are successful, the teams need timely feedback, signaling if their changes do or do not result in improvement. This feedback most frequently occurs by defining and collecting key process and outcome measures and plotting them over time. For example, care teams testing approaches to reducing surgical site infections (SSIs) may gauge success using short-term changes in process measures, including reliable administration of presurgical antibiotics and the longer-term outcome of SSI.

Teams need to apply a rigorous method to inform them if changes from one data point to the next are simply chance or whether the data indicate that meaningful improvement is occurring. Without such a method, overreaction to one data point may occur. For example, 1 month with a low rate of SSIs does not necessarily suggest ongoing and sustained performance at this new level.

Based on Shewhart's Theory of Variation, statistical process control (SPC) chart methodology is standard practice for visualizing, interpreting, and learning from process and outcome improvement measures, plotted over time.[2,3] Shewhart described two types of variation in data: "common cause"—innate to the system, like random week-to-week variation—and "special cause," which is not part of the routine system, signaling something important changed and possibly improved. In general, once there are at least 20 data points, SPC methods plot improvement measures over time, with a centerline (typically the mean) and upper and lower limits.[4,5] In health care, five "control chart rules" (Fig. 28.1) signal if the data are consistent with common (random) or special cause (something has changed) variations.[6]

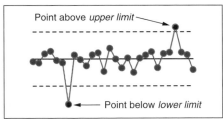

Rule 1: Any point below the *lower limit* or above the *upper limit* (Any point greater than 3σ below or 3σ above the centerline)[a]

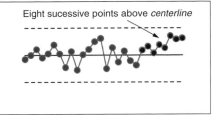

Rule 2: Eight successive points below or above the *centerline*

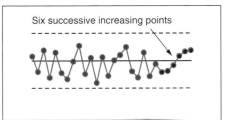

Rule 3: Six or more successive increasing or decreasing points

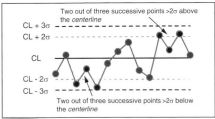

Rule 4: Two out of three successive points greater than 2σ above or 2σ below the *centerline*

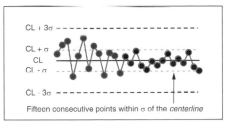

Rule 5: Fifteen successive points within σ either side of the *centerline*

Fig. 28.1 Rules for signaling special cause. In total, more than five rules have been developed for signaling special cause variation; however, in health care, the five rules described are most commonly used.[6] SPC, statistical process control. [a]Sigma (σ) is a measure of variation between successive data points. Each type of SPC chart has a specific method for calculating σ. σ differs from a standard deviation by measuring the variability of a process *over time* instead of the overall variation in the *static* distribution in the data.[4]

Displaying 30-Day Readmission Rates Using a P-Chart

SPC methodology can be illustrated in an example of 30-day readmissions after cardiac surgery. For 2015 and 2016, in a large academic hospital, of 5229 patients undergoing cardiac surgery, 835 (15.9%) were readmitted within 30 days of surgery. Fig. 28.2A shows monthly readmission rates plotted over time around this centerline of 15.9%. The figure shows that readmissions varied from 11.8% in September 2015 to 20.4% in September 2016. Fig. 28.2B shows the data displayed as a P-chart, a specific type of SPC chart, showing monthly readmission rates, a centerline, and upper and lower limits. To calculate the limits, a value, sigma (σ) is calculated indicating month-to-month variation. The upper and lower limits are placed three times sigma (3σ) either side of the centerline. For 2015 to 2016, all the points are within the limits, suggesting readmission rates are consistent with random (common cause) variation, and no change in the underlying process occurred.

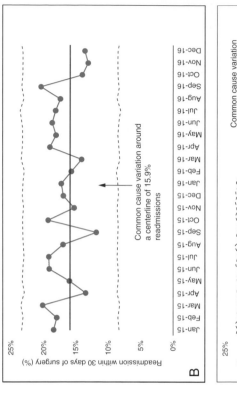

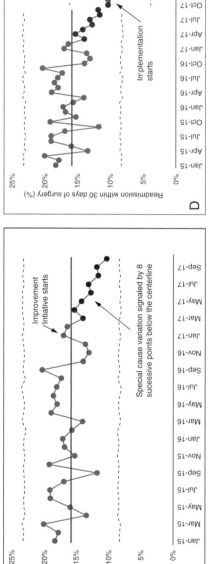

Fig. 28.2 A, Readmission within 30 days of surgery for 2015 to 2016. B, Readmission within 30 days of surgery for 2015 to 2016 displayed as a P-chart. C, Readmission within 30 days of surgery for 2015 to 2017 displayed as a P-chart. D, Readmission within 30 days of surgery for 2015 to 2019 displayed as a P-chart.

At the start of 2017, the hospital prioritized reducing 30-day readmissions after cardiac surgery. They formed a multidisciplinary cardiac care team who tested several changes during 2017. The hospital continued to plot readmissions rates as a P-chart. As can be seen in Fig. 28.2C, during 2017, the readmission rate started, with some fluctuations, to reduce, remaining within the upper and lower limits. By October 2017, the hospital experienced eight successive months with a readmission rate below the centerline, signaling special cause variation from rule 2 (see Fig. 28.1). In other words, this data pattern was inconsistent with random variation and something had changed in the care system.

After the special cause signal in October 2017, the hospital team implemented the changes they had been testing. As can be seen in Fig. 28.2D, since September 2017, the monthly readmission rate has varied around 10.1%, with only random variation in monthly rates.

The SPC methodology, led the hospital to conclude that during 2015 to 2016, monthly readmission rates were stable around 15.9% per month. During 2017, after the improvement work began, readmissions reduced, and subsequent changes implemented within the system resulted in readmission rates stabilizing around 10.1% per month.

Displaying Postsurgical Pain Scores Using an I-Chart

As summarized in Fig. 28.3, the specific SPC chart depends on the type of measure.[7] For example, SSIs or postsurgical readmissions are made up of a numerator and denominator and are typically displayed as a monthly rate on a P-chart. We can display individual patient postsurgical pain scores over time using an I-chart.

The perioperative team at one hospital was interested in examining the self-reported 0 to 10 Numeric Rating Scale (NRS) pain scores of patients 4 hours after thoracic surgery.[8] Fig. 28.4A shows an I-chart displaying the 50 individual pain scores varying around a centerline of 7.2, with lower and upper limits of 5.1 and 9.3. A perioperative pain improvement team was formed aiming to reduce postoperative pain. Changes to surgical anesthetic medications and postsurgical medications were tested from the 55th patient onward, and progress displayed as on the I-chart.

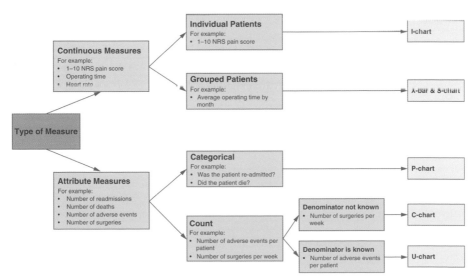

Fig. 28.3 Common types of statistical process control charts.

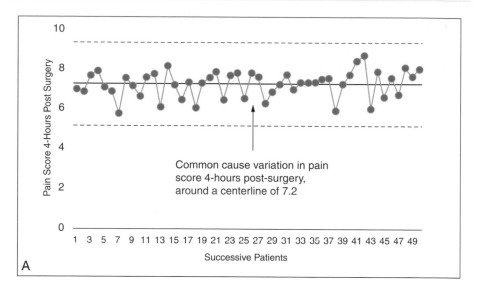

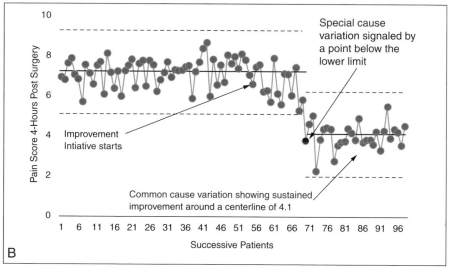

Fig. 28.4 A, Pain score 4 hours after thoracic surgery displayed as an I-chart. B, Pain score 4 hours after thoracic surgery displayed as an I-chart before and after initiating an improvement initiative.

For patient 70, the team introduced a standardized postsurgical order form. Their 6-hour pain score of 3.7 was less than the lower limit (5.1), signaling special cause (Rule 1, Fig. 28.1). The care team continued to test the standardized postsurgical order form, with pain scores for subsequent patients stabilizing around a new centerline of 4.1, with lower and upper limits of 2.0 and 6.2 (see Fig. 28.4B).

In this example, the hospital applied SPC methodology to identify that patient-reported pain scores were stable, averaging around 7.2, with the improvement initiative resulting in a reduction to 4.1. The hospital went on to implement the new processes into the standard system of care and continued to use an I-chart to monitor whether the improvement was sustained.

Displaying Occurrences of Hematoma After Breast Augmentation Surgery Using a G-Chart

Some adverse-events can be very rare, and although presented as a rate, displaying them as a P-chart is not appropriate and a G-chart, displaying cases between events, can be used. Hematoma after breast augmentation, a rare event occurring in 2% to 4% of cases, can be used to illustrate the use of a G-chart.[9] Between 2018 and 2019, a surgical center conducted 1391 breast augmentation procedures, with 28 (2.01%) cases experiencing a hematoma. Nevertheless, the surgical team felt that in the last month, they had experienced more hematomas than usual. A G-chart was used to display the number of cases between hematomas. A G-chart assumes a specific type of distribution, akin to using a geometric mean, to calculate the centerline. Moreover, a G-chart only includes an upper limit because the formula for the lower limit often produces negative values, which are impossible in time between calculations. Fig. 28.5 shows the G-chart with a centerline of 35.8 days and an upper limit of 208.2 days. All the data points are below the upper limit, suggesting that hematoma occurrences over this 2-year period are consistent with random variation, and no changes in the underlying system had occurred.

In this example the surgical team used a G-chart to look at variations in the occurrence of hematomas after breast augmentation. They concluded that the time between hematomas was consistent with random variation, and they would continue to monitor hematomas using a G-chart to assess future performance.

The examples presented here represent a high-level introduction to the use of SPC methodology in perioperative care. Numerous examples of the use of SPC charts to drive improvement exist, such as the reduction of SSIs in a diabetic population, the improvement of opioid management in pediatric tonsillectomy and adenotonsillectomy surgery patients, and the prevention of perioperative hypothermia in patients with major burns.[10–12] Additionally, SPC charts are also being used to monitor the performance of existing processes and systems (e.g., monitoring cardiac surgery outcomes).[13,14]

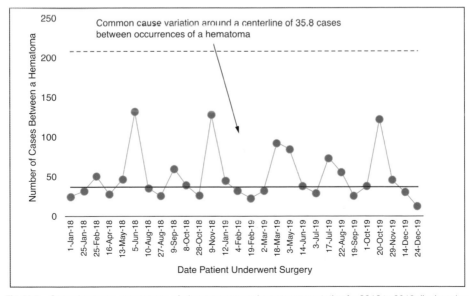

Fig. 28.5   Cases between occurrences of a hematoma post breast augmentation for 2018 to 2019 displayed as a G-chart.

Moreover, more detailed descriptions of how to construct and interpret SPC charts, including some nuances not covered in this chapter, are available.[4,15] For example, there are descriptions of how to stratify data by patient characteristics (including gender, income, race, and, ethnicity), deal with trends, and adjust for large sample sizes.[16–19] As SPC methods have become more mainstream, most major statistical packages now include SPC functions within their standard releases. Nevertheless, many of these functions are relatively basic and lack the ability to readily change the centerline once special cause variation has signaled. The code-oriented statistics package "R" currently has several open-source functions available that allow for changes in the centerline and other adaptations not covered in this chapter.[20] Additionally, several spreadsheet-type plugins and macros are commercially available, providing a straightforward approach to generating SPC charts for perioperative data.

The lasting power of Shewhart's Theory of Variation applied through SPC charts is to provide a practical, rigorous, and intuitive method for teams at the point of care to visualize and learn whether the variation in process and outcome measurers they experience day-to-day is simply common-cause random variation around a stable process or whether it is some special-cause variation because of a change in the process. The aforementioned examples demonstrate how this powerful visual tool can be readily applied to drive improvement in the perioperative field.

References

1. Langley GJ, Moen RD, Nolan KM, Nolan TW, Norman CL, Provost LP. *The Improvement Guide.* 2nd ed. Jossey Bass Wiley; 2009.
2. Shewhart WA. *Economic Control of Quality of Manufactured Product.* New York: D Van Nostrand Company; 1931 [Reprinted by ASQC Quality Press, 1980].
3. Tennant R, Mohammed MA, Coleman JJ, Martin U. Monitoring patients using control charts: a systematic review. *Int J Qual Health Care.* 2007;19:187–194.
4. Provost LP, Murray S. *The Health Care Data Guide: Learning From Data for Improvement.* John Wiley & Sons; 2011.
5. Shewhart WA, Deming WE. *Statistical Methods From the Viewpoint of Quality Control.* Washington, DC: The Graduate School, U.S. Department of Agriculture; 1939 [Republished by Dover Publications, 1986].
6. Lloyd R. *Quality Health Care: A Guide to Developing and Using Indicators.* 2nd ed. Jones & Bartlett Learning; 2019.
7. Groom R, Likosky DS, Rutberg H. Understanding variation in cardiopulmonary bypass: statistical process control theory. *J Extra Corpor Technol.* 2004;36(3):224–230.
8. Jensen MP, Turner JA, Romano JM, Fisher LD. Comparative reliability and validity of chronic pain intensity measures. *Pain.* 1999;83:157–162.
9. Masuda S, Fujibayashi S, Takemoto M, et al. Incidence and clinical features of postoperative symptomatic hematoma after spine surgery: a multicenter study of 45 patients. *Spine Surg Relat Res.* 2019;4(2):130–134.
10. Ehrenfeld JM, Wanderer JP, Terekhov M, Rothman BS, Sandberg WS. A perioperative systems design to improve intraoperative glucose monitoring is associated with a reduction in surgical site infections in a diabetic patient population. *Anesthesiology.* 2017;126(3):431–440.
11. Franz AM, Dahl JP, Huang H, et al. The development of an opioid sparing anesthesia protocol for pediatric ambulatory tonsillectomy and adenotonsillectomy surgery—a quality improvement project. *Pediatric Anesthesia.* 2019;29(7):682–689.
12. Rogers AD, Saggaf M, Ziolkowski N. A quality improvement project incorporating preoperative warming to prevent perioperative hypothermia in major burns. *Burns.* 2018;44(5):1279–1286.
13. Rogers CA, Reeves BC, Caputo M, Ganesh JS, Bonser RS, Angelini GD. Control chart methods for monitoring cardiac surgical performance and their interpretation. *J Thorac Cardio Surg.* 2004;128(6):811–819.
14. Woodall WH. The use of control charts in health-care and public-health surveillance. *J Qual Technol.* 2006;38(2):89–104.
15. Wheeler DJ, Chambers DS. *Understanding Statistical Process Control.* SPC Press; 1986.
16. Nolan T, Perla RJ, Provost L. Understanding variation, 26 years later. *Qual Prog.* 2016;49(11):28–37.

17. Perla RJ, Provost SM, Parry GJ, Little K, Provost LP. Understanding variation in covid-19 reported deaths with a novel Shewhart chart application. *Int J Qual Health Care.* 2020. https://doi.org/10.1093/intqhc/mzaa069.
18. Tsironis LK, Dimitriadis SG, Kehris E. Monitoring operating room performance with control charts: findings from a Greek public hospital. *Int J Qual Health Care.* 2021;33(1):mzaa167.
19. Shackley DC, Whytock C, Parry G, et al. Variation in the prevalence of urinary catheters: a profile of National Health Service patients in England. *BMJ Open.* 2017;7(6).
20. Knoth S. spc: statistical process control—calculation of ARL and other control chart performance measures. https://cran.r-project.org/web/packages/spc/index.html. Accessed May 2021.

CHAPTER 29

Process Mapping

Carolyn Johnston, BM BCh, MA (Oxon), FRCA

KEY POINTS

- Process maps provide a useful tool to help understand a system and stimulate improvement ideas.
- Process maps are a visual representation of a process or pathway broken down into the constituent steps and options along the pathway.
- Creating a process map should involve key stakeholders across the process.
- A perioperative process map is most useful if it includes patients to give important insights into how the process works and scrutiny of whether individual steps add "value" to their care.

Background

Most patient care is designed or described in "pathways" of care, and most healthcare processes can be mapped out in a linear or graphical form described as a *process map.*

Process maps lay out the steps in a process in a visual format and can be extremely useful to give an overview of an entire pathway or process, allowing the viewer to scrutinize each step looking for elements that could be improved. A process map defines the start and end of the process, any decisions in the process, any delays, and interconnections or dependencies on other processes. These points in the process are represented by standard symbols on the map (Fig. 29.1). The flow of the process is indicated by arrows.

Process maps can be high level, or extremely detailed, depending on the intended purpose for the process mapping exercise.

Process maps are a useful tool in many improvement methodologies but are commonly associated with "Lean" and the concept of "value."[1,2] Creating a process map focused on patient value is called "value stream mapping."[3,4]

The process mapping exercise is a helpful early step to understand the system, convene a group of stakeholders to focus on the problem, and create a project team. It is often the first time that some team members have taken a high-level overview of something they do every day. A process mapping session is a good opportunity to build a multidisciplinary team and to think about the range of stakeholders that may need to be engaged to generate improvement ideas.

The creation of the process map also provides an opportunity to highlight the differences between "work as done" (what actually happens and is laid down on the map), "work as disclosed" (what staff members describe as their work), and "work as prescribed" (what the formal written policy or guideline says should be done). The differences between these types of work are an important aspect of human factors and ergonomics.[5]

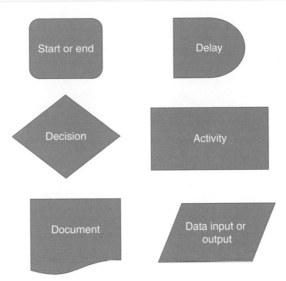

Fig. 29.1 Some of the symbols used to denote activities in a process map.

To Create a Process Map

It is helpful to produce the map as a team exercise to ensure that as many views as possible are used to describe the process from a variety of perspectives, including medical, nursing, and other healthcare professionals and administrators. Also try to include junior and senior members of staff because their perspective will be different. It is also very important to have the patient perspective on the process, if at all possible.

- First, agree on the start and end point of the process and on the scope and level of detail. This can be difficult because there are few healthcare processes that stand alone, and most processes have complex interdependencies.
- Brainstorm the steps in the process. Some people may find it helpful to list them in order, or you can brainstorm all the steps and then place them in sequence afterward.
- Note any points of choice or divergence and mark them as a decision point.
- Any point where there is significant disagreement about the process, or if the team is unsure about the process, can be clarified by either asking more stakeholders to contribute or observing the process in real time and recording the observations.
- If there are data to support particular steps, they can be used to annotate the map. It is often helpful to include waiting times because process maps are often used to highlight and eliminate unnecessary waits.

A high-level process map is given in Fig. 29.2. Each step could be developed in a great deal more detail, such as by listing out each step in the patient triage process.

When reviewing the process map, note any redundant steps, or steps that add little value or no value to the patient. Can the process be redesigned to eliminate these steps or simplify the process?

Look at the process for any other "wastes." For example, steps that are unreliable or have significant associated waiting or unnecessary transport of people or equipment. Can the process be redesigned to improve these?

There are many proprietary process mapping tools, but a common approach with healthcare teams is to simply use sticky notes on a wall or cards on a table (Fig. 29.3). Be sure to make a dated

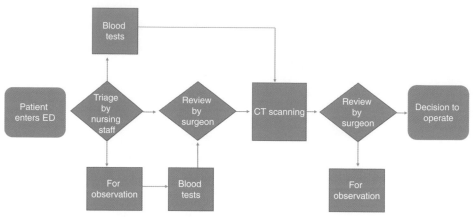

Fig. 29.2 A high-level process map of an emergency surgical attendance to the emergency department. The improvement team should consider the optimum timing of blood tests, computed tomography (CT) scanning, and surgical review to give best value to the patient and to reach the "decision to operate" as quickly as possible.

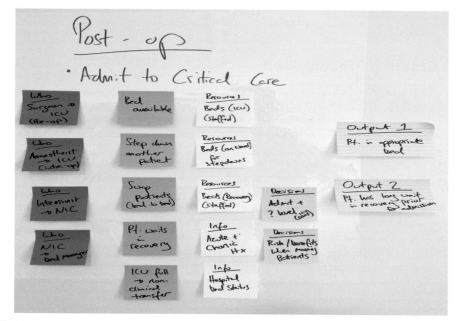

Fig. 29.3 A photograph of the practical development of a process map for discharge of a patient after surgery to intensive care unit (ICU) using sticky notes. Individuals who may be involved in the process are listed, as are steps, resources, decisions that must be made, and possible outcomes.

record of the map; in the future, you may return to this for comparison after you have made some changes to the process.

For work that involves a number of subprocesses or people working in parallel, the map can be arranged in "swim-lanes." These are parallel maps laid out so that the timing of individual sub processes or workers is clear. These are useful to coordinate workers with different roles within a task (Fig. 29.4).

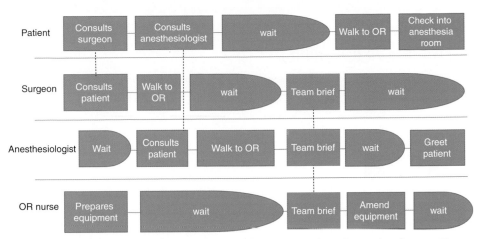

Fig. 29.4 A high-level "swim-lane" process map of the staff and patient tasks on the morning of surgery. Changing the tasks or processes of anyone on the map will have a knock-on impact on the others.

References

1. *Institute for Healthcare Improvement. Going Lean in Health Care. IHI Innovation Series White Paper.* Cambridge, MA: IHI; 2005. www.IHI.org.
2. Jones D., Mitchell A. *Lean Thinking for the NHS.* Vol. 51. NHS Confederation, 2006. https://www.leanuk. org/wp-content/uploads/2020/03/Lean-Thinking-in-the-NHS-Daniel T Jones and Alan-Mitchell.pdf. Accessed September 3, 2021.
3. Marin-Garcia JA, Vidal-Carreras PI, Garcia-Sabater JJ. The role of value stream mapping in healthcare services: a scoping review. *Int J Environ Res Public Health.* 2021;18:951.
4. King R. Virginia Mason Institute. Why is a value stream map important for transforming patient care and decreasing costs? https://www.virginiamasoninstitute.org/why-is-a-value-stream-map-important for transforming-patient-care-and-decreasing-costs/ Accessed September 3, 2021.
5. Shorrock S, Williams C, eds. *Human Factors and Ergonomics in Practice: Improving System Performance and Human Well-Being in the Real World.* CRC Press; 2016.

Further Reading

Boaden R, Harvey G, Moxham C, Proudlove N. *Quality Improvement: Theory and Practice in Healthcare.* NHS Institute for Innovation and Improvement; 2008.

CHAPTER 30

Driver Diagrams

Harry Soar, MB ChB, FRCA ■ Claire Cruikshanks, MB ChB, FRCA

KEY POINTS

- A driver diagram demonstrates the factors underlying a particular outcome.
- It can offer a visual representation of the "theory of change" underpinning the improvement work.
- A driver diagram is useful for generating change ideas that directly link to a desired outcome.
- It is a simple but effective tool to develop and communicate a quality improvement project with team members.
- It can help organize the work that needs to be done.

Introduction

A driver diagram is a simple but powerful improvement tool. It is a concise, visual description of the contributing or "driving" factors that lead to the ultimate goal of an improvement project.[1] Consisting of an overall aim, with associated primary and secondary drivers, the driver diagram demonstrates how different factors logically contribute toward achieving the aim. Collaboratively created and widely shared, a driver diagram can be an excellent way of communicating the overall strategy of a project and serve as a point of reference for teams to ensure efforts are occurring in the key areas related to the stated goal.[2,3] A driver diagram illustrates the theory of change for an area of improvement, and if the theory is sound, the change ideas that address the primary and secondary drivers will lead to improvement.[4,5]

Why make a driver diagram?

- To clarify the key factors or "drivers" that underpin your aim
- To create a visual improvement strategy
- To help communicate your theory of change

Creating a Driver Diagram

Creating a driver diagram starts by gathering a team of people (often termed "stakeholders") who have a good understanding of the current system. Involving staff from a variety of roles will bring different information and perspectives to the topic. This diversity will lead to a more coherent and comprehensive understanding of the system and the factors that underlie an improvement goal. Ideally, in projects focused on improving patient care, a patient representative should be included in the stakeholder group.

SETTING AN AIM

The diagram begins with an aim.[6] This is the overall goal of the improvement project. At this stage, it is worth considering what really matters to the patients you are serving. It might be that outcomes considered important to the team differ from those considered important by the service users.[7] Involving patients through co-production, discussion, and the garnering of feedback through surveys may be helpful.[8]

To give clarity and focus to your aim, consider using the SMART format[9]:

- **S**pecific
- **M**easurable
- **A**chievable
- **R**elevant
- **T**ime-based

Using isolated words like "improving" or "reducing" does not give enough information to those wanting to understand the goal of your improvement effort.

For example, "We aim to reduce waiting times at the preoperative assessment clinic" is not specific enough.

Providing specific details in an aim statement gives clarity to all team members on what you are trying to achieve. A more complete aim statement might look like the following:

"We aim to reduce waiting times (that is from booking in at reception to being seen by the clinician) at the preoperative assessment clinic at St. Elsewhere Hospital by 75% by March 1, 2024."

PRIMARY AND SECONDARY DRIVERS

Once the overall aim is set, the team works together to create the rest of the driver diagram. This process usually involves a brainstorming session, where the team writes down all the areas that require improvement to achieve the stated aim.[10] At this stage the team need not worry about how these improvements will be achieved; just outlining the factors that require attention to achieve the goal is enough. The boundaries of the system to be worked in should also be defined. Is this for a hospital or for only surgical units?

Once this brainstorming process is complete, there may be some overlap and common themes that emerge among the ideas. These common themes are termed "primary drivers" (sometimes also termed "key drivers") and are the main factors that if worked on should lead to the stated aim. By reviewing the rest of the ideas, further links are made, and the team may find smaller and more defined areas for improvement that naturally link to the primary drivers. These are termed "secondary drivers." It may be that a third level of contributory factors that underlie the secondary drivers are discussed; these are unsurprisingly named "tertiary drivers" or change ideas.[11] To tidy up the diagram, it may be helpful to discuss whether some of the drivers should be removed if they are wrong, immaterial to the aim, or duplicated (Fig. 30.1).[12]

Using a Driver Diagram

CHANGE IDEAS

"All improvement requires change, but not every change will result in improvement."[13]

A driver diagram is a great place to start when thinking of change ideas. The diagram illustrates what the team believes are the underlying issues in the given area for improvement. Testing a change

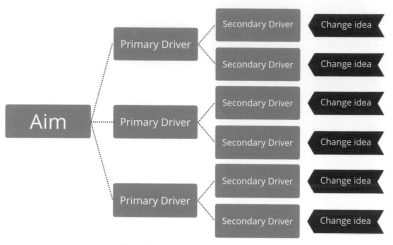

Fig. 30.1 Driver diagram concept.

idea that directly addresses one of the drivers is therefore a logical place to start. The best change ideas are generated by those people who have a profound understanding of how the system works currently, and therefore a range of voices from a variety of multidisciplinary team members is helpful.[14] Brainstorming again at this phase of the driver diagram development as a group will help generate a range of change ideas. These change ideas are the suite of changes that will form your improvement strategy.

It is important to prioritize change ideas and focus the team's efforts where it is most valuable. To do this, consider:

- Which ideas are the most viable?
- Which ideas would have the largest impact?
- Which ideas have a preferable effort-to-impact ratio?
- Which ideas are in your circle of control?

Rather than choosing a very complex, expensive, or time-consuming idea, choosing an idea that is within your circle of control, is inexpensive, and needs few permissions may represent "lower hanging fruit" for improvement.[6]

The driver diagram is not set in stone and can be changed. By testing change ideas and measuring their effect on the outcome, it may be that some drivers are less important than the team first thought. The theory of change (and the driver diagram) can be adjusted accordingly (Fig. 30.2).[4]

COMMUNICATION

A driver diagram is an effective way to communicate change ideas and to demonstrate an improvement strategy. To engage with stakeholders and create a sense of ownership over a proposed change idea, people need to understand the reason for a change. The theoretical concepts underpinning the change idea can be termed a "theory of change"[5] (See Chapter 21 on the Programme Theory of Change). The driver diagram can help offer a visual representation of this theory.[4] It links the ultimate desired outcome to the underlying drivers and therefore justifies testing a change idea. Driver diagrams very quickly allow an understanding of the rationale behind a change idea, and therefore people outside the core team are more likely to be supportive of the change.[5]

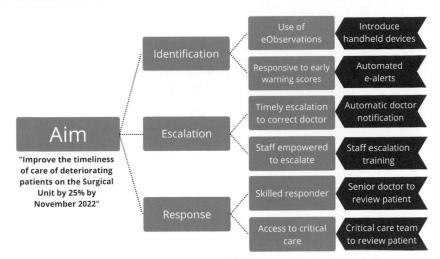

Fig. 30.2 Example of a driver diagram: "Timely care of deteriorating patients."

The diagram can be used at ongoing improvement meetings as a reference point to help keep team efforts on track. Current activities can be checked against the strategy outlined in the diagram to see if they are addressing the agreed-upon drivers and helping work toward the original improvement goal.

Conclusion

The driver diagram is an essential tool for any improvement project. It illustrates the improvement strategy, communicates the theory of change, and connects actions to overall aims. They are simple to create and have multiple benefits.

References

1. Institute for Healthcare Improvement. Driver diagram. http://www.ihi.org/resources/Pages/Tools/Driver-Diagram.aspx. Accessed June 1, 2021.
2. Xu W, Huang Y, Bai J, Varughese AM. A quality improvement project to reduce postoperative adverse respiratory events and increase safety in the post-anesthesia care unit of a pediatric institution. *Paediatr Anaesth.* 2019;29(2):200–210. https://doi.org/10.1111/pan.13534.
3. Caruso TJ, Trivedi S, Chadwick W, et al. A quality improvement project to reduce combination acetaminophen-opioid prescriptions to pediatric orthopedic patients. *Ped Qual Safety.* 2020;5(3):e291.
4. Driver diagrams. https://improvements.hpft.nhs.uk/start-an-improvement-project/driver-diagrams/. Accessed June 1, 2021.
5. Davidoff F, Dixon-Woods M, Leviton L, Michie S. Demystifying theory and its use in improvement. *BMJ Qual Safety.* 2015;24(3):228–238.
6. Quality Improvement, East London NHS Foundation Trust. Driver diagrams. https://qi.elft.nhs.uk/resource/driver-diagrams/. Accessed June 1, 2021.
7. Elwyn G, Nelson E, Hager A, Price A. Coproduction: when users define quality. *BMJ Qual Safety.* 2020;29(9):711–716.
8. Realpe A, Wallace LM. What Is Co-Production? *The Health Foundation;* 2010. http://www.qi.elft.nhs.uk/wp-content/uploads/2017/01/what_is_co-production.pdf.

9. TIPSQI. Step 5c—Defining the project: SMART aims. https://tipsqi.co.uk/guide-5c/. Accessed June 1, 2021.

10. Peden CJ. Improvement basics: driver diagrams. In: Chereshneva M, Johnston C, Colvin JR, Peden CJ, eds. *Raising the Standards: RCoA Quality Improvement Compendium.* 4th ed. The Royal College of Anaesthetists; 2020. https://www.rcoa.ac.uk/sites/default/files/documents/2020-08/21075%20RCoA%20Audit%20Recipe%20Book_Combined_Final_25.08.2020_0.pdf. Accessed 1 June 2021.

11. Perioperative Quality Improvement Programme. Driver diagrams—tool kit. https://pqip.org.uk/FilesUploaded/How-to%20Driver%20Diagrams%20PQIP.pdf. Accessed June 1, 2021.

12. NHS Institute for Innovation and Improvement. An example of a Driver Diagram. https://www.england.nhs.uk/improvement-hub/wp-content/uploads/sites/44/2018/06/An-example-of-driver-diagrams-1.pdf. Accessed June 1, 2021.

13. *The Improvement Guide: A Practical Approach to Enhancing Organizational Performance.* 2nd ed. https://learning.oreilly.com/library/view/the-improvement-guide/9780470549032/. Accessed June 1, 2021.

14. Lothian Quality. Lens of profound knowledge. https://qilothian.scot.nhs.uk/pc-resource-lens-of-profound-knowledge. Accessed June 1, 2021.

CHAPTER 31

Care Bundles for Perioperative Improvement

Carol J. Peden, MB ChB, MD, FRCA, FFICM, MPH

KEY POINTS

- Care bundles provide a means of grouping a small number of evidence-based components together for a defined patient group or setting of care to facilitate a desired and improved outcome.
- The processes, when grouped into a bundle, should have a synergistic impact compared with individual use.
- The processes in the care bundle should be delivered regularly and highly reliably.
- An effective bundle should have all or no responses (e.g., in the central line insertion bundle, the answer to the question "Was the patient appropriately draped?" can only be yes or no).
- For effective implementation of a care bundle to occur, teamwork and communication are central, and culture change may be necessary.
- Care bundles are not the same as "bundled care"; the latter term is applied in the United States to care management and associated funding across the continuum of care for a defined procedure, such as a total joint replacement.

Background

The concept of a care bundle was developed in 2001 by the Institute of Healthcare Improvement (IHI) to improve management and decrease harm in intensive care unit (ICU) patients who were on ventilators.[1] This bundle is now well recognized as the "care of the ventilated patient" bundle. The central line bundle was also developed as part of the same project, "Idealized Design of the Intensive Care Unit," in which the two topic areas (ventilators and central lines) were chosen because they were recognized to have high rates of patient harm and to have clear evidence-based practices, which if applied reliably, could lead to improved outcomes. The need to group key processes together to lead to better outcomes than would occur if the processes were delivered singly was recognized during the IHI ICU project. Teams were required to work together to create solutions that would facilitate reliable delivery of all components of the bundle.

In addition to the central line bundle and the care of the ventilated patient bundle,[2,3] another application of care bundles familiar to perioperative clinicians is found in the "Surviving Sepsis" campaign.[4,5] Increasing bundle compliance in the Surviving Sepsis campaign has been associated with decreasing mortality.[4] Short, clear, and concise bundles are easier to implement, and the Surviving Sepsis bundle approach has evolved from two bundles to a simpler 1-hour bundle.[5] Evolution and adaption of a bundle over time as new evidence emerges should occur because bundles form only one part of an improvement approach, which must include measurement and behavioral change.

Why Do Bundles Work?

Measurement is a key component of bundle implementation, and in the IHI ICU project, it was rapidly recognized that standard components of care were not being delivered reliably.[1] That has been my experience when working on bundle implementation both in my own units and on collaborative projects around the world. The realization by the care team that essential processes of care do not occur as reliably as assumed is an important one. There then must be a cultural acknowledgment that providing reliable care is hard, and other tools and techniques such as frequent measurement and feedback on performance are required to ensure high reliability. This contrasts to the familiar approach often used in medicine, which believes that knowing more and working harder will be enough.

When beginning to work toward high reliability with a given bundle, it may be appropriate to work on each process individually, then, as each component becomes highly reliable, teams can consider aiming for high reliability with the whole bundle. This is challenging and will usually require the development of aids, such as prompts that can be delivered through the electronic health record (EHR) and redundancies. An example of an aid used to help delivery of a bundle is the "Boarding Card," a checklist developed to increase key bundle adherence in an emergency laparotomy bundle.[6]

Analysis of the "Michigan Keystone" project, a statewide scale up of an ICU collaborative[7] including implementation of the central line insertion bundle, showed that success depended on much more than defining care components and grouping them in a bundle.[8] Bundle implementation was accompanied by implementation of a Comprehensive Unit-Based Safety Program (CUSP) with a focus on teamwork and learning from safety events and an ICU reporting system. The statewide implementation became a social process with chief executive officer (CEO) sign-up required and pressure for ICUs to join a community of around other 100 ICUs working on the problem. The central line infection issue was reframed as a social problem (i.e., not just a technical list of actions that might fix a harm but a dynamic issue that requires consideration of how the interventions will be delivered reliably). A culture change was fostered to move to expectation of high performance and zero tolerance of infection. Some discipline was involved, with ICUs being required to openly disclose their infection rates, a process that drove further improvement. Culture change is complex and local, and a similar approach to reduce central line infection with bundle implementation in the UK was not so effective. Local rates were already low, and work had been ongoing for some time on central line infection. Also, the project was viewed as government enforced and so it was much harder to generate a community with the type of study design used. Nevertheless, the single most important factor for success that emerged was the degree of agreement and multidisciplinary working that was present between medical and nursing staff on an individual unit.[9]

Components that should be considered in development of a bundle are shown in Fig. 31.1.

Examples of Bundle Application in Perioperative Care

A care bundle was designed to improve care in high-risk patients undergoing emergency laparotomy and was termed the ELPQuIC bundle, which stands for the Emergency Laparotomy Pathway Quality Improvement Care bundle.[10,11] This bundle was designed to ensure that high-impact, evidence-based care components, which were frequently not delivered reliably, were provided to this group of surgical patients. The components were developed after reviewing the evidence, considering the patient pathway and gaps in care, and ensuring multidisciplinary team consensus. A pilot project showed a significant reduction in risk-adjusted mortality, and delivery of all bundle elements improved. This pilot was then scaled up with bundle implementation across 28 hospitals in a large study entitled the Emergency Laparotomy Collaborative (ELC).[12] This study showed a reduction in mortality and length of stay (compared with the preintervention group and with

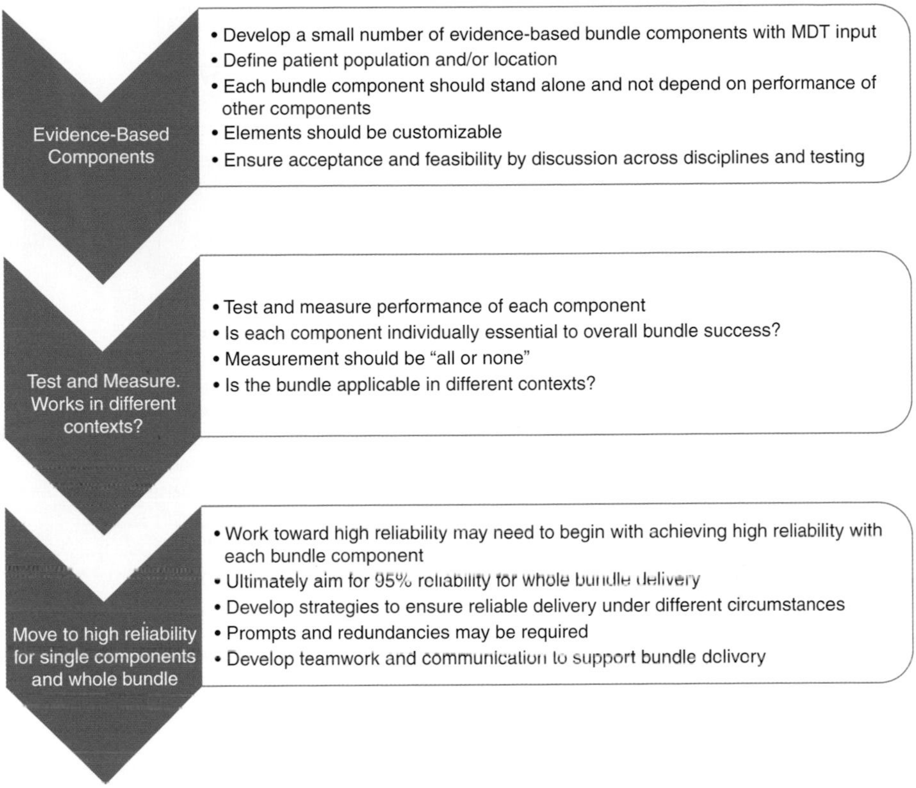

- Develop a small number of evidence-based bundle components with MDT input
- Define patient population and/or location
- Each bundle component should stand alone and not depend on performance of other components
- Elements should be customizable
- Ensure acceptance and feasibility by discussion across disciplines and testing

Evidence-Based Components

- Test and measure performance of each component
- Is each component individually essential to overall bundle success?
- Measurement should be "all or none"
- Is the bundle applicable in different contexts?

Test and Measure. Works in different contexts?

- Work toward high reliability may need to begin with achieving high reliability with each bundle component
- Ultimately aim for 95% reliability for whole bundle delivery
- Develop strategies to ensure reliable delivery under different circumstances
- Prompts and redundancies may be required
- Develop teamwork and communication to support bundle delivery

Move to high reliability for single components and whole bundle

Fig. 31.1 Key components in development of a care bundle. *MDT,* multidisciplinary team.

national data) and a significant improvement in the delivery of the majority of processes. With this larger project, it took time for change to be seen, and bundle implementation was supported by regular data feedback, coaching in leadership, and change management for teams, with multiple opportunities for mutual and synergistic learning across the collaborative. The ELPQuIC bundle as applied in ELC is shown in Fig. 31.2.

Another area in the perioperative arena where the concept of care bundles has been applied is in the prevention of postoperative pulmonary complications (PCCs). PCCs are common in postoperative patients and yet there is less literature and discussion about them than with postoperative cardiac complications. One large single-center study of the application of a bundle of processes called I-COUGH, evaluated through the National Surgical Quality Improvement Program (NSQIP) database, showed a reduction in the incidence of pneumonia and unplanned intubation.[13] This program emphasized education and standardization as part of the implementation strategy, so that every patient, regardless of surgical team, unit, or procedure, received the evidence-based care. The multidisciplinary team was involved in design and implementation of the bundle throughout. The authors noted that maintenance of their results required constant reinforcement of the I-COUGH principles, audit, and feedback. In line with enhanced recovery principles, patient and family education about the importance of I-COUGH, began preoperatively. A recent Canadian study applying I-COUGH in high-risk hepatectomy and Whipple's patients showed a significantly reduced incidence of postoperative pneumonia and consequently costs.[14] Again, this study used the NSQIP database and emphasized the importance of the multidisciplinary team, patient and family engagement and education, and standardized staff and patient materials.

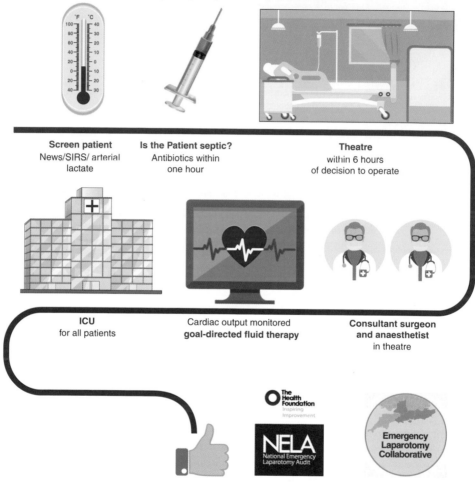

Fig. 31.2 The six ELPQuIC bundle components[10,11] applied in the Emergency Laparotomy Collaborative.[12] (From Peden C, Aggarwal G, Quiney N, et al. 1040 The emergency laparotomy collaborative: scaling up an improvement bundle for high risk surgical patients. *BMJ Open Quality.* 2017;6.)

ABCDEF Bundle in Intensive Care

The Society of Critical Care Medicines ICU Liberation, or ABCDEF, bundle[15] may not be used directly in the perioperative arena; however, it will be applied to many patients who are managed in intensive care after surgery. This care bundle is complex, with six component parts:

A: **A**ssess, Prevent, and Manage Pain

B: **B**oth Spontaneous Awakening Trials (SATs) and Spontaneous **B**reathing Trials (SBTs)

C: **C**hoice of Analgesia and Sedation

D: **D**elirium: Assess, Prevent, and Manage

E: **E**arly Mobility and Exercise

F: **F**amily Engagement and Empowerment

Each component of this bundle requires a number of steps, and thus reaching high reliability (95% of performance of all bundle components) is extremely hard. Nevertheless, even small improvements in overall bundle performance can lead to better outcomes. A paper evaluating more than 15,000 ICU patients who received the bundle showed a significant and dose-related improvement in important outcomes, such as mortality, next-day ventilation, and discharge to a destination other than home. Patients who received more of the ABCDEF bundle elements each day had a large and significantly improved likelihood of surviving.[16]

Bundles can show a dose response curve. Although high reliability is desired, a number of studies have shown that the more bundle components that are implemented, and with increasing fidelity, a related improvement in outcomes is seen.[10,12,16]

What Care Bundles Are Not?

In the United States, the Centers for Medicare and Medicaid Services (CMS) Innovation Center introduced a concept to drive care toward value and address the fragmented care caused by fee-for-service payments for separate steps in patient care pathways. This approach was trialed as the "bundled payments for care initiative" (BPCI) between 2013 and 2017. This bundled payment approach is very different from a care bundle because it is focused on incentive alignment across a very wide patient pathway, including multiple providers (e.g., hospitals, post-acute care providers, physicians, and other practitioners). This approach has had some success in the perioperative arena, particularly with joint replacements, driving down the use of postacute care facilities and implant costs.[17,18]

Some improvement approaches have been termed care bundles but include multiple steps and components and are more akin to checklists or protocols. Any considered approach to defining key components of care for improvement is likely to be helpful, but it is worth remembering that the further away from the original bundle concept of three to five key interventions a pathway is moved, the harder it will be to implement with high reliability.

Meta-Analysis

A meta-analysis of the effect of care bundles concluded that the implementation of care bundles may be an effective strategy to improve patient outcomes compared with usual care but noted that the quality of evidence was low. Nevertheless, the authors noted that a significant limitation in their analysis was grouping multiple different care bundles tackling different conditions and in different settings together. The important point was made that future studies should focus on the explicit and transparent reporting of implementation approaches for care bundles and particularly the fidelity of adherence to a particular strategy. The commonest methods used in implementation were audit and feedback, education, and reminders.[19]

References

1. Resar R, Griffin FA, Haraden C, Nolan TW. *Using Care Bundles to Improve Health Care Quality.* IHI Innovation Series white paper, Institute for Healthcare Improvement; 2012. www.IHI.org.
2. Eom JS, Lee MS, Chun HK, et al. The impact of a ventilator bundle on preventing ventilator-associated pneumonia: a multicenter study. *Am J Infect Control.* 2014;42(1):34–37.
3. Pronovost PJ, Needham D, Berenholtz SM, et al. An intervention to decrease catheter related bloodstream infections in the ICU. *NEJM.* 2006;355:2725–2732.

4. Levy MM, Rhodes A, Philips GS, et al. Surviving Sepsis Campaign: association between performance metrics and outcomes in a 7.5-year study. *Crit Care Med.* 2015;43(1):3–12.
5. Levy MM, Evans LE, Rhodes A. The Surviving Sepsis Campaign Bundle: 2018 update. *Crit Care Med.* 2018;46(60):997–1000.
6. Richards SK, Cook TM, Dalton SJ, Peden CJ, Howes TE. The 'Bath Boarding Card': a novel tool for improving pre-operative care for emergency laparotomy patients. *Anaesthesia.* 2016;71(8):974–976.
7. Lipitz-Snyderman A, Steinwachs D, Needham DM, et al. Impact of a statewide intensive care unit quality improvement initiative on hospital mortality and length of stay: retrospective comparative analysis. *BMJ.* 2011;342, d219.
8. Dixon-Woods M, Bosk CL, Aveling EL, Goeschel CA, Pronovost PJ. Explaining Michigan: developing an ex post theory of a quality improvement program. *Milbank Q.* 2011;89(2):167–205.
9. Dixon-Woods M, Leslie M, Tarrant C, Bion J. Explaining Matching Michigan: an ethnographic study of a patient safety program. *Implement Sci.* 2013;20(8):70.
10. Huddart S, Peden CJ, Swart M, et al. Use of a pathway quality improvement care bundle to reduce mortality after emergency laparotomy. *Br J Surg.* 2015;102(1):57–66.
11. Quiney N, Huddart S, Peden C, Dickinson M. Use of a care bundle to reduce mortality following emergency laparotomy. *Br J Hosp Med (Lond).* 2015;76(6):358–362.
12. Aggarwal G, Peden CJ, Mohammed MA, et al. Emergency laparotomy collaborative. *JAMA Surg.* 2019;20: e190145.
13. Cassidy MR, Rosenkranz P, McCabe K, Rosen JE, McAneny D. I COUGH: Reducing postoperative pulmonary complications with a multidisciplinary patient care program. *JAMA Surg.* 2013;148(8):740–745.
14. Mahama G, Vigneswaran L, Silva A, et al. A bundled approach to care: reducing the incidence of post-operative pneumonia in patients undergoing hepatectomy and Whipple procedures. *Can J Surg.* 2021;64(1):E9–E13.
15. Marra A, Ely E, Pandharipande P, Patel M. The ABCDEF bundle in critical care. *Crit Care Clin.* 2017; 33(2):225–243.
16. Pun B, Balas M, Barnes-Daly M, et al. Caring for critically ill patients with the ABCDEF bundle: results of the ICU Liberation Collaborative in over 15,000 adults. *Crit Care Med.* 2019;47(1):3–14.
17. NEJM Catalyst. What are bundled payments? *NEJM Catalyst.* 2018. https://catalyst.nejm.org/doi/full/10.1056/CAT.18.0247.
18. Navathe AS, Troxel AB, Liao JM, et al. Cost of joint replacement using bundled payment models. *JAMA Intern Med.* 2017;177(2):214–222.
19. Lavallée JF, Gray TA, Dumville J, Russell W, Cullum N. The effects of care bundles on patient outcomes: a systematic review and meta-analysis. *Implement Sci.* 2017;29;12(1):142.

CHAPTER 32

Human Factors in Perioperative Care: General Principles

Peter McCulloch, MB ChB, MA, MD, FCRSEd, FRCS

KEY POINTS

- Human factors (HF) is a scientific discipline that uses observation and analysis of work processes to identify opportunities for improvement and design interventions to implement these.
- HF differs from standard quality improvement (QI) in its reliance on systematic analysis of work using standardized tools and in its focus on the humans in the system.
- HF shares with QI a belief in the importance of co-design of changes with the frontline workers and iterative improvement using rapid tests of change.
- HF uses insights into cognitive, perceptual, and social aspects of teamwork to identify ways of making it easy to do things the right way and designing out error.
- HF considers team culture and relationships with higher management in its analysis and provides general principles for dealing with both, which are relevant to multidisciplinary relationships within the operating room and ward teams and with hospital management.

Human factors (HF) is a discipline that studies work systems involving human beings, including their interactions with each other and with the systems, processes, and technology they use. It can be applied to both efficiency and safety in perioperative care. It shares several features with classic quality improvement (QI) programs but differs particularly in emphasis on expert analysis of work systems using a portfolio of standardized tools, models, and measures. This analysis permits a richer understanding of the system, which can help design more elegant and insightful solutions to problems than might be developed using iterative modification of ideas proposed by frontline workers. One aspect of HF that has attracted considerable interest is team training to increase awareness of the cognitive, perceptual, and communication limitations of humans. This appears to enhance engagement with QI initiatives, but the evidence that it improves patient safety on its own is weak. The classic model of HF system analysis has recently been challenged by a new paradigm (Safety II), which emphasizes the need for trade-offs between efficiency, safety, and other objectives. Whereas classic HF analysis sought to identify and fix faults in the system, Safety II seeks to enhance the resilience of the system (i.e., its ability to respond dynamically to changes) and therefore places greater emphasis on learning from success. At present, it is not clear whether or when Safety II produces more satisfactory outcomes than classic HF, and the development of a hybrid approach incorporating elements of both appears to be an interesting potential way forward.

What Do We Mean by Human Factors?

There is a significant degree of overlap between HF and other disciplines involved in QI, but the term is often used incorrectly in health care. The World Health Organization (WHO) definition[1] states: "Human factors examines the relationship between human beings and the systems they work in, focusing on improving efficiency, safety, creativity, productivity and job satisfaction." The overlap with QI disciplines is obvious, the differences perhaps less so. Both QI and HF use a systematic approach to analyzing and rationalizing systems and processes and solving problems. Both advocate close cooperation with frontline staff in devising solutions. HF, however, emphasizes expert professional techniques in systems analysis, whereas QI approaches often rely on frontline workers for both data collection and understanding of the system. The Toyota Production System,[2] for example, used no HF professionals but looked to the frontline worker for both diagnosis and solution of problems. This is potentially risky because frontline staff without systems analysis training may misunderstand complex systems problems, resulting in ineffective initiatives.

Practical Suggestion: If you can afford it, hire an HF specialist to analyze your work process and help you plan your QI approach.

The other obvious distinction between QI and HF is the attention given to humans as sources of both problems and solutions. QI systems create a goal and expect staff to achieve it, with relatively little consideration of their motivation. HF places more importance on studying the humans and their interactions with each other, the system, and the technology they have to deal with. It concerns itself with cognitive, perceptual, and psycho-social issues such as fatigue, hierarchy, and tunnel vision during crisis situations. This provides a richer understanding of the system than standard QI approaches. It is, however, very difficult to compare the effectiveness of HF and QI in improving either quality or safety because of the substantial overlap in their methods and the overriding importance of staff engagement as a success factor for both types of project. Our group conducted a program of safety improvement experiments with surgical operating room (OR) teams, comparing and combining a "Lean" QI approach and a more HF-based systems improvement approach with an approach based purely on teamwork training. We found little difference between the redesign approaches of the two systems, but convincing evidence that the team training acted as an adjuvant to both, whilst having little effect on its own.[3,4]

The type of team training used in this work, Crew Resource Management (CRM), has been widely advocated in health care and formed the basis for programs such as MedTeams. Its early popularity led many healthcare professionals to associate HF only with this type of team training, focusing on cognitive, perceptual, and communications problems. Although it remains popular, the literature does not present a convincing case for patient benefit. Four systematic reviews have shown a small improvement in outcomes,[5–8] but this is entirely because of the effect of a single very large Veterans Administration (VA) study,[9] which was biased by an important methodological error. The study compared VA hospitals after training with those that had not yet had it during the roll-out of a system-wide implementation, but the order in which sites received the training was based on "readiness."

Practical Suggestion: Team training based on HF can enhance engagement with QI programs, so it may be worth considering as an adjunct.

Standard Human Factors Approach to Analysis of Work

HF interventions often begin with ethnographic observation, where the observer tries not to interfere with normal work patterns or team interactions. Photo, video, and documentary evidence may be used, and interviews help build up a picture of how workers see things. The data are used to develop an algorithmic model of the work system, represented by a whole process map plus models of key tasks known as "Cognitive and Hierarchical Task Analyses." Another HF approach, often used after safety incidents, is to model the influences on work and its outcomes in terms of several dimensions, using a system such as the Systems Engineering Initiative for Patient Safety (SEIPS) model.[10] Key problem areas in a process can be highlighted using Failure Modes and Effects Analysis (FMEA) techniques. FMEA goes through an existing description, such as a hierarchical task analysis, in detail, considering at each step the various ways (modes) in which the step could fail and the likelihood and severity of the effects of such a failure. Multiplying the likelihood by the severity estimate for each step gives a kind of "heat map" of risk within the process (Table 32.1 is an example).

In the currently popular modified version of HF (Safety II, see later), these techniques are replaced by models based largely on qualitative analysis of interviews with frontline staff, such as the Functional Resonance Analysis Method (FRAM). FRAM describes the connections between the "functions" in a process and their nature, classifying these links into six "aspects": input, output, precondition, resource, control, and time (Fig. 32.1). Safety II is principally concerned with identifying variability in processes and its causes, rather than specifically focusing on risk and error.

Practical Suggestion: FMEA and FRAM provide complementary insights into processes, which can help identify areas for change.

Approach to Improvement

Analysis of the system leads to recommendations for change. The goal in health care, as in other safety critical industries, is to produce highly reliable systems in which harm is minimized, but efficiency, effectiveness, and worker well-being are also desirable objectives, and HF seeks solutions that achieve multiple objectives simultaneously. Some QI systems place great importance on objective measurement as the key driver for improvement, whereas HF tends to regard the impressions and opinions of staff as at least equally important. The core QI methodology of Plan Do Study/ Check Act (PDSA/PDCA) cycles is often less formal in HF projects, but the principle of continuous rapid feedback and iteration is retained (Box 32.1). HF specialists also recognize the need for engagement at all levels of the organization for successful change management and, therefore, regularly communicate with senior managers and other important stakeholders.

Focus on Humans

The origins of HF were often concerned with making tasks more convenient, comfortable, and safe. The humans working in the system are regarded as both an essential component and as individuals whose safety and satisfaction should be prioritized. HF solutions are designed around the humans using them, making them easy to use and preventing errors by design whenever possible. This includes consideration of aspects like individual fatigue and the culture of work teams. The salience of work culture and team relationships in disasters, both within health care[11] and in other industries (e.g., Chernobyl, Deepwater Horizon, Korean Airlines) is clear. Changing culture is complex and difficult, but if analysis suggests that it is necessary, it is self-defeating to ignore it, because engagement with systems change will remain anemic in the face of adverse cultural attitudes. Neither HF nor other disciplines involved with change management have developed a reliably successful approach to culture change, and only general principles can be proposed with any confidence. These include leadership that sets clear goals; trust between leadership and workforce; and careful design of roles and responsibilities to empower and incentivize facilitation of necessary change.

Practical Suggestion: Always aim for solutions that make it easy to do it right and impossible to do it wrong.

Safety I and Safety II: Humans as the Solution

A more nuanced approach to improving the quality of work and work processes has arisen in the HF community in recent years. The "Safety II" movement relies on the work of writers such as

TABLE 32.1 ■ A Failure Modes and Effects Analysis (FMEA) Applied to the Accurate Recording and Prescribing of a High-Risk Perioperative Medication (A Parkinson's Disease Medication)[a]

Step Description	Failure Modes	Consequences	Risk Evaluation	Possible Causes	Control Risk/Control Measures
Patient attends preoperative assessment clinic	No medication list Inaccurate medication list No medication history available	Unable to establish accurate medication history No documentation of medications	Severity — Minor 2; Likelihood — Likely 4; = 8 Low-risk	Did not receive preoperative information letter No current medication list available Patient forgot to bring in Poor historian	Patients sent preoperative letter with information regarding medication Carer involvement Nursing home medication sheet available Information from nurse specialist to preoperative clinic Nurses may contact primary care for information
Patient attends preoperative assessment clinic	No patient advice on withholding medication preoperative	Patient inappropriately withholds or takes medication on day of operation	Severity — Major 4; Likelihood — Possible 3; = 12 Medium risk	Insufficient medication history to advise patient Insufficient knowledge of nurse Inadequate information sent to patient preoperative	Letter to patient from preoperative
Patient admitted to admission suite	No medication history available	No/inaccurate medication chart Missed doses Potential deterioration in condition Patient anxiety	Severity — Major 4; Likelihood — Likely 4; = 16 High risk	Consequences of incomplete preassessment process	Patient/carer may bring in medication/medication list

Patient admitted to admission suite	No responsibility taken for writing medication chart	Anesthetist not aware of medication regime — Patient misses doses — increased anxiety Delay in medication chart being written until on postoperative floor Potential deterioration in condition	Severity — Major 4; Likelihood — Almost certain 5; = 20 High risk	None
Patient admitted to admission suite	Surgeon unaware of Parkinson's disease condition and medication regime	Inappropriate management of patient in theatre/postanesthesia care unit (PACU)	Severity — Major 4; Likelihood — Possible 3; = 12 Medium risk	Consequences of incomplete preassessment process No documentation	None

RISK SCORE	RATING
1 — 4	Insignificant
5 — 9	Low
10 — 15	Medium Risk
16 — 24	High
25	Extreme

SEVERITY
1 — Negligible
2 — Minor
3 — Moderate
4 — Major
5 — Catastrophic

LIKELIHOOD
1 — Rare
2 — Unlikely
3 — Possible
4 — Likely
5 — Almost certain

aEach step is analyzed for the likelihood of the occurrence happening and then given a risk score for the consequences should that likelihood occur. This provides a structure around which to plan an approach, which takes into account not only the risk of the problem but also the likelihood of occurrence.

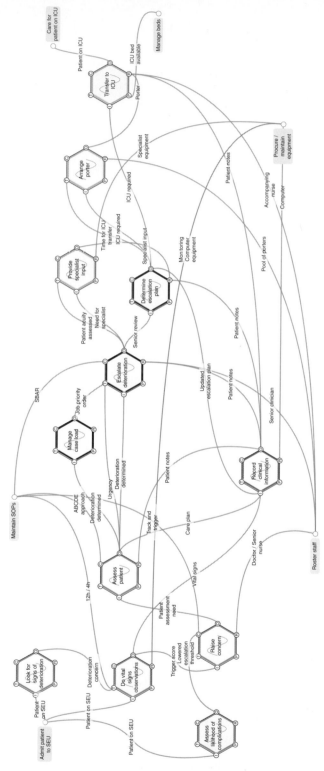

Fig. 32.1 An example of a FRAM analysis diagram: This shows the process of responding to deterioration in surgical patients. *FRAM*, Functional Resonance Analysis Method.

BOX 32.1 ■ PDCA Cycles

In a study of high levels of patient falls on a neurosurgery unit, observation revealed a high percentage occurred when patients attempted to reach a toilet unassisted during the night. The solution selected was to include "Do you need the toilet?" in the intentional rounding (IR) routine carried out at regular intervals by nursing staff.

Intervention

Cycle 1 Changes:
- IR introduced and trialed on a 26-bed area of the ward
- IR training video and drop-in days for staff to learn about IR
- IR log sheet for each patient with stamps for staff to stamp their rounds

Staff Feedback (n = 5):
- Increased workload (80%)
- Unsure if helpful (56% said it was helpful)
- IR unachievable (75% said no/unsure)
- Unsure whether IR increased patient satisfaction or safety (56%; 56%)

Cycle 2 Changes:
- IR log sheet as per Cycle 1
- Extended training and opportunities for staff to come ask about IR
- Prompt cards introduced (clear set of tasks for rounding)
- Trialed on same area of ward

Staff Feedback (n = 7):
- No effect on workload (71%)
- Helpful and achievable (92%; 83%)
- Believed IR increased patient satisfaction and safety (92%; 92%)

Cycle 3 Changes:
- Training drop-in days for new log sheet
- IR log sheet per ward area rather than per patient (except for High Care area)
- Alternating rounding hours for nurses and care support workers (CSWs)
- Trialed on the entire 75-bed ward

Staff Feedback (n = 7):
- No effect on workload (67%)
- Helpful and achievable (78%; 78%)
- Believed IR increased patient satisfaction and safety (67%; 89%)

Cycle 4 Changes:
- Staff given the choice of two options:
  - IR sheet per patient
  - IR sheet per ward area
- Trialed on the entire 75-bed ward
- Staff choose option the per patient sheet

Final Improvement:

IR sheet per patient was used, where staff marked when patient was seen.

IR, Intentional rounding; *PDCA*, Plan Do Check Act.

Amalberti, Hollnagel, and Shorrock,[12–14] arguing that the reality of work process is always different from the theoretical model developed by management. This difference between "work as imagined" and "work as done" should not be regarded as a fault because it usually results from adaptation by workers to allow faster or more efficient work based on their intimate knowledge of the system. Most workplaces—including in health care—constantly require workers to make trade-offs between competing objectives. In complex systems, the outcomes of such choices always have an element of unpredictability because of the influence of unknown variables. This quality of "emergence" makes the creation of an error-free perfect system impossible, and means that choices will always have unpredictable results, undermining the "root cause analysis" approach to error. The Safety II prescription for optimizing system function—very familiar to those involved in organizing emergency surgery—is to maximize "resilience" (the ability of the system to adapt rapidly). Considerable emphasis is put on learning from success and from failure. Although Safety II analysis clearly has validity, current guidance on how to implement it for practical improvement is underdeveloped and vague, and empirical evidence of its superiority is lacking. Our current experience in attempting to use Safety II in a program of action research in surgery (RESPOND [Rescue for Emergency Surgery Patients Observed to uNdergo acute Deterioration]) is providing interesting insights into the challenges of operationalizing its precepts. Using Safety I and Safety II models together seems to provide a more complete description of work systems than either approach alone. This author recommends that, until operational approaches to Safety II intervention are better defined and validated, it should be used as a high-level conceptual guide in concert with tools and methods from the Safety I repertoire.

Practical Suggestion: Keep the Safety II approach in mind when designing the change you want. Aim for more flexibility and resilience in the face of challenges.

References

1. World Health Organisation. Patient safety curriculum guide: multi-professional edition, 2011. https://www.who.int/publications/i/item/patient-safety-curriculum-guide-multi-professional-edition. Accessed June 21, 2021.
2. Ohno T. *Toyota Production System: Beyond Large Scale Production.* Cambridge, MA: Productivity Press; 1988.
3. McCulloch P, Morgan L, Flynn L, et al. *Safer delivery of surgical services: a programme of controlled before-and-after intervention studies with pre-planned pooled data analysis.* Southampton (UK): NIHR Journals Library; 2016. PMID: 27977092.
4. Flynn LC, McCulloch PG, Morgan LJ, et al. The Safer Delivery of Surgical Services Program (S3): explaining its differential effectiveness and exploring implications for improving quality in complex systems. *Ann Surg.* 2016;264(6):997–1003.
5. McCulloch P, Rathbone J, Catchpole K. Interventions to improve teamwork and communications among healthcare staff. *Br J Surg.* 2011;98(4):469–479.
6. Gordon M, Darbyshire D, Baker P. Non-technical skills training to enhance patient safety: a systematic review. *Med Educ.* 2012;46(11):1042–1054.
7. Hughes AM, Gregory ME, Joseph DL, et al. Saving lives: a meta-analysis of team training in healthcare. *J Appl Psychol.* 2016;101:1266–1304.
8. Costar DM, Hall KK. Improving team performance and patient safety on the job through team training and performance support tools: a systematic review. *J Patient Saf.* 2020;16(3S(suppl 1)):S48–S56.
9. Neily J, Mills PD, Young-Xu Y, et al. Association between implementation of a medical team training program and surgical mortality. *JAMA.* 2010;304(15):1693–1700.
10. Carayon P, Schoofs Hundt A, Karsh BT, et al. Work system design for patient safety: the SEIPS model. *Qual Saf Health Care.* 2006;15(suppl 1):i50–i58.
11. Francis R. Mid Staffordshire NHS Foundation Trust Public Inquiry. *Report of the Mid Staffordshire NHS Foundation Trust Public Inquiry.* HC (Series) (Great Britain. Parliament. House of Commons), 947, 2012–13. London: The Stationery Office; 2013.
12. Morel G, Amalberti R, Chauvin C. Articulating the differences between safety and resilience: the decision-making process of professional sea-fishing skippers. *Hum Factors.* 2008;50(1):1–16.
13. Hollnagel E, Woods DD, Leveson N. *Resilience Engineering: Concepts and Precepts.* Aldershot, England: Ashgate Publishing; 2007.
14. Shorrock S, Williams C, Williams C. Human Factors and Ergonomics in Practice [Internet]. Shorrock S, Williams C, editors. Taylor & Francis Group, 6000 Broken Sound Parkway NW, Suite 300, Boca Raton, FL 33487-2742: CRC Press; 2016.

CHAPTER 33

Human Factors and Perioperative Improvement: Handover Checklists and Protocols for Safe and Reliable Care Transitions

Caoimhe C. Duffy, MD, MSc, CPPS, FCAI   ■   Meghan B. Lane-Fall, MD, MSHP, FCCM

KEY POINTS

- A checklist is a complex sociotechnical intervention that requires careful attention to instrument design, implementation, and identification of essential task-oriented skills.
- Successful implementation of checklists must leverage human factors engineering and implementation science principles to promote "stickiness," or habit formation, and to mediate successful culture change.
- Creating a standardized handover checklist and following a structured process for handover increases the accuracy of information transferred, increases positive clinician perception of handover quality, and may improve patient outcomes.

Handover Checklists

Handovers are the exchange of information and responsibility of a patient from one provider or team to another at transition points in that patient's care pathway. They are frequent in the perioperative period and are susceptible to communication breakdowns.[1] Poor communication at the time of a handover is associated with information transmission errors, adverse advents, and preventable clinical errors.[2-5]

A checklist is a cognitive aid designed to support recall under both routine and stressed conditions.[6] More than a simple tool, a checklist is a complex sociotechnical intervention that requires careful attention to instrument design, implementation, and identification of essential task-oriented skill sets.[7] A successful checklist in the perioperative domain requires both an established safety culture and significant collaborative input and proactive leadership from surgeons and other operating room (OR) professionals.[8,9] In health care, the seminal studies by Gawande and colleagues[10] and Pronovost et al.[11] demonstrated the value of checklists in driving patient quality and safety improvement programs. One of the most high-profile examples of perioperative checklists is the World Health Organization's (WHO's) Surgical Safety Checklist (SSC) developed as part of their 2006 "Safe Surgery Saves Lives" campaign. Although the initial implementation study demonstrated an association between SSC adherence and a reduction in postoperative mortality, the generalizability of the SSC has subsequently been called into question, with validation studies meeting with varying success.[9,12–14] This demonstrates that successful implementation of checklists requires more than just a well-designed checklist and must leverage human factors engineering and implementation science principles to promote "stickiness" (habit formation) and to mediate successful culture change.

The perioperative environment is complex and dynamic, with frequent interruptions and staff changes. Breakdown in multidisciplinary teamwork in the OR is reported as one of the most common contributory factors toward the occurrence of wrong-site surgeries and other surgical adverse events.[8] High-quality structured perioperative checklists facilitate clear communication and teamwork, embed patient-level risk-estimation, and verbalize mitigation planning for identified risks (introductions, discussion of patient risk factors, concerns). Checklists act to familiarize team members with one another. Sharing names and roles of individuals in the OR is one of the most effective methods for promoting an individual's sense of participation and responsibility, increasing the probability of speaking up if they perceive an issue.[15]

Systematic review reveals that safety checklists improve both perceived and observed teamwork and communication in the OR.[8] A poorly designed or implemented checklist, however, can have a deleterious impact. A growing surgical evidence base demonstrates that safety checklists are associated with improved adherence to appropriate clinical practices (e.g., antibiotic administration, deep venous thrombosis [DVT] prophylaxis) and a reduction in morbidity and mortality.[8,16,17] Nevertheless, association does not imply causation, and it is difficult to ascertain from the literature the true impact of checklists. Checklists are often implemented as part of a multifaced strategy to improve care, making it difficult to determine whether improvements are secondary to the checklist or other changes (e.g., improved communication, enhanced safety culture).[17] A systematic review of surgical checklist implementation demonstrated four key components (Fig. 33.1). These include institutional support, frontline staff involvement and support, training staff on checklist use, and continuously reviewing and auditing for process improvement.[17]

Handover Protocols

There is a lack of clear evidence for best practices related to handovers and limited evidence for the association of handovers with clinical outcomes.[18] Creating a standardized handover checklist and following a structured process for handover increases the accuracy of information transferred, increases positive clinician perception of handover quality, and may improve patient outcomes.[2,4,5] The checklist combined with the structured process can be considered a *handover protocol*. The handover checklist should act as a template, with no mandatory items included. The process should specify which clinicians are expected to take part, and the way that they are expected to engage with each other. The protocol should simultaneously be consistent but flexible enough to accommodate variability in patient needs. In this way, the handover process can be individualized to every patient.[2] The literature on standardized handover processes is limited by the absence of input from clinicians caring for mixed surgical populations, decreasing the utility in real-world practice.[2]

It is vital to develop handover structures that are complementary to clinician workflow and sensitive to organizational context. The receiving clinician plays a critical role in guiding the handover process. Providing a pre-handover notification and an undistracted time-frame for handover have been cited as crucial in patient handover to the intensive care unit (ICU).[2]

Education and training alone are insufficient, but they are essential elements of affecting behavior.[18] Handover of care between providers can occur at multiple time-frames within the perioperative period. There are several recommendations in the literature that are common to all perioperative handovers[5,18,19] (Box 33.1).

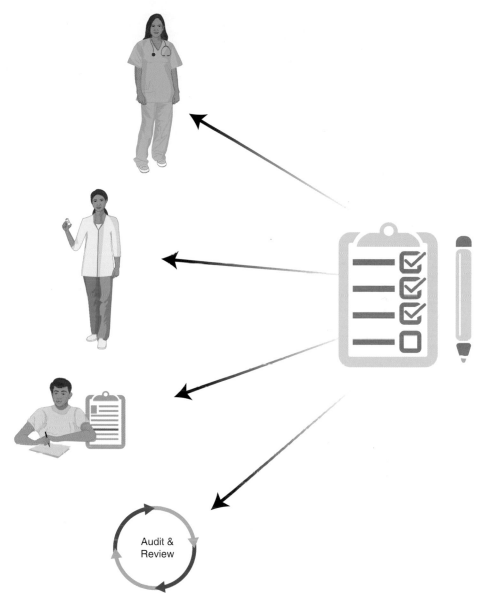

Fig. 33.1   Key components of successful checklist implementation A systematic review of surgical checklist implementation demonstrated four key components: Institutional support, frontline staff involvement and support, training staff on checklist use, and continuously reviewing and auditing for process improvement.[17]

BOX 33.1 ■ Recommendations for Implementing a Structured Handover in the Perioperative Period[18,19]

1. Early key stakeholder involvement is vital both for the development and implementation of handover checklists and protocols.
2. Standardize the handover process across the institution, allowing for area-specific adaption and alteration.
3. Before beginning the transfer of information, all urgent tasks should be completed. Notify the receiving staff in advance of the handover so that they are prepared to receive and create a distraction-free time frame for the handover to occur.
4. The handover should be structured to make information transfer easy. Ensure that only patient-specific discussion occurs during the verbal handover. Cognitive aids should be encouraged and available to use during the handover. Providers should be given the opportunity to ask and answer questions and all relevant team members should be present for the entire duration of handover.
5. Staff education and training on the handover process is essential although insufficient in isolation.

References

1. Lazzara EH, Keebler JR, Simonson RJ, Agarwala A, Lane-Fall MB. Navigating the challenges of performing anesthesia handoffs and conducting anesthesia handoff research. *Int Anesthesiol Clin.* 2020;58:32–37.
2. Lane-Fall MB, Pascual JL, Massa S, et al. Developing a standard handoff process for operating room-to-ICU transitions: multidisciplinary clinician perspectives from the Handoffs and Transitions in Critical Care (HATRICC) study. *Jt Comm J Qual Patient Saf.* 2018;44:514–525.
3. Agarwala AV, Nurudeen S, Haynes AB. Perioperative checklists and handoffs: implementation and practice. *Adv Anesth.* 2015;33:191–217.
4. Nagpal K, Abboudi M, Fischler L, et al. Evaluation of postoperative handover using a tool to assess information transfer and teamwork. *Ann Surg.* 2011;253:831–837.
5. Segall N, Bonifacio AS, Schroeder RA, et al. Can we make postoperative patient handovers safer? A systematic review of the literature. *Anesth Analg.* 2012;115:102–115.
6. Geeraerts T, Le Guen M. Checklists and cognitive aids in simulation training and daily critical care practice: simple tools to improve medical performance and patient outcome. *Anaesth Crit Care Pain Med.* 2018;37:3–4.
7. Catchpole K, Russ S. The problem with checklists. *BMJ Qual Saf.* 2015;24:545–549.
8. Russ S, Rout S, Sevdalis N, Moorthy K, Darzi A, Vincent C. Do safety checklists improve teamwork and communication in the operating room? A systematic review. *Ann Surg.* 2013;258:856–871.
9. Weinger MB. Time out! Rethinking surgical safety: more than just a checklist. *BMJ Qual Saf.* 2021;30:613–617.
10. Haynes AB, Weiser TG, Berry WR, et al. A surgical safety checklist to reduce morbidity and mortality in a global population. *N Engl J Med.* 2009;360:491–499.
11. Pronovost P, Needham D, Berenholtz S, et al. An intervention to decrease catheter-related bloodstream infections in the ICU. *N Engl J Med.* 2006;355:2725–2732.
12. Treadwell JR, Lucas S, Tsou AY. Surgical checklists: a systematic review of impacts and implementation. *BMJ Quality & Safety.* 2014;23:299–318.
13. Bergs J, Hellings J, Cleemput I, et al. Systematic review and meta-analysis of the effect of the World Health Organization surgical safety checklist on postoperative complications. *Br J Surg.* 2014;101:150–158.
14. Haugen AS, Søfteland E, Almeland SK, et al. Effect of the World Health Organization checklist on patient outcomes: a stepped wedge cluster randomized controlled trial. *Ann Surg.* 2015;261:821–828.
15. Scott E, Lindow SW, Duffy CC. Assessment of operating room team members' ability to identify other team members in the operating room, a quality improvement exercise. *Ir J Med Sci.* 2022;191(1):491–493. https://doi.org/10.1007/s11845-021-02521-6.

16. Patel J, Ahmed K, Guru KA, et al. An overview of the use and implementation of checklists in surgical specialities—a systematic review. *Int J Surg.* 2014;12:1317–1323.
17. Treadwell JR, Lucas S, Tsou AY. Surgical checklists: a systematic review of impacts and implementation. *BMJ Qual Saf.* 2014;23:299–318.
18. Agarwala AV, Lane-Fall MB, Greilich PE, et al. Consensus recommendations for the conduct, training, implementation, and research of perioperative handoffs. *Anesth Analg.* 2019;128:e71–e78.
19. Barbeito A, Agarwala AV, Lorinc A. Handovers in perioperative care. *Anesthesiol Clin.* 2018;36:87–98.

CHAPTER 34

Checklists for Safer Perioperative Care

Yun-Yun K. Chen, MD ■ Alexander F. Arriaga, MD, MPH, ScD

KEY POINTS

- Perioperative safety checklists exist for both routine (e.g., safety pause before case start) and nonroutine situations (e.g., perioperative critical events).
- Insight from the implementation sciences has been used to determine the best strategies to determine how to foster use of perioperative checklists, when indicated.
- Perioperative safety checklists can benefit not only the patient but also healthcare professionals at the individual, team, and system level.

Why Is This Important In Perioperative Medicine?

The global volume of surgery continues to rise, with an annual estimate of 234 million operations annually in 2008 to over 313 million in 2016.[1,2] Available safety data suggests the incidence of perioperative crises (e.g., massive hemorrhage, cardiac arrest) to be around 145 per 10,000 cases, such that millions of crisis events may occur annually.[2] Despite these data, these crises are considered rare at the level of the individual perioperative clinician. A clinician's preparedness with best practices for nonroutine high-stress critical events can determine the difference between life and death for a patient,[3] but there is literature to support that adherence to best practices during a critical event may be suboptimal.[3] Because of potential downstream effects of a crisis event on the wellness of a healthcare professional, extensive literature supports that debriefing after a critical event may benefit the individual, team, environment, and overall healthcare system.[2] Nevertheless, in various medical disciplines studying nonsimulation critical events, proximal critical event debriefing takes place only a fraction of the time.[2]

Perioperative safety checklists and cognitive aids are used to prevent, manage, and deal with the aftermath of such crises. These include routine checklists for safety pauses, crisis checklists for critical events, checklists for debriefing after critical events, and checklists for perioperative handoffs.[4,5] The aim of this chapter is to provide a brief overview of perioperative checklists and cognitive aids, discuss the evidence behind these checklists, and provide some practical guidance for perioperative clinicians. We hope this overview will facilitate the informed healthcare professional on how and when to use perioperative checklists with the goal of improving safety for both our patients and perioperative clinicians.

Evidence Base, Discussion, and Important Relevant References

The story of perioperative safety checklists and cognitive aids in medicine have existed for at least a century, with much associated work in safety and human factors taking place across various high-stakes industries such as aviation.[6] Goldhaber-Fiebert and Macrae provide helpful terminology regarding crisis checklists: "[Emergency manuals] are context-relevant sets of cognitive aids, such as crisis checklists, that are intended to provide professionals with key information for managing rare emergency events. Synonyms and related terms include crisis checklists; emergency checklists; and cognitive aids, a much broader term, although often used to describe tools for use during emergency events specifically."[7]

In 2006 the use of safety checklists to reduce catheter-related bloodstream infections in the intensive care unit (ICU) was seen as a success for patient safety.[8] Since then, there has been vast work specifically on routine surgical safety checklists for use during key pause points in perioperative care, with observed reductions in morbidity and mortality in a global population.[1] These studies have been followed by numerous studies, editorials, systematic reviews, and other publications on the effect of surgical safety checklists (or interventions heavily involving these checklists) on reducing morbidity and mortality and improving perioperative outcomes. In one systematic review, surgical checklists were associated with decreased surgical complications, increased detection of potential safety hazards, and improved communication among operating staff.[9] There have also been publications that have either called into question the value of these checklists or have simply emphasized that checklists work best when they are part of a sociocultural solution to improve the overall culture of safety of a clinical environment.[10,11] In this regard, the value of a thoughtful implementation strategy cannot be overemphasized.

Checklists are less effective when they are provided but not actually used, used out of context, or implemented in a suboptimal fashion.[12] It is important to understand the basic principles of crisis management for specific perioperative critical events to develop and implement cognitive aids and manuals.[13] Because of the relative rarity and unpredictable nature of crisis events, much of the research on this topic has been done via medical simulation. In one multi-institution, simulation-based randomized controlled trial, the use of crisis checklists for perioperative critical events resulted in a nearly 75% reduction in failure to adhere to critical steps in management.[3] This has been followed by other similar studies showing the benefit of crisis checklists in other settings, including in the ICU and the emergency department.[4] There is a growing amount of research now involving the study of actual events. In one study of actual critical events, the use of emergency manuals was associated with catching errors of omission and process improvements.[14] Critical events can entail an intense and time-sensitive cognitive load for perioperative providers. Accordingly, there has been notable work on the design of cognitive aids for critical events, including collaborative work that included expertise from the Human Systems Integration Division from the National Aeronautics and Space Administration (NASA).[15] Similar to efforts for routine surgical safety checklists, there has been much emphasis on the importance of modifying the cognitive aid and having an effective implementation plan when bringing crisis checklists to one's institution.[7] An operating room emergency checklist implementation toolkit was developed that reviews essential implementation principles such as getting buy-in; creating a multidisciplinary team; customizing the checklists to local settings/needs; training staff; using the checklists; and ongoing monitoring, measurement, and improvement.[16]

Perioperative handoff checklists and cognitive aids for intraoperative or postoperative hand-offs have also been an area of study to improve communication and prevent significant harm, such as postoperative complications and mortality.[17] For a more in-depth discussion on hand-overs, see the dedicated chapter in this book (see Chapter 33). A recent systematic review and meta-analysis was published on interventions for operating room to ICU handoffs, which references over 20 studies that evaluated interventions comprising information transfer/communication checklists and protocols such as visual aids and training sessions.[18] Some examples of handoff mnemonics include PATIENT (Procedure, Patient; Anesthesia, Antibiotic, Airway, Allergies; Temperature; Intravenous/invasive lines; End tidal carbon dioxide [ventilation]; Narcotics; Twitches) for intraoperative handoffs for anesthetized patients and IPASS (Illness severity, Patient summary, Action list, Situation awareness and contingency plans, Synthesis by receiver) for postoperative handoffs to postoperative care units.[5,17] There has also been observed success with the use of standardized handoff protocols with cognitive aids, as was seen with the Handoffs and Transitions in Critical Care (HATRICC) study.[19] When implemented with leadership involvement and proper educational and hands-on training of all team members, implementation of handoff checklists and cognitive aids appears to improve communication between teams and outcomes for patients.[5,17,18]

The aftermath of a critical event can impact not only the patient but also the entire medical team involved in the critical event. Therefore the development of cognitive aids for perioperative critical event debriefing is an active area of research. In recent publications by Arriaga et al.: (1) proximal, or "hot," debriefing is "debriefing at the point of care shortly after a critical event or the associated operation/procedure" and is differentiated from (2) distal/"cold" debriefing once members have had more time to process an event, or (3) routine debriefing after every single case, as has been seen in surgical safety checklists for use during safety pause points.[2,20] There is unfortunately a large gap between the promoted benefits of proximal critical event debriefing (including education, learning, quality assurance, and clinician wellness) and the actual occurrence of debriefing after critical events.[2] Various debriefing tools for different healthcare settings have been developed and the beginnings of a cognitive aid specific to perioperative proximal critical event debriefing is shown in Fig. 34.1. As noted in the figure, elements to consider for brief, proximal debriefing after perioperative critical events include (summarized by the mnemonic "WATER")[4]:

Welfare check (assessing if team members are okay to continue providing care)
Acute/short-term corrections
Team reactions and reflection
Education
Resource awareness and longer-term needs.

Practical Guidance

When considering perioperative checklists, it is helpful to know what specific checklists/cognitive aids already exist, as part of deciding on a plan for customization (or new development), implementation, and ongoing measurement. As implementation was previously discussed, some practical resources where specific checklist examples can be found include the following: the routine surgical

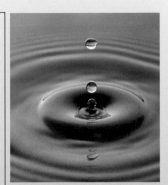

Potential elements for debriefing just after a perioperative event include (but are not limited to):

1. Welfare check:
   - Assessing if team members are ok to continue providing care
2. Acute/Short-term corrections:
   - Matters to be addressed before next case ?
   - Clinical/patient care needs ?
3. Team Reactions and Reflection:
   - Summarize case and listen to team member reactions
   - Plus/Delta: Matters that went well and matters that could be improved
4. Education:
   - Lessons learned from the event and the debriefing
5. Resource Awareness and longer-term needs:
   - Improve awareness of local peer-support and employee assistance resources
   - Assess if any follow-up needed (e.g. safety/QI report)

While a drop of water may seem small in time and space, it can have a substantial ripple effect.

Fig. 34.1 Elements to consider for debriefing just after a perioperative critical event. These elements are not meant to be comprehensive. Customization to local culture and available resources is essential.[2,20] The responsibility for interpretation/application lies with the reader. *QI*, Quality improvement. (Image from Restivo D. Water drop impact on water surface. https://commons.wikimedia.org/wiki/File:Water_drop_impact_on_a_water-surface_-_(5).jpg. Accessed February 13, 2021. With permission via Creative Commons; From Chen YK, Arriaga A. Crisis checklists in emergency medicine: another step forward for cognitive aids. *BMJ Qual Saf.* 2021; 30(9):689–693. https://doi.org/10.1136/bmjqs-2021-013203. With permission.)

safety checklist studied globally by Haynes et al., which was published as a supplementary appendix to their article in the *New England Journal of Medicine*, with more recent editions/adaptations readily available online[1]; illustrative examples of crisis checklists and emergency manuals, as shown in Figs. 34.2 and 34.3; and a long list of available cognitive aids, which can be found online, such as at the Emergency Manuals Implementation Collaborative website (https://www.emergencymanuals.org). Recent review articles with different examples of handoff and debriefing tools have also been mentioned and referenced regarding evidence of real-time critical events.[2,17,18] When implemented appropriately within a specific institution, perioperative checklists have the potential to improve quality measures such as communication and patient care outcomes.

Acute massive bleeding

START

1. **Call for help and a code cart**
   ▲ **Ask:** *"Who will be the crisis manager?"*

2. **Open IV fluids** and **assess for adequate IV access**

3. **Turn FiO₂ to 100%** and **turn down volatile anesthetics**

4. **Call blood bank**
   ▲ Activate massive transfusion protocol
   ▲ Assign 1 person as primary contact for blood bank
   ▲ Order blood products (in addition to PRBCs)
     • 1 FFP : 1 PRBC
     • If indicated, 6 units of platelets

5. **Request rapid infuser** (or pressure bags)

6. **Discuss management plan between** surgical, anesthesiology, and nursing teams

7. **Call for surgery consultation**

8. **Keep patient warm**

9. **Send labs**
   CBC, PT/PTT/INR, fibrinogen, lactate, arterial blood gas, potassium, and ionized calcium

10. **Consider …**
    ▲ Electrolyte disturbances (hypocalcemia and hyperkalemia)
    ▲ Uncrossmatched type O-neg blood if crossmatched blood not availbale
    ▲ Damage control surgery (pack, close, resuscitate)
    ▲ Special patient populations (see considerations below)

DRUG DOSES and treatments

HYPOCALCEMIA treatment

Give calcium to replace deficit
(calcium chloride or calcium gluconate)

HYPERKALEMIA treatment

1. Calcium gluconate	• 30 mg/kg IV
- or -	
Calcium chloride	• 10 mg/kg IV
2. Insulin	• 10 units regular IV with 1–2 amps D50W as needed
3. Sodium bicarbonate if pH < 7.2	• 1–2 mEq/kg slow IV push

SPECIAL PATIENT POPULATIONS

OBSTETRIC:
• Empirical administration of 1 pool of cryoprecipitate (10 cryo units)
• Check fibrinogen (goal is 200 mg/dL)

< 100 mg/dL	Order 2 more pools of cryoprecipitate
100 – 200 mg/dL	Order 1 more pool of cryoprecipitate

TRAUMA:
Give either…
• Antifibrinolytic tranexamic acid: 1000 mg IV over 10 minutes followed by 1000 mg over the next 8 hours

– or –

• Aminocaproic acid: 4–5 g in 250 mL NS/RL IV over first hour followed by a cont nuing infusion of 1 g in 50 mL NS/RL IV per hour over 8 hours

NON-SURGICAL UNCONTROLLED BLEEDING despite massive transfusion of PRBC, FFP, platelets and cryo:
• Consider giving Recombinant Factor VIIa: 40 mcg/kg IV
  – Surgical bleeding must first be controlled
  – **use with CAUTION** in patients at risk for thrombosis
  – **DO NOT use** when pH is < 7.2

Fig. 34.2 Hemorrhage crisis checklist. (From Ariadne Labs. Operating room crisis checklists. https://www.ariadnelabs.org/safe-surgery-safe-systems/surgical-safety/.)

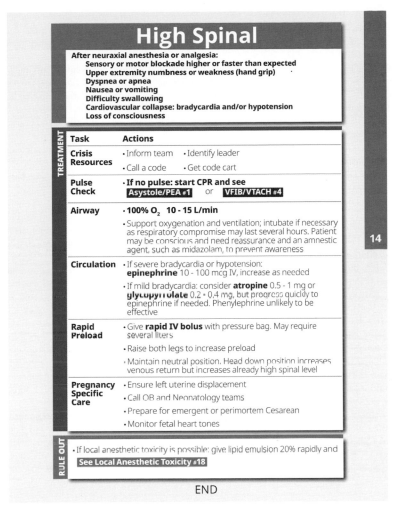

Fig. 34.3 Emergency manual entry for total spinal anesthesia. (From Stanford Anesthesia Cognitive Aid Program, *Emergency Manual: Cognitive aids for perioperative crises, Version 4, 2021. See http:// emergencymanual.stanford.edu for latest version. Creative Commons BY-NC-ND [https://creativecommons. org/licenses/by-nc-nd/4.0/legalcode]. *Goldhaber-Fiebert SN, Austin N, Sultan E, Burian BK, Burden A, Howard SK, Gaba DM, Harrison TK.)

References

1. Haynes AB, Weiser TG, Berry WR, et al. A surgical safety checklist to reduce morbidity and mortality in a global population. *N Engl J Med.* 2009;360:491–499.
2. Arriaga AF, Szyld D, Pian-Smith MCM. Real-time debriefing after critical events: exploring the gap between principle and reality. *Anesthesiol Clin.* 2020;38:801–820.
3. Arriaga AF, Bader AM, Wong JM, et al. Simulation-based trial of surgical-crisis checklists. *N Engl J Med.* 2013;368:246–253.
4. Chen YK, Arriaga A. Crisis checklists in emergency medicine: another step forward for cognitive aids. *BMJ Qual Saf.* 2021;30(9):689–693.

5. Agarwala AV, Lane-Fall MB, Greilich PE, et al. Consensus recommendations for the conduct, training, implementation, and research of perioperative handoffs. *Anesth Analg.* 2019;128:e71–e78.

6. Hepner DL, Arriaga AF, Cooper JB, et al. Operating room crisis checklists and emergency manuals. *Anesthesiology.* 2017;127:384–392.

7. Goldhaber-Fiebert SN, Macrae C. Emergency manuals: how quality improvement and implementation science can enable better perioperative management during crises. *Anesthesiol Clin.* 2018;36:45–62.

8. Pronovost P, Needham D, Berenholtz S, et al. An intervention to decrease catheter-related bloodstream infections in the ICU. *N Engl J Med.* 2006;355:2725–2732.

9. Treadwell JR, Lucas S, Tsou AY. Surgical checklists: a systematic review of impacts and implementation. *BMJ Qual Saf.* 2014;23:299–318.

10. Urbach DR, Govindarajan A, Saskin R, Wilton AS, Baxter NN. Introduction of surgical safety checklists in Ontario. *Canada N Engl J Med.* 2014;370:1029–1038.

11. Bosk CL, Dixon-Woods M, Goeschel CA, Pronovost PJ. Reality check for checklists. *Lancet.* 2009;374:444–445.

12. Leape LL. The checklist conundrum. *N Engl J Med.* 2014;370:1063–1064.

13. Gaba DM, Fish KJ, Howard SK, Burden AR. *Crisis management in anesthesiology.* 2nd ed. Philadelphia, PA: Elsevier/Saunders; 2015.

14. Goldhaber-Fiebert SN, Bereknyei Merrell S, Agarwala AV, et al. Clinical uses and impacts of emergency manuals during perioperative crises. *Anesth Analg.* 2020;131:1815–1826.

15. Clebone A, Burian BK, Watkins SC, et al. The development and implementation of cognitive aids for critical events in pediatric anesthesia: The Society for Pediatric Anesthesia critical events checklists. *Anesth Analg.* 2017;124:900–907.

16. Hannenberg AA. Cognitive aids in the management of critical events. *Anesthesiol Clin.* 2020;38(4):789–800. https://doi.org/10.1016/j.anclin.2020.08.002.

17. Abraham J, Pfeifer E, Doering M, Avidan MS, Kannampallil T. Systematic review of intraoperative anesthesia handoffs and handoff tools. *Anesth Analg.* 2021;132(6):1563–1575. https://doi.org/10.1213/ANE.0000000000005367.

18. Abraham J, Meng A, Tripathy S, Avidan MS, Kannampallil T. Systematic review and meta-analysis of interventions for operating room to intensive care unit handoffs. *BMJ Qual Saf.* 2021;30(6):513–524. https://doi.org/10.1136/bmjqs-2020-012474.

19. Lane-Fall MB, Pascual JL, Peifer HG, et al. A partially structured postoperative handoff protocol improves communication in 2 mixed surgical intensive care units: findings from the Handoffs and Transitions in Critical Care (HATRICC) prospective cohort study. *Ann Surg.* 2020;271:484–493.

20. Arriaga AF, Sweeney RE, Clapp JT, et al. Failure to debrief after critical events in anesthesia is associated with failures in communication during the event. *Anesthesiology.* 2019;130:1039–1048.

Social Aspects of Change in Perioperative Care and the Importance of Context

Graham P. Martin, MA(Oxon), MSc, PhD

KEY POINTS

- The importance of context to the fate of healthcare improvement is well acknowledged but inconsistently studied and understood.
- Social scientific methods and theories offer an important resource for understanding contextual and social influences.
- Conceptual frameworks help to provide a structured approach to anticipating and accounting for a wide range of contextual influences in planning, delivering, and evaluating improvement.
- The complexity of the social world means that these influences are not always consistent or predictable; complexity theory offers pragmatic guidance for achieving scientifically informed change.

Social Aspects of Change in Perioperative Care and the Importance of Context

For any clinician working in perioperative care, the importance of the peculiarities and personalities of their own hospital to the fate of improvement initiatives will be self-evident. What works well in one hospital or department may falter in another. Context matters. Yet the move toward more systematically seeking to anticipate, study, and understand the impact of social context as a part of improvement or research efforts is a relatively recent development. This chapter briefly traces the history of the study of context in improvement research and offers some examples of where and how context matters. It outlines some of the key tools that have been used to make sense of context, before suggesting key points for practitioners seeking to account for local context in improvement efforts.

Context and Perioperative Improvement

As discussed elsewhere in this book, much of the thinking behind process improvement in health care can be traced to methods and ideas originally developed in other sectors. The work of key figures in engineering and the manufacturing industry, such as Deming and Shewhart, remains an important foundation of many of the improvement methods used in health care today. In perioperative care in particular, there have been efforts to learn from the successes achieved in fields such as civil aviation, with its enviable safety record and widespread use of improvement approaches that attend to both processes (e.g., Standard Operating Procedures) and people (e.g., efforts to mitigate the negative impacts of hierarchy). For both health care in general and perioperative care in particular, these efforts to transfer approaches and interventions from other contexts have brought some notable successes. But at both levels, the differences between the healthcare setting and the contexts from which these approaches are drawn also mean that there are important constraints on transferability.

At the level of health care as a whole, there is increasing recognition of the limitations of applying approaches developed largely in the manufacturing industry—where quality is largely determined on a production line or similar, before the product reaches the consumer—to service sectors such as health care, where outcomes are co-produced in the interaction between producer (clinician) and consumer (patient).[1] In perioperative care specifically, the differences between clinics, operating rooms, and intensive care units, and settings such as aviation, are evident, and can be consequential for what improvement interventions transferred from one to the other can do. Thus while concepts such as the "authority gradient"[2] and interventions such as checklists have clear relevance to perioperative settings,[3] the specifics of context matter for whether and how they work. Building the completion of a checklist into complex healthcare processes may be a more challenging task than incorporating it into structured pre-flight procedures,[4] and the particular social and professional dynamics of perioperative care teams will also affect how a checklist is received and carried out.[5]

Differences of context within health care are also important. Although interventions such as checklists are often seen as having universal application—as reflected in the World Health Organization's advocacy of the Surgical Safety Checklist across low-, middle-, and high-income settings[6]—their impact is often variable. Evaluations of the implementation of the checklist and similar tools across different contexts have highlighted the challenges of incorporating it into routine work, ensuring consistent use, and securing a culture in which the importance of such activity is embraced.[7] Other interventions designed to improve the quality of perioperative care often have similarly mixed results, with context a crucial mediator. For example, a recent evaluation of an intervention designed to improve speed of treatment for patients requiring emergency cholecystectomy in the United Kingdom had a notably inconsistent impact,[8] with a process evaluation highlighting leadership clarity, organizational capacity, and ability to learn from data and experience, among other things, as crucial influences.[9]

Making Sense of Social and Contextual Influences on Perioperative Improvement

Context, then, is vital, but systematic study of the role of context in influencing improvement interventions in perioperative care is relatively novel. There are perhaps three broad reasons for this. First, there has been a tendency to underestimate the complexity both of interventions themselves and the contexts in which they are being implemented. Far from being a simple additional step that can be slotted into existing processes, routines, and organizational cultures unproblematically, improvement tools such as checklists constitute "a complex social intervention with an expectation of interaction and cooperation between surgeons, anaesthetists and nurses."[7] Second, there has been a tendency to relegate matters of context to the category of noise or random variation, rather than foregrounding them as something to be explained. This relates in part to the fact that the gold standard evaluation approach in pharmaceutical research, the randomized controlled trial (RCT), is often also seen as a gold standard in health services research. When using RCTs to evaluate the effectiveness of organizational interventions such as improvement initiatives, variation in context (like variation in human bodies) can become something to be nullified (e.g., through sampling criteria and sample sizes) rather than something to be explained or understood.[10] Third, and connected, it is only relatively recently that health services research has come to embrace the theories and methods offered by disciplines in the social sciences that offer analytical purchase on contextual influences on change. Although the value of mixed-methods approaches to evaluating improvement interventions and incorporating process evaluation, qualitative methods, and (sometimes) sociological and psychological conceptual frameworks is now broadly recognized, they are still sometimes seen as optional extras. In their absence, evaluations of improvement interventions may be able to identify their inconsistent impact across settings, but can do little to explain it.

Getting from an acknowledgment that context matters toward an understanding of *how* it matters is thus crucial. Besides the methodological tools and empirical evidence they bring, one important contribution of the social sciences is a more detailed consideration of what we mean by social and contextual influences, and how best to conceptualize them in planning and evaluating improvement interventions.[11] Various frameworks cataloging social and contextual influences have been developed, offering conceptualizations that can be helpful in planning, delivering, and evaluating improvement work. Many of these have their roots in the psychological and behavioral sciences[12]; some draw on fields such as sociology and science and technology studies.[13] One relatively simple, but transparently constructed and comprehensive, framework for accounting for context is the Consolidated Framework for Implementation Research (CFIR; Fig. 35.1).[14] Frameworks of this kind are often used to inform process evaluations of improvement interventions but can also offer a valuable resource for those planning change, for example, by helping improvement leads to anticipate the influences that are likely to be most important to the success or failure of their work.

Practical Implications

Of course, it is one thing for professional research teams, with six- or seven-digit budgets for developing, piloting, and evaluating interventions, to seek to systematically account for the influence of context on improvement interventions. For a typical improvement team in an acute hospital,

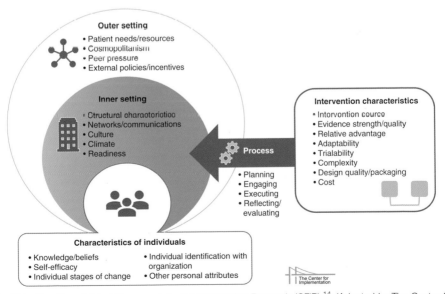

Fig. 35.1 The Consolidated Framework for Implementation Research (CFIR).[14] (Adapted by The Center for Implementation, Toronto, Canada.)

without access to multidisciplinary research expertise, dedicated budgets, or often even protected time, it is quite a different prospect. Nevertheless, many of the tools and approaches used to understand context have relevance for even the smallest perioperative improvement project.

As a starting point, frameworks such as CFIR offer a structured way of thinking through the likely influences on the success of a project. They can help those leading improvement identify the key stakeholder groups whose attitudes and behavior could make or break an improvement effort, as well as help in thinking through strategies for evaluation—including aspects of change beyond the primary intended outcome that might merit some form of data collection, qualitative or quantitative. Anticipating these influences may result in more nuanced interventions and associated program theories of change (describing how and why they are expected to work), and provides a basis for rapidly reviewing progress and early modification as necessary.[15] It is important, however, to acknowledge the complexity of contextual influences and to avoid the trap of simply identifying a list of "barriers" and "facilitators" to success. Influences on improvement are rarely so straightforward or linear. They may interact with one another in difficult-to-predict ways, and simultaneously help and hinder implementation. The role of medical professionalism, to take one example, in the success of a perioperative improvement initiative is unlikely to be singular: at once, it may be a resource invoked in resisting change and a rationale for change; it may impede cross-professional teamwork and help to locate responsibility for effective delivery; it may encourage collaboration across organizations, and it may give rise to competition between units, for better or worse.[16]

This complexity undoubtedly makes the task of understanding and acting on social and contextual influences on change all the harder. The world is a complex place, and while the theory, evidence, and methods of social science offer useful predictive and explanatory tools, not everything that happens is easily predicted or readily understood. Sometimes, social influences on change appear less a matter of consistent patterns of behavior and more a matter of random occurrence. Proponents of complexity theory offer helpful explanations for the unpredictability of social influences, and for why implementing the same intervention in seemingly near-identical contexts can result in very different outcomes.[17] They also provide useful guidance on how to respond as practitioners and researchers of improvement—for example, by combining methods of scientific inquiry with insights that arise from intuition, and by seeking to draw on the knowledge of people across various positions in the system to be changed.[18] This combination of prior evidence, empirical data, and the implicit wisdom that comes from improvement practice perhaps offers the best foundation for understanding the role of context, planning improvement interventions that account for it, and learning from practice to adapt plans for the better.

References

1. Batalden M, Batalden P, Margolis P, et al. Coproduction of healthcare service. *BMJ Qual Saf.* 2016; 25(7):509–517.
2. Cosby KS, Croskerry P. Authority gradients in medical error. *Acad Emerg Med.* 2004;11(12):1341–1345.
3. Clay-Williams R, Colligan L. Back to basics: checklists in aviation and healthcare. *BMJ Qual Saf.* 2015; 24(7):428–431.
4. Catchpole K, Russ S. The problem with checklists. *BMJ Qual Saf.* 2015;24(9):545–549.
5. Aveling E-L, McCulloch P, Dixon-Woods M. A qualitative study comparing experiences of the surgical safety checklist in hospitals in high-income and low-income countries. *BMJ Open.* 2013;3(8): e003039.
6. Haynes AB, Weiser TG, Berry WR, et al. A surgical safety checklist to reduce morbidity and mortality in a global population. *N Engl J Med.* 2009;350(5):491–499.
7. Bergs J, Lambrechts F, Simons P, et al. Barriers and facilitators related to the implementation of surgical safety checklists: a systematic review of the qualitative evidence. *BMJ Qual Saf.* 2015;24(12):776–786.

8. Bamber JR, Stephens TJ, Cromwell DA, et al. Effectiveness of a quality improvement collaborative in reducing time to surgery for patients requiring emergency cholecystectomy. *BJS Open [Internet].* 2019. https://bjssjournals.onlinelibrary.wiley.com/doi/abs/10.1002/bjs5.50221.

9. Stephens TJ, Bamber JR, Beckingham IJ, et al. Understanding the influences on successful quality improvement in emergency general surgery: learning from the RCS Chole-QuIC project. *Implement Sci.* 2019; 14(1):84.

10. Martin GP, O'Hara J, Waring J, Pettersen-Gould K, Macrae C. Large-scale mixed-methods evaluation of safety programmes and interventions. In: *Inside Hazardous Technological Systems: Methodological Foundations, Challenges and Future Directions.* London: CRC Press; 2021:169–186.

11. Bate P, Robert G, Fulop N, Øvretveit J, Dixon-Woods M. *Perspectives on Context.* London: The Health Foundation; 2014.

12. Cane J, O'Connor D, Michie S. Validation of the theoretical domains framework for use in behaviour change and implementation research. *Implement Sci.* 2012;7(1):37.

13. Murray E, Treweek S, Pope C, et al. Normalisation process theory: a framework for developing, evaluating and implementing complex interventions. *BMC Med.* 2010;8(1):63.

14. Damschroder LJ, Aron DC, Keith RE, Kirsh SR, Alexander JA, Lowery JC. Fostering implementation of health services research findings into practice: a consolidated framework for advancing implementation science. *Implement Sci.* 2009;4:50.

15. Davidoff F, Dixon-Woods M, Leviton L, Michie S. Demystifying theory and its use in improvement. *BMJ Qual Saf.* 2015;24(3):228–238.

16. Martin GP, Armstrong N, Aveling E-L, Herbert G, Dixon-Woods M. Professionalism redundant, reshaped, or reinvigorated? Realizing the "third logic" in contemporary health care. *J Health Soc Behav.* 2015;56(3):378–397.

17. Plsek PE, Greenhalgh T. The challenge of complexity in health care. *BMJ.* 2001;323(7313):625–628.

18. Reed JE, Howe C, Doyle C, Bell D. Simple rules for evidence translation in complex systems: a qualitative study. *BMC Med.* 2018;16(1):92.

CHAPTER 36

Stakeholder Engagement

Della M. Lin, MS, MD, FASA

KEY POINTS

- Psychological safety and "humble inquiry" are the foundation and scaffolding for successful, productive, learning teams.
- A strong team is even stronger when interpersonal relationships are valued.
- Mental rehearsal and planning an engagement strategy *before* important meetings are important skills.
- Understand the importance of continuous engagement and take steps to ensure it happens, such as by using regular feedback and celebrating success.
- Consider the acronym "BAM" (belief, adaptation, mutual accountability) to create an environment for effective stakeholder engagement.

How do we avoid these common quality improvement epitaphs…?

"Great idea that never saw the light of day."
"We followed the best and brightest ideas that worked elsewhere… didn't work here."
"Started OK, but couldn't roll with the punches."

The process map discussed in a previous chapter (see Chapter 29) gives insight into identifying the key stakeholders that make up a team for action and successful implementation. Once identified, creating an environment where the stakeholder team is engaged and stays engaged is a critical leadership skill in quality improvement. What follows is a framework of tips for success and pitfalls to avoid—foundational always events, team design, mental rehearsal, and *continuous* engagement.

Foundational Always Events

The most critical experience for an engaged stakeholder group is psychological safety. Amy Edmondson, an organizational learning scholar who described psychological safety, defines it as "a climate in which people… feel comfortable sharing concerns and mistakes without fear of embarrassment or retribution."[1] Candor is expected. It is essential at a group level to nurture an environment of new ideas and productive dissent.

The leader shapes and role-models this environment by promoting a culture of psychological safety and humble inquiry. Edgar Schein, arguably the father of organizational culture, coined the term "humble inquiry." It is about "asking questions and building a relationship based on curiosity."[2] It implies that there is no one expert "telling" the group what to do. Questions are not asked to test answers but are asked in a true spirit of inquiry.

These two elements—psychological safety and humble inquiry—are the foundation and scaffolding for successful, productive, learning teams where every voice is valued. What emerges is the collective wisdom—a clearer and wiser signal separated from the noise. From this emerges collective ownership.

Team Design—More Than Stakeholders

A strong team is even stronger when interpersonal relationships are valued. There are three important caveats to consider.

IGNORE MAVENS AT YOUR PERIL

In every department, there are a few individuals who are considered highly influential scholars. These individuals spread ideas by collecting, translating, and sharing information. They are called "mavens" (derived from a Yiddish word for someone who accumulates knowledge). Consider who these people are in the perioperative environment. Avoiding key (often) informal communication channels offered through these individuals can be a critical pitfall. Ideally, make mavens part of the quality improvement communication channel. If the influencer is not supportive of the initiative, sit down with the individual with "humble inquiry." Most importantly, do not avoid the conversation.

IDENTIFY THE SOURCE/RISK OF "MONOVOXOPLEGIA"

Break down the word "monovoxoplegia" into its parts to reveal the term's definition coined by Dr. James Reinertsen (personal communication).[3] A single…voice…paralyzes. Recall a likely scenario from your past with a room full of people. After discussion on an issue, one lone person (usually in the back) raises a hand (or not) and states emphatically, "It won't work!" The grandstanding remark is commonly embellished with how many years they have been in medicine and how we may have tried something like this before to no avail. The result is the same. The discussion and any progress come to a screeching stop.

It is important to identify the source of monovoxoplegia. If this person is a maven who has been unintentionally ignored, find time for "humble inquiry" as previously described and outlined more in the next section. Candor, including constructive opinions and differing perspectives, are a hallmark of psychological safety. When leading meetings, however, be clear that using "monovoxoplegia" is against meeting ground rules. Although differing opinions should be welcome, they are not welcome in a grandstanding manner that paralyzes all further conversation.

PERSONIZING

Edgar Schein advises that humble inquiry at the 1:1 level is about "personizing." Taking the time to be curious about what matters to each person in the group shines a light on motivation and new ideas. One technique for this is shadowing. For example, shadowing the central processing staff for a couple of hours with an open inquiring attitude can shine a light on communication challenges while working on an initiative to standardize supplies or an effort to minimize instrument breakage. If the quality improvement effort is about on-time starts, shadowing the preoperative staff shines a light on the multiple morning workflows, conflicting decision making, and potential chaos.

Mental Rehearsal—More Than Finding a Meeting Time and Agenda

An important skill in world-class performance is exercising mental rehearsal. Athletes and performing artists rigorously use this skill to optimize success. Members of the perioperative team, such as surgeons and anesthesiologists, are also known to use this skill in preparation for particularly challenging cases.

This technique is similarly useful before meetings and when planning overall engagement strategy. Who is in the room? How is the room set up? What ground rules need to be set? Will the team already be on the same page, and if not, how will you navigate to that common vision? What might be the responses to potential conflicts or sensitive statements? What might be the reaction to a presentation? How does the meeting start? How does it end?

Here are two examples of mental rehearsal before going into a meeting:

- Does the lead presentation pass the "grandmother test"?
    - Sir Richard John Roberts, Nobel Laureate in Physiology/Medicine, advises that "the grandmother test ensures that people of all fields understand what you are doing."[4] Would someone else who is not in your field of expertise be able to take the remarks and convince their friend about the worthiness of this effort? The larger the number of stakeholders, the more important this test becomes. The lead message should be clear and translatable to anyone in the organization.
- What are some questions that can be pre-scripted to ensure open dialog? A few suggestions include:
    - What puzzles you about what is being suggested?
    - What else do we need to know? How do we find out?
    - How do we connect the dots?

Continuous Engagement

It is vitally important to recognize how critical it is to maintain *continuous* engagement. Each intervention is only a mini-milestone. Do not assume that these mini-milestones are the end-game. For example, implementation of a new electronic order set for an enhanced recovery pathway is a mini-milestone with milestones that precede and follow. A pitfall would be to make the order set the end-game.

- **Regular, timely feedback** is essential. This can be as frequent as weekly and should not be any further spaced apart than quarterly. Feedback allows team members to realize how they have made a difference and also allows for any necessary early course corrections .
- **Visible learning boards**. Learning boards can be in the form of poster boards, but learning boards that are dynamic in real time are most effective. These visible boards track initiatives from the idea to the intervention; from process metrics to outcome metrics; and from smaller individual improvements to collaborative team improvements. Learning boards can also track the journey through the lens of a patient's experience or a team member's experience.
- **Celebrating failures**. This aspect of continuous engagement nurtures trust and nurtures the learning system. It sends a message that we learn from everything—successes and failures alike. Failures, in fact, can arguably tell us more because they help provide clarity and an understanding of the working boundaries.
- **Never stop personizing.** Continue to invest in relationships and take the time to understand how the effort is affecting individual team members as it matures.

Pulling it Together

It does not require special superhero powers to create an environment for effective stakeholder engagement. Nevertheless, the acronym **BAM** summarizes important key features:

B: Believe. Invite stakeholders onto your team that really believe in the work. Team members that are there simply because they are the token surgeon/nurse/anesthesia team member are a recipe for disappointment. Make the time to develop personizing relationships and understand the "What's in it for me (WIIFM)" for each member of the team.

A: Adaptation. Every quality initiative will require local adaptation. Ignoring this is akin to putting a square peg into a round hole. The amount of adaptation will depend on the level of certainty and complexity of the effort. Even the simplest of interventions will likely require some local adaptation. For example, if your perioperative area is planning to standardize medication labels across the system, the concept may seem quite simple. The intervention will promote patient safety. Nevertheless, the sociotechnical understanding of existing workflows and preexisting color labels makes even the simplest of interventions more complex in implementation.

M: Mutual accountability. Two accountability challenges frequently occur with the implementation of quality initiatives. The first challenge is that our teams are not static… people come and go. The handover in the transition can be suboptimal; important information and to-dos get lost in the cracks. The second accountability challenge compounds the first. It occurs when we fall prey to the pitfall of accountability silos—designating certain tasks to just one individual.

The most successfully engaged quality improvement teams embrace mutual accountability and design overlapping roles. These actions move the team from one made up of individuals focused on advocacy to a team focused on the common goal. What emerges is reliability and resilience for the quality initiative.

Establishing foundational "always" events, thoughtfully designing the team, exercising mental rehearsal, mindfully practicing continuous engagement, and using the BAM acronym will enable successful engagement and avoid an early project gravestone.

The Ultimate Stakeholder: The Patient

The most critical of mutual accountabilities… is the patient. All of these tips are empty and meaningless if we forget the patient in the process of stakeholder engagement.

Progressive quality improvement teams invite patients as partners in the design and implementation of quality improvement efforts. Finding the right patients for your team is as important as finding other stakeholders for the team.[5] Importantly, patients have a unique lens. They build forward momentum, with little tolerance for stalling.

It can never be stressed enough… the ultimate stakeholder is the patient.

Acknowledgments

Humble thanks to Jeff Cooper, John Corman, Denise Dubuque, Robert Eubanks, Gary Kaplan, Michael Leonard, Carol Peden, Liana Peiler, Edgar Schein, and Michael Rosen for their insights and collective wisdom in shaping this chapter.

References

1. Edmondson A. *The Fearless Organization.* Hoboken, NJ: John Wiley and Sons; 2019.
2. Schein E, Schein P. *Humble Inquiry, Second Edition: The Gentle Art of Asking instead of Telling.* Oakland, CA: Berrett-Koehler Publishers, Inc; 2021.
3. Reinertsen JL, Bisognano M, Seven Pugh MD. *Leadership Leverage Points for Organization—Level Improvement in Health Care.* 2nd ed. Cambridge, MA: Institute for Healthcare Improvement; 2008.
4. Nobel Laureate Richard J. Roberts: what makes us listen to science? https://www.youtube.com/watch?v=PIeHqZslifw. Accessed July 31, 2021.
5. Institute for Patient and Family-Centered Care. https://www.ipfcc.org/. Accessed July 31, 2021.

CHAPTER 37

Techniques for Creating Urgency

Della M. Lin, MS, MD, FASA

KEY POINTS

- Urgency is not always about going fast. Provide some breathing room and allow the team to co-create their own ideas for success.
- The ideal temperature for forward change is in the "productive range of distress," not too hot and not too cold.
- The combination of data and stories is unbeatable. They create human impact.
- Consider the acronym: STAT (**S**tories, ideal **T**emperature, **A**ction more affordable than inaction, and **T**empo) when designing urgency into change initiatives.

Acknowledge that clinical leaders, including physician leaders, are reluctant to make people uncomfortable. We do not see conflict as a way to problem solve. Leaders must embrace conflict and be willing to create a sense of urgency.
— Gary Kaplan, MD, Chairman and CEO, Virginia Mason[1]

Change is messy. Clinicians are not drawn to messiness and conflict.

We know that change depends on a compelling vision, a burning platform, and creating urgency. If these are so known, why do more than 70% of change initiatives fail?

The acronym *STAT* gives insight into four considerations in a toolkit for creating urgency.

S: Stories

The combination of data and stories is unbeatable. They create human impact.

Creating urgency requires a willingness to surface our defects and errors. It requires the combination of logos, ethos, and pathos. The natural tendency in perioperative medicine is to lean into our scientific method for discovery. By default, logos is prioritized as the data and rationality for change. Medicine also naturally leans into doing what is right: the ethos. The will to change is driven by an ethical force—the ethos of changing the status quo when the status quo is not right.

Pathos draws the emotion. Telling stories illustrates the human experience behind the gap: a preventable harm, a frustrating inefficiency, and a workaround. Patient stories are particularly impactful. Describing the experience and surfacing the defects or errors from the patient's eyes pivots the focus to patient-centered care. This then enables everyone to rally.

T: Temperature

The ideal temperature for forward change is in the "productive range of distress," not too hot and not too cold.

This phrase is described by Ron Heifetz. Trained as a surgeon, Heifetz co-developed the highly regarded adaptive framework for leadership,[2] an extremely helpful framework for steering urgency and change.

Heifetz and Marty Linsky describe the distinction between technical challenges and adaptive change. Technical challenges are solved by existing know-how and problem-solving techniques. Adaptive challenges and change are complex, ambiguous, and often without a blueprint. Adaptive change requires transformation. The "solution" for adaptive change emerges within the people because the people themselves evolve through change from the status quo.

Most of our significant quality improvement challenges are a mixture of both. Solving the challenge technically is seductive and avoids difficult conflict but fizzles in the long term.

Embracing the more difficult adaptive change requires acknowledging and providing space for conflict. Conflict in the form of passionate opinions and beliefs—this "productive range of distress"—is a key and often necessary part of change. Handled well, not too hot and not too cold, it is the constructive fuel for the engine of urgent progress.

To maintain forward urgency is to manage the temperature; keep the heat high enough to motivate people. This requires creating psychologically safe places where constructive conflict can percolate. Similarly, over-percolating can result in a disastrous explosion. A leader needs to know when to bring the temperature down, reduce the chaos and bring the discussion back into the productive range. When the change is too uncomfortable, fear, false urgency, and apathy can prevail.

- Fear requires chunking the change down to a bite-size piece, even allowing for a short-term technical challenge win.
- "False urgency" is described by John Kotter[3] as frantic, energetic activity—running constantly between meetings and presentations. He cautions that this unfocused activity is draining and destructive: a "howling wind of activity" that builds nothing. The perioperative environment is one that is particularly focused on action. We should be particularly wary of false urgency.
- Apathy signals disengagement and indifference. One might assume that the person who is passionately vocal against an initiative is the hardest challenge. That loud individual is "the enemy." Instead, recall the adage, "The opposite of love is not hate; it is indifference." The reframe is that the loud individual is showing passion and that passion can turn into a potential source of support. Deftly enabling—instead of suppressing—the "*productive* range of distress" enables the individual to emerge as part of the solution.

A: Action

Make **ACTION** more **AFFORDABLE** than inaction. There are many nuances to make action the easier thing to do.

- Design forcing functions where the defaults are the desired action. Instead of trumpeting out a new order set in hopes that a busy clinician will find them and "opt in," encourage default order-set utilization where "opting out" is the less convenient/less affordable step. For example, instead of trying to remember to activate order sets that limit medications such as diphenhydramine and gabapentin in the elderly, design the default where these medications cannot be ordered in the drop-down menu for patients older than 70. A clinician who feels this medication is necessary can order it with extra keystrokes.
- Align the effort across the organization or service line. Locate the initiative's source of urgency. If it is coming from the frontline, align the administration with the same will for change. Similarly, if the source of urgency is coming from administration, align the passion and "why" from the frontline.
- Consider dyad and triad leadership. Perioperative leadership teams have formed dyad partnerships (physician leader and administrative leader) and triad partnerships (physician leader, nurse leader, and administrative leader). These leadership partnerships have been

described as "the secret sauce." They are visible and transparent in their aligned message. They use their different peer influences to connect with various team members. Importantly, they vet contrasting perspectives, debate opinions, and entertain "what-if's" with each other. What emerges is a message others can accept as one that has been wisely scrutinized and evaluated.

T: Tempo

Urgency is not always about going fast. Sustaining the tension of urgency is analogous to a dance—the "active space" between partners. There are both forward steps and backward steps. Provide breathing room and allow the team to co-create their own ideas for success.

Proper attention to tempo can be challenging, especially when we are passionate about a particular change. We own the compelling vision and the burning platform, and it may be difficult to understand what is taking everyone else so long to come on board.

Heifetz and Linsky[2] provide another leadership skill embodied in their metaphor of moving back and forth between the balcony and the dance floor. Going to the balcony requires taking a step back and gaining a long view of the activities below. Being on the dance floor requires going to where the action is and being more than an observer. Going back and forth gains an understanding of how the imagined work and reality actually overlap. This skill helps a leader to know when to accelerate and when to slow down (Box 37.1).

Urgency is about tension. Keeping the tension creates momentum to move from the status quo. As perioperative leaders, consider the STAT toolkit to create urgency by optimizing the use of:

- **S**tories with human impact,
- the productive **T**emperature of "distress,"
- affordable aligned **A**ction, and
- **T**empo

BOX 37.1 ■ Case Vignette: Hawaii's Central Line Associated Bloodstream Infection Collaborative and STAT[4,5]

There was a vision for all of Hawaii to partner with the Johns Hopkins Armstrong Institute (under the leadership of Dr. Peter Pronovost) and be part of a national collaborative to eliminate preventable central line–associated bloodstream infections (CLABSIs). At the time, Hawaii's state mean CLABSI rate already met national benchmarks. There was no historical statewide improvement infrastructure and no state public reporting mandate to support the vision. In other words, there was no natural urgency to participate in the collaborative.

The state had 17 hospitals with intensive care units (ICUs; adult, pediatric, and neonatal). Hospitals ranged from small critical access to larger academic-affiliated community hospitals. They ranged from smaller combined surgical/medical ICUs without dedicated ICU physicians to specialty-specific ICUs (e.g., burn, trauma, neurology, neonatal). Some hospitals had dedicated quality improvement staff; many did not. Most hospitals were in a competitive marketplace with each other.

How did STAT aid in creating urgency? How did it nurture a common belief from inevitable infections to preventable infections?

Stories: We used stories to make the data have faces. Peter Pronovost told the story of Josie King on the national level. At the local level, we had family members participate and tell their stories. We reported the decreasing infection rate not only as a statistic but also in the number of prevented infection lives, and more importantly, the number of lives saved. We shared stories of small successes, not just with data, but in how these successes "burst the bubbles" of isolation across the state and made work easier, shareable and...fun!

BOX 37.1 ■ Case Vignette: Hawaii's Central Line Associated Bloodstream Infection Collaborative and STAT (continued)

<u>**Temperature:**</u> The leads for the different hospital teams across the state were uniquely different (e.g., a medical intensivist, a surgical intensivist, an ICU nurse, a nurse educator, an infectious disease improvement clinician). We enabled the productive conversation—"the productive range of distress"—with opportunities such as field visits to each other's units and a common web page enabled with forum discussions. It was critical that we nurtured and normalized *across* team dialog. These efforts were foundational toward normalizing asking for help. Members of the collaborative gave and received mutual support and trust. When it was time to celebrate the collaborative's success, team member remarks included, "It's no longer one man down, we are bringing everyone up!"; "Everyone makes a difference"; "Everyone communicates, and staff feel safe and compelled to speak up"; and "No need to reinvent the wheel."

<u>**Making Action Affordable and Easy:**</u> At the executive level, incentives were created at the health plan level to encourage hospital participation. At the team level, a statewide summit was held every 6 months, creating energy and enthusiasm and accelerating the pace for action. At the frontline ground level, we created forcing function insertion and dressing change kits, where all needed supplies were bundled and accessible in a cart or a kit. Adopting the evidence-based bundle (e.g., using full drapes instead of small rectangular drapes, sterile capping the end of infusion lines instead of looping the end to an infusion port) became the *easier* opt-in default.

<u>**Tempo:**</u> We established a *relentless* drumbeat of weekly messaging during the collaborative. These messages provided a means to share tools, set challenges, and provide feedback. Some weeks, the message was an inspirational quote (e.g., "It is good to have an end to journey toward; but it is the journey that matters, in the end"—*Ursula Le Guin*). Sometimes it was a practical challenge (e.g., test a new tool on three patients by next week!). The goal was to always keep a tension (the dance space). Within that space, every team was allowed to speed up and slow down as needed.

Over the 2-year length of the collaborative, the statewide CLABSI rate dropped 80%. Hawaii was recognized as having the lowest statewide standardized infection ratio (SIR) in the nation, an achievement that was sustained for 3 years beyond the end of the collaborative.

Acknowledgments

Humble thanks to Jeff Cooper, John Corman, Denise Dubuque, Robert Eubanks, Gary Kaplan, Michael Leonard, Carol Peden, Liana Peiler, Edgar Schein, and Michael Rosen for their insights and collective wisdom in shaping this chapter.

References

1. Kaplan, G. Chairman and CEO, Virginia Mason. Personal communication.
2. Heifetz RA, Linsky M. *Leadership on the Line: Staying Alive through the Dangers of Change.* Boston: Harvard Business Review Press; 2017.
3. Kotter J. *A Sense of Urgency.* Boston: Harvard Business Review Press; 2008.
4. Lin DM, Weeks K, Bauer L, et al. Eradicating central line-associated bloodstream infections statewide: the Hawaii experience. *Am J Med Qual.* 2012;27(2):124–129.
5. Lin DM, Weeks K, Holzmueller C, Pronovost PJ, Pham JC. Maintaining and Sustaining the On the CUSP-STOP BSI Model in Hawaii. *Jt Comm J Qual Patient Saf.* 2013;39(2):51–59.

CHAPTER 38

Leadership in Perioperative Quality

Lee A. Fleisher, MD ■ Carol J. Peden, MB ChB, MD, FRCA, FFICM, MPH

KEY POINTS

- The leader can help set the culture and the vision for the organization.
- Effective leadership creates "psychological safety" for all team members to perform optimally.
- Classic change models are described with the key first step being creating urgency.
- In perioperative care, urgency came originally from the demonstration of patient harm.
- Effective leadership is key to creating an environment for innovation.

To ensure high-quality care for patients, coordination among team members is critical. Over the past decade, we have learned that simply knowing the best approach to care is insufficient to achieving the goal of best outcomes. We now know that implementation of strategies at a local level is critical, as has been demonstrated by the variability in the effectiveness of strategies such as the World Health Organization (WHO) safe surgery checklist.[1–3] Institutional culture has been shown to be one of the key factors in success or failure of any quality improvement (QI) initiative. Culture is, in large part, created by leadership. Leadership does not always mean the authority figure but can include all members of the team. In many high-risk industries, the importance of a "just culture" has become clear, and everyone needs to be able to speak up or errors occur.[4] A leader can help set the culture and the vision for the organization and help create an environment of psychological safety where all team members can feel it is "safe" to express ideas, ask questions, and admit mistakes (Fig. 38.1).[5]

This chapter will outline some key attributes for leadership in perioperative QI.

Leadership and Change Management

QI requires change and, until recently, medicine resisted change. Fortunately, practitioners of medicine and allied professions have recognized the need to change beginning with the publication of a series of Institute of Medicine (IOM) reports, which began with *To Err Is Human.*[6] In that report, anesthesiology was recognized as the specialty that has focused on patient safety with a goal of achieving Six Sigma outcomes. However, perioperative QI has a much longer tradition. A surgeon, Ernest Codman, was at the forefront of using data to benchmark outcomes.[7] Over 100 years ago, Codman said, "Hospitals, if they wish to be sure of improvement, must find out what their results are, must analyze their results, and must compare their results with those of other hospitals." Unfortunately, his ideas were not well accepted by his colleagues at the time (i.e., resistance to change), which led him to resign from the Massachusetts General Hospital, but his ideas were later accepted and eventually led to the founding of The Joint Commission.

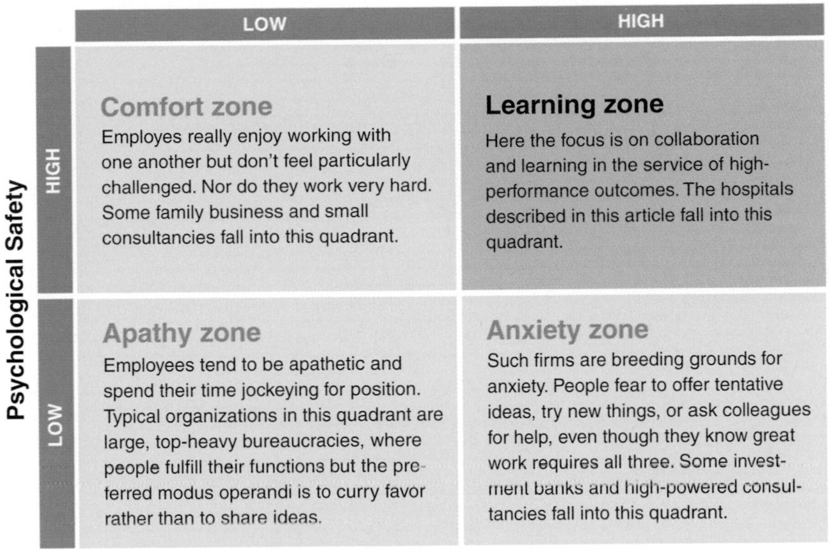

	LOW	HIGH
Psychological Safety — **HIGH**	**Comfort zone** Employes really enjoy working with one another but don't feel particularly challenged. Nor do they work very hard. Some family business and small consultancies fall into this quadrant.	**Learning zone** Here the focus is on collaboration and learning in the service of high-performance outcomes. The hospitals described in this article fall into this quadrant.
Psychological Safety — **LOW**	**Apathy zone** Employees tend to be apathetic and spend their time jockeying for position. Typical organizations in this quadrant are large, top-heavy bureaucracies, where people fulfill their functions but the preferred modus operandi is to curry favor rather than to share ideas.	**Anxiety zone** Such firms are breeding grounds for anxiety. People fear to offer tentative ideas, try new things, or ask colleagues for help, even though they know great work requires all three. Some investment banks and high-powered consultancies fall into this quadrant.

Fig. 38.1 Accountability for meeting demanding goals. (Adapted from Edmondson AC. The competitive imperative of learning. *Harv Bus Rev.* 2008;86(7–8):60–67, 160.)

John Kotter, a Harvard Business School Professor, has written extensively on leading change through an eight-step process.[8,9] The first step is creating a sense of urgency. For anesthesiology, publications demonstrating high mortality directly related to provision of anesthesiology and the associated malpractice costs created a sense of urgency and led to the work of the Closed Claims Study and creation of the Anesthesia Patient Safety Foundation.[10] *To Err Is Human* created the sense of urgency for all of medicine. It is critical to use data to create that sense of urgency. Kotter's other eight steps are listed in Box 38.1.

The leader is responsible for building the coalition and developing the strategic vision. Importantly, the ability to push a vision forward against a clear barrier is very difficult. Therefore it is important for the leader or team to remove barriers.

Kotter went on to develop his model, recognizing the increasing need for speed and agility in leading complex organizations and the need to empower a network of achievers within the organization.[11] This approach applies well to health care, and within that, perioperative care. His developed network has employees from all levels of the organization providing organizational knowledge, relationships, credibility, and influence. This network with a "volunteer army" can harness local creativity and innovation, which can be so important when an in-depth understanding of front-line

---

BOX 38.1 ■ The Eight-Step Process For Leading Change

1. Create a sense of urgency
2. Build a guiding coalition
3. Form a strategic vision and initiatives
4. Enlist a volunteer army
5. Enable action by removing barriers
6. Generate short-term wins
7. Sustain acceleration
8. Institute change

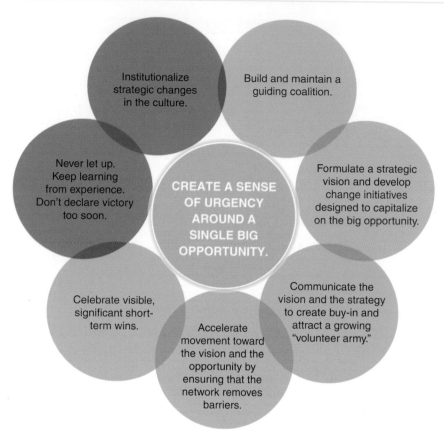

Fig. 38.2 The eight accelerators: The processes that enable the strategy network to function. (Adapted from Kotter JP. Accelerate! *Harv Bus Rev.* 2012;90[11]:44–52, 54–58, 149.)

challenges are needed, as in perioperative care. The volunteers are motivated by an emotional engagement to change, such as a surgeon being passionate about improving patient safety. Kotter's Accelerate model recognizes that leadership can be more fluent, dynamic, and dispersed than in the eight-step model. The key steps of the evolved Accelerate model are shown in Fig. 38.2.

Leadership and Innovation

QI frequently requires developing innovative solutions to quality-of-care problems. Innovation requires hypothesis testing to determine the best solution. Adam Grant recently published a book titled *Think Again.* In the book, he argues, "Thinking again can help you generate new solutions to old problems and revisit old solutions to new problems."[12] Leaders should help teams use data to determine which QI interventions are associated with better outcomes and which ones are not working. The leader can then help the team lean into those that work and help the team stop doing those things that do not work.

Psychological Safety

For teams to be effective problem solvers, the leader must ensure that the team has both a strong sense of accountability and psychological safety. Amy Edmondson, another Harvard Business School professor, defined team psychological safety as "a shared belief held by members of a team that the team is safe for interpersonal risk taking." She defines three key components: (1) Frame the work as a *learning problem,* not an execution problem; (2) acknowledge your *own fallibility;* and (3) model *curiosity.*[13] The figure (see Fig. 38.2) demonstrates this by framing the upper right hand corner of high psychological safety and high accountability as the learning zone. In a recent perspective, Edmondson and colleagues at Penn wrote, "Practice, collaboration, experimentation, feedback solicitation, and reflection on mistakes should be encouraged and not seen as a route to punishment. A culture of psychological safety could allow students and trainees to overcome learning anxieties and defensiveness, reduce stress, engage in positive learning behaviors, and ultimately mitigate the high rates of physician burnout."[14]

Summary

In summary, leadership is critical to establish a culture consistent with QI. In this chapter, we have outlined some of the key characteristics to establish a just culture and learning environment. For further related reading in this book, see Chapters 18, 36, 37, and 62.

References

1. Haynes AB, Weiser TG, Berry WR, et al, Safe Surgery Saves Lives Study Group. A surgical safety checklist to reduce morbidity and mortality in a global population. *N Engl J Med.* 2009;360:491 499.
2. de Vries EN, Prins HA, Crolla RM, et al, SURPASS Collaborative Group. Effect of a comprehensive surgical safety system on patient outcomes. *N Engl J Med.* 2010;363:1928–1937.
3. Urbach DR, Govindarajan A, Saskin R, Wilton AS, Baxter NN. Introduction of surgical safety checklists in Ontario, Canada. *N Engl J Med.* 2014;370:1029–1038.
4. James R. *Managing the risks of organizational accidents.* Ashgate Publishing; 1997.
5. Edmondson AC. *The Fearless Organization: Creating Psychological Safety in the Workplace for Learning, Innovation, and Growth.* Hoboken, NJ: John Wiley & Sons; 2018.
6. Kohn LT, Corrigan JM, Donaldson MS. *To Err Is Human: Building a Safer Health System.* Washington, DC: Institute of Medicine; 2000.
7. American College of Surgeons. Ernest Codman. https://www.facs.org/about-acs/archives/pasthighlights/codmanhighlight. Accessed January 31, 2022.
8. Kotter JP. What leaders really do. *Harv Bus Rev.* 1990;68:103–111.
9. Kotter JP, Schlesinger LA. Choosing strategies for change. *Harv Bus Rev.* 1979;57:106–114.
10. Lee LA, Domino KB. The Closed Claims Project. Has it influenced anesthetic practice and outcome? *Anesthesiol Clin North Am.* 2002;20:485–501.
11. Kotter JP. Accelerate! Harvard Business Review; 2012. https://hbr.org/2012/11/accelerate. Accessed January 31, 2022.
12. Grant A. Think Again: *The Power of Knowing What You Don't Know.* Viking; 2021.
13. Garvin DA, Edmondson AC, Gino F. Is yours a learning organization? *Harv Bus Rev.* 2008;86:109–116. 134.
14. Swendiman RA, Edmondson AC, Mahmoud NN. Burnout in surgery viewed through the lens of psychological safety. *Ann Surg.* 2019;269:234–235.

CHAPTER 39

Establishing and Running Quality Collaboratives: The Michigan Experience

Michael Englesbe, MD

KEY POINTS

- Healthcare quality is high, and costs are low in Michigan.
- The Continuous Quality Improvement (CQI) platform is a statewide learning health system that informs a physician-led, value-based reimbursement scheme.
- The quality agenda in Michigan is outsourced to the physician community and bolstered by a robust value-based scheme that is informed by high-quality registry data that is actionable.
- Financial incentives are important drivers of quality improvement but rarely motivate clinicians to practice change.
- It is unclear whether the CQIs can have success using their quality improvement methods to address gaps in health equity and poor health behaviors, but that is the next challenge.

Approximately 20 years ago, healthcare purchasers in Michigan engaged with the state's dominant private payer to make the strategic decision to invest in a portfolio of collaboratives. This created a statewide learning health system known as the Continuous Quality Improvement Collaboratives (CQIs). The goal of the collaborative work is to drive value and improve health care for patients, clinicians, payers, and purchasers.

The CQIs were born out of efforts to improve perioperative care but have grown to more than 20 specialty or disease-based CQIs. Quality of care is high in Michigan, and costs are the lowest in the United States.[1] As a result, many health systems, payers, and regional healthcare organizations have asked the CQI portfolio to share the framework. In this context, we identify the key domains for developing a successful CQI program within a region.

Funding of the Collaborative Portfolio

Doing CQI work requires a significant investment. In Michigan, the CQI platform is funded by many tens of millions of dollars because detailed and continuous CQI work requires dedicated, full-time, expert support in clinical implementation, statistics, change management, and administration. The collaborative coordinating centers boast a staff of more than 200 full-time employees that dedicate their efforts to improve the value of care in the state of Michigan. This has been a good investment for the large statewide private payer.[2]

The most common question asked by stakeholders outside of the state of Michigan is, "How is all of this paid for?" In short, reimbursement for hospitals and physicians over the past 20 years in

Michigan has been held relatively flat with an increasing proportion of payment put at "risk" via value-based reimbursement and pay-for-performance endeavors. This large resource pool of clinical dollars from the statewide private payer funds the infrastructure, including the CQIs, to engage clinical stakeholders, drive change, and measure performance.

Establishing Trust

The general view in the state of Michigan is that health plans compete and health systems compete, but nurses and doctors do not. As clinicians, we are trained to evaluate evidence, commit to continuous quality improvement, and share best practices. This positive culture has been relatively easy to maintain across the CQI even though all the major health systems and all the clinicians are involved. There is a general rule that CQI data cannot be used for strategic advantage in the healthcare marketplace, nor for direct marketing around high performance. We have never had a breach of this trust. Most impressive is the cardiac surgery group in the state of Michigan. They share identified surgeon and hospital outcomes, review every mortality, and continuously question the appropriateness and technical decisions made by colleagues in an open forum. This sounds threatening, but it is a remarkably collegial and productive community, committed to clinical excellence. The funder does not attend these types of meetings and has never tried to direct business toward high-performing sites; they remain committed to try to help every patient in the state of Michigan have access to the highest quality of care, no matter where they seek care.

Setting the Quality Improvement Agenda With Good Data

The core of any CQI is that nurses and doctors set the patient-centered quality improvement (QI) agenda. Traditionally, many QI initiatives within clinics and operating rooms are guised as efficiency-driven efforts to optimize financial outcomes. Other improvement work driven by measures often related to regulatory influences may assign accountability to stakeholders with little leverage over complex patient experiences. As a result, clinicians can be difficult to engage and may resist change, and efforts fail.

Within this context, the best QI efforts must start with what matters to the patient the most and with reliable and actionable data (Fig. 39.1). All stakeholders can rally around patient-centered care, and it is the best theme for performance measures. These themes will help "win the hearts" of the busy clinical staff. Then, high-quality and robust clinical data must drive the change. Next-level quality measures, such as cancer-specific margin data after surgical resection, appropriateness of percutaneous coronary intervention procedures, and patient-reported empirical data on outcomes (such as regret after surgery and pain control), provide exciting opportunities. Moreover, if you bring specific cancer margin data to cancer surgeons, they will fully engage, own the workflow, and provide significant effort to improve these important cancer outcomes. If you bring QI data to surgeons around clinical outcomes that are important but that those surgeons have less control over, such as urinary tract infection and length of stay in the hospital, you will get less engagement.

A good example of this is perioperative opioid prescribing. First, the CQI facilitators used a story and emotions to engage the physicians and nurses. A compelling and emotional narrative around overprescribing and surgeon behavior and the opioid epidemic was carefully made. Second, the CQIs brought good data to drive the change. They developed site- and provider-specific prescribing reports and a robust system of patient-reported outcomes to ensure the change was patient-centered. Finally, the CQIs developed clear pathways for change informed by evidence and clinical experts. Continuous data feedback and iterative learning facilitated this learning health system and, as a result, very rapid practice change was made across a statewide population of physicians.[3,4]

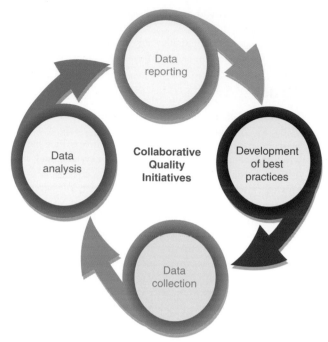

Fig. 39.1   Collaborative quality initiatives. The best quality improvement efforts must start with what matters to the patient the most and with reliable and actionable data.

Leveraging Incentives

Under the CQI model in Michigan, the physician community sets a QI agenda, which ultimately informs value-based reimbursement and pay-for-performance programs. These specialty-based initiatives are pragmatic and evidence-based. Performance benchmarks and criteria for hospital and provider participation are set by the CQIs and by the clinical community. These organizations acknowledge that effective QI must respect the tribal nature of medicine. Said another way, orthopedic surgeons will listen most to other orthopedic surgeons about how to improve orthopedic surgery.

Incentives must align with change that clinicians or hospitals can make. They must also be informed by clinical data that patients and providers care about. An example of a good quality measure is the one mentioned previously—cancer margin status after colorectal cancer surgery. In Michigan, there is an approximately 7% positive margin rate for colorectal cancer resection; this is too high. Some hospitals can achieve a near 0% positive margin rate, suggesting an opportunity for improvement.

One colorectal cancer surgeon said, "I wake up in the morning thinking about my positive margin rate. It is fundamental to how I serve my patients, and it is my identity." The measure is high stakes, and it is easy to get buy-in from surgeons and hospitals to engage. High-performing sites design the key steps and behaviors related to high-performance. Adjustments are made for "uncontrollable" risk, such as patient access to care and health equity, because these issues are critical for overall care in Michigan but are poorly suited to a specific quality-based financial incentive. Said again, we do not want to penalize surgeons and hospitals who serve at-risk populations, and we do not want to lose groups because they feel they have no leverage to make the needed changes in care.

There are three key steps in this program. Step 1 is making sure each site is measuring margin status the same way; this includes engagement from surgical pathology. Step 2 is to communicate the imperative, including patient stories and setting an aspirational goal of 0% positive margin rate for Michigan. Step 3 is sharing evidence-based pathways for care and establishing process and outcome measures that will inform the financial incentive program. These measures should be based on a mix of relative improvement and benchmarked outcomes.

Incentives are complex issue for providers. A common sentiment when discussing financial incentives is "We do the work, and the hospital gets the incentive" or "I am not sure where the incentives go but not to me." In short, incentives are key for organizational buy-in but rarely motivate clinicians to practice change. The incentives enable an organization (hospital or physician organization) to focus on a domain for improvement and dedicate infrastructure to support the change, but the compelling, patient-centered narrative is the most important lever to motivate change for administrators and providers. Effective change requires both financial incentives and a compelling narrative focused on patients.

Summary

The CQI model for regional care is good for patients, providers, payers, and purchasers.[5-7] Many cultural hurdles must be overcome around trust and funding, but once a robust learning health system is in place, the utility to the served population is large, and the return on investment is robust. The platform allows for care transformation. The next steps for the CQI portfolio include focusing on the foundational health of the population. It is unclear whether the CQIs can have success using their QI methods to address gaps in health equity and poor health behaviors, but that is the next challenge.

References

1. White C, Whaley CM. Prices paid to hospitals by private health plans are high relative to Medicare and vary widely. *Rand Health Q.* 2019;9(2):5.
2. Sheetz KH, Englesbe M. Expanding the quality collaborative model as a blueprint for higher-value care. *JAMA Health Forum.* 2020;1(5), e200413.
3. Brown CS, Vu JV, Howard RA, et al. Assessment of a quality improvement intervention to decrease opioid prescribing in a regional health system. *BMJ Qual Saf.* 2021;30:251–259.
4. Vu JV, Howard RA, Gunaseelan V, Brummett CM, Waljee JF, Englesbe MJ. Statewide implementation of postoperative opioid prescribing guidelines. *N Engl J Med.* 2019;381:680–682.
5. Campbell DA, Englesbe MJ. How can the American College of Surgeons-National Surgical Quality Improvement Program help or hinder the general surgeon? *Adv Surg.* 2008;42:169–181.
6. Campbell DA, Englesbe MJ, Kubus JJ, et al. Accelerating the pace of surgical quality improvement: the power of hospital collaboration. *Arch Surg.* 2010;145:985–991.
7. Campbell DA, Krapohl GL, Englesbe MJ. Conceptualizing partnerships between private payers and medicare for quality improvement initiatives. *JAMA Surg.* 2018;153:4–5.

CHAPTER 40

Excellent Perioperative Patient Experience

Thomas H. Lee, MD

KEY POINTS

- Patient experience in the perioperative setting is increasingly important, driven by the growing complexity of medicine and aging of the population.
- The same principles of high reliability that have markedly improved safety can be used to improve patient experience.
- Key focuses should be coordination, empathy, communication, and cleanliness.

Patient experience has become an increasingly important focus in health care over the last 20 years, but its relevance and implications for perioperative care are just becoming understood. The easing of patients' fears and anxiety as they undergo procedures has always been a goal for clinicians, but the critical nature of this goal became more obvious during the COVID-19 pandemic, when care was disrupted in so many ways. Without the familiarity of "business as usual" procedures of perioperative care, patients and their families were unnerved, and clinicians had to use principles of high reliability to preserve safety but also to ensure that care was coordinated and empathic—before, during, and after surgery.

The lessons learned in perioperative care during the COVID-19 pandemic should not be forgotten once the crisis passes. This chapter will therefore present a brief history of the emergence of patient experience as an important dimension of quality, a summary of data on factors that help increase patients' trust in their care, and some principles for improvement.

A Brief History of Patient Experience

Patient experience is a relatively new focus for health care, and when the field first developed, its goals and terminology were different from today. "Patient satisfaction" emerged as a concern of hospital managers in the 1980s with the goal of reducing malpractice litigation. At that time, it was common for clinicians to assert that quality was not something that could be defined or measured and that it was basically fine, with the exception of occasional unfortunate events, which were usually considered unforeseeable and unpreventable. Many clinicians believed in that era that the most important way to protect quality was to preserve the autonomy of good, hard-working doctors.

The event that set change in motion was the publication at the beginning of this century of the Institute of Medicine (IOM) reports *To Err Is Human*[1] and *Crossing the Quality Chasm*.[2] The IOM reports revealed that quality was *not* just fine and that work to improve quality was an imperative for clinicians and their organizations. The most conspicuous focus of the IOM reports was patient safety, but the reports also asserted that care should be timely, effective, efficient, equitable, and patient-centered. In its recommendations, the IOM defined goals, including:

- That health care should be responsive to patients' needs at all times (24 hours a day, 7 days a week)
- That clinicians and patients should communicate effectively and share information
- That clinicians should cooperate, communicate, and coordinate their efforts

Shortly after these reports, the term "patient satisfaction" began to give way to "patient experience." This change reflected the realization that being a patient was qualitatively different from being a "consumer" whose expectations could be "satisfied." Patients were people who were frightened and often in pain; the goal was to reduce their suffering. Their experiences were, in fact, an important outcome of care.[3] Fig. 40.1 provides a structure to incorporate the patient's voice and what matters to them into health care.[3]

What Matters to Patients

In the two decades since the IOM reports, extensive data on many millions of patients have been collected to capture the nuances of patients' experiences, allowing analyses of what matters most to them. These analyses have been performed by Press Ganey in all the major settings of care—inpatient, outpatient, ambulatory surgery, emergency departments—and the conclusions are similar. Patients may not be able to judge the technical quality of care, but five issues are consistent independent drivers of their trust in their care (as reflected in their "likelihood to recommend" the providers)[4]:

1. Confidence in their clinicians
2. Coordination
3. Empathy
4. Communication
5. Cleanliness

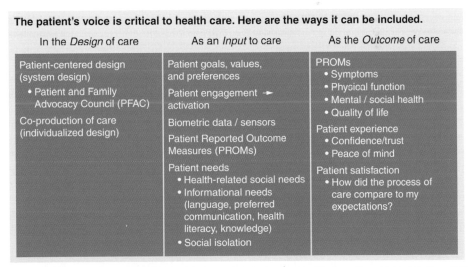

The patient's voice is critical to health care. Here are the ways it can be included.

In the *Design* of care	As an *Input* to care	As the *Outcome* of care
Patient-centered design (system design) • Patient and Family Advocacy Council (PFAC) Co-production of care (individualized design)	Patient goals, values, and preferences Patient engagement → activation Biometric data / sensors Patient Reported Outcome Measures (PROMs) Patient needs • Health-related social needs • Informational needs (language, preferred communication, health literacy, knowledge) • Social isolation	PROMs • Symptoms • Physical function • Mental / social health • Quality of life Patient experience • Confidence/trust • Peace of mind Patient satisfaction • How did the process of care compare to my expectations?

Fig. 40.1 A structure to incorporate the patient and family voice into health care. (From Mohta NS, Prewitt E, Volpp KG, et al. Insights roundtable report: measuring what matters and capturing the patient voice. *NEJM Catalyst*. 2017. https://catalyst.nejm.org/doi/full/10.1056/CAT.17.0380.)

After these variables are taken into account, other issues (e.g., waiting time) are not independent drivers of "likelihood to recommend" in virtually every analysis and every organization. Patients do not like to wait, of course, but data consistently demonstrate that if communication about the reasons for delay is good, the delays do not damage patients' confidence in their care.

Cleanliness has emerged as a more important driver of patient trust with the COVID-19 pandemic. Patients and their families are more aware of the risk of infection than in the past, so they are unnerved by restrooms that are not clean or body fluids that are allowed to remain on gowns and sheets.

How to Improve

Improvement of perioperative patient experience relies on extending the same high reliability principles that transformed safety in anesthesia and (less completely) the rest of medicine in recent decades.[5] Key steps include:

1. Committing to goals that reflect an aversion to failure (e.g., Zero Harm in safety)
2. Measurement, followed by analysis of data, and creating systems to respond to resulting insights
3. Creating a culture with a commitment to improvement
4. Fostering "norms" of behavior that support goals

Particularly essential in perioperative care is attention to coordination of care. Of course, teamwork is essential to patient safety, but the goal is deeper than preventing physical harm. Clinicians should recognize that when it is obvious to patients that their caregivers do not actually know each other (e.g., when it is not clear who will be doing what to them), it is unnerving. Patients draw reassurance from knowing that their caregivers know each other, work together all the time, and like and trust each other. Conveying that reassurance is most readily accomplished, of course, by having caregivers actually be organized as true teams.

Coordination and communication within the perioperative team and with the patient is essential for one level of excellence, but deeper excellence requires extension of these values to other clinicians involved in patients' care and to their families. The importance of these two "satellite" groups is growing for two irresistible reasons. First, medical progress has meant increasing numbers of clinicians are involved in the care of most patients, and they tend to have narrow focuses, leading to chaos that frightens patients and is dispiriting for clinicians. Real efforts to ensure communication and coordination with outpatient physicians, for example, is something that helps ease fear for patients.

Patients' families are increasingly a focus because of demographic trends, such as the aging of the population combined with the high standards of the Baby Boom generation. The conversation between an individual physician and the patient is often just the first step in needed communication.

For this reason, "Zoom Family Meetings" have become increasingly common,[6] with adoption accelerating during the COVID-19 pandemic when so many people became more comfortable with web-based interactions. A valuable part of such meetings is for clinicians to have 15 minutes to discuss patients' issues before patients and their families are "admitted" to the "room." In this era when clinicians often are interacting more with the electronic record than with each other, the difference between doing a competent job as an individual and an excellent job as a team becomes immediately obvious when caregivers are "face-to-face" in a Zoom room. Including outpatient physicians in such conferences is particularly valuable for bolstering the confidence of patients and their families and for addressing issues and concerns related to postprocedure care.

A final principle for improvement of perioperative patient experience is adoption of the first line of Tolstoy's novel, *Anna Karenina*, which reads, "Happy families are all alike; every unhappy family is unhappy in its own way." The Anna Karenina Principle as applied to health care means that every patient's care should include certain features (i.e., coordination, good communication, showing empathy).

On the other hand, reliable practicing of these "always events" should be accompanied by the same type of aversion for patient experience "never events" akin to safety failures (i.e., doing all that can be done to prevent the myriad types of failures that can undermine patients' confidence that they are getting excellent care). For example, when patients witness problems like the wrong food being brought to them, they cannot help but wonder "what else can't they get right!"

In summary, extending the same principles of high reliability learned through patient safety to patient experience provides a familiar path forward for improvement of perioperative patient experience. Just as performing the preoperative checklist and excellent hand hygiene are norms in virtually every surgical setting today, the same should be true for ensuring that patients and their families are treated with respect and experience care that is coordinated and well-communicated. Just as perioperative teams detect and learn from every safety event, they should detect and learn from every instance in which care disappoints patients and their families.

References

1. Kohn LT, Corrigan JM, Donaldson MS, eds. *To Err Is Human: Building a Safer Health System*. Washington, DC: National Academies Press; 2000.
2. *Committee on Quality of Health Care in America: Crossing the Quality Chasm: A New Health System for the 21st Century*. Washington, DC: National Academies Press; 2001.
3. Mohta NS, Prewitt E, Volpp KG, et al. Insights roundtable report: measuring what matters and capturing the patient voice. *NEJM Catalyst*. 2017. https://catalyst.nejm.org/doi/full/10.1056/CAT.17.0380.
4. Lee TH. *An Epidemic of Empathy in Healthcare*. New York: McGraw Hill; 2016.
5. Gandhi TK, Feeley D, Schummers D. Zero harm in health care. *NEJM Catalyst*. 2020. https://catalyst.nejm.org/doi/abs/10.1056/CAT.19.1137.
6. Lee TH. Zoom family meeting. *N Engl J Med*. 2021;384:1586–1587.

CHAPTER 41

An International Perspective on Training and Setting Standards in Perioperative Medicine

Monty G. Mythen, MBBS, MD, FRCA, FFICM, FCAI (Hon)

KEY POINTS

- Perioperative medicine/care is multidisciplinary and covers the whole pathway from moment of contemplation of surgery to full recovery.
- Perioperative medicine and perioperative care are synonymous in many countries (but not all). Base training (e.g., nurse, physician, or physiotherapist) will be a factor in determining scope of practice and thus training, but the knowledge base is common.
- A common curriculum has been codified and published (open source) by the International Board of Perioperative Medicine. This was based on preexisting training programs and taught Masters (MSc).
- Standards are largely from professional bodies (e.g., Colleges/Associations) but are being extended and complemented by younger perioperative-focused organizations (e.g., the UK Centre for Perioperative Care, The Perioperative Quality Initiative, and The African Perioperative Research Group).

The Importance of Training and Standards in Perioperative Medicine

A BRIEF HISTORY

In 1996 an editorial was published in the journal *Anesthesiology* titled "Anesthesia and Perioperative Medicine—A Department of Anesthesiology Changes Its Name."[1] In the editorial, Alpert et al. explain the rational for the switch from "anesthesiology" to "anesthesia" and the addition of "perioperative medicine" (POM). They cite two previous Rovenstine lectures (the eponymous invited plenary lecture usually delivered at the annual meeting of the American Society of Anesthesiologists) by Greene (1992) and Saidman (1994) that explored the journey to departments of "perioperative and pain medicine," dropping anesthesia completely. In an editorial published in 1995, Rosenthal went so far as to say, "With the many changes in health care delivery, the future survival of anesthesiology as a specialty may well depend on the acceptance that perioperative involvement, rather than sole intraoperative anesthesia practice, is the purview of the anesthesiologists."[2] There was a growing minority opinion that the future of anesthesiology was going to be increasingly outside the operating room.

The organization Evidence-Based Perioperative Medicine (EBPOM) was formed in 1997.[3] EBPOM is a:

> not for profit collaborative project between a number of UK and international academic institutions that exists to promote the examination, discussion and application of evidence-based medicine to perioperative care. Its aim is to improve the outcome of patients undergoing surgery, through creating a forum for research development, practical acquisition of essential skills, and dissemination of evidence-based perioperative knowledge.

Since then (i.e., up to 2021), many departments have changed their names to include POM, fellowships have been advertised,[4] and new sections have appeared in the main anesthesia journals (*BJA*; *Anesthesiology*; *Anesthesia and Analgesia*; *Anaesthesia*). There is a new journal of POM,[5] and postgraduate training programmes are on offer.[6]

A tipping point was in 2014, when the UK's Royal College of Anaesthetists launched the POM program[7] to "facilitate the delivery of best preoperative, intraoperative, and postoperative care through implementation of evidence-based medicine to reduce variation and improve postoperative outcomes." A network of POM leads was established through the UK's National Health Service (NHS), and Guidelines for the Provision of Anaesthetic Services from the Royal College of Anaesthetists were published. The anaesthetic higher specialist curriculum approved by the UK's General Medical Council was revised to include specific competencies in POM and an advanced POM training section.[8] This information is all open source and can be found via the Internet.[7,8]

Many quite rightly point out that POM has existed for as long as surgery, and that it is a core component of being a surgeon.[9] "Internists" or "hospitalists" specializing in POM are commonplace in many US centers,[10] and services specializing in prehabilitation,[11] surgery schools,[12] and teams dedicated to the needs of the frail elderly surgical patient and so on were emerging at the time.[13] The UK thus moved to the formation of a new "Centre for Perioperative Care" (CPOC) that is multidisciplinary and supported by multiple professional colleges and societies.[14] The first group of appointed leaders (CPOC Directors) are from anesthesia, surgery, and geriatrics. POM in much of the world is synonymous with perioperative care.

There is understandably no internationally agreed on common path to training in POM. Nevertheless, a postgraduate qualification (e.g., a university-awarded certificate, diploma, or Masters) combined with a clinical fellowship is now quite common.[15] A selection of international fellowships can be found with an Internet search or on the website of the Trainees in Perioperative Medicine (TRIPOM).[16] Many are open to and encourage overseas applicants. A common curriculum has been codified and published (open source) by the International Board of Perioperative Medicine (IBPOM).[17] The IBPOM curriculum was based on preexisting training programs and taught Masters (MSc) and has four broad sections:

1. General topics and introduction;
2. Preoperative assessment and planning;
3. Postoperative assessment and management;
4. Improvement science, research, and value for perioperative medicine

The learning objectives are that on completion of the IBPOM syllabus, the learner would be expected to:

1. Demonstrate a patient-centered approach to the integrative multidisciplinary care of patients contemplating or undergoing surgery.
2. Demonstrate expertise in the clinical management of patients in the perioperative period (i.e., preoperative, intraoperative, acute postoperative, and postoperative transition of care periods).

3. Ensure that perioperative services are fully integrated, consistent, and reliable and make efficient use of resources.
4. Partner with colleagues in other disciplines, including primary care, surgeons, hospitalists, rehabilitation, geriatricians, nurses, and allied health professionals.
5. Demonstrate an advanced understanding of the importance and functioning of the preadmission process and/or clinic.
6. Educate the perioperative physician to risk stratify and optimize care of the patient in the perioperative period.
7. Develop the expertise to take a lead in collaborative decision making about the suitability of high-risk patients for surgery.
8. Collaboratively manage the patient in the perioperative period (in particular, high-risk surgical patients with acute or chronic medical comorbidities that require optimization and management to improve patient outcomes).
9. Obtain the managerial skills to lead a multidisciplinary perioperative management team.
10. Be equipped with research skills to understand POM research.
11. Provide teaching to colleagues of all grades (levels) and specialties.

Despite wide global variation in resources available for the delivery of health care, there is published evidence of new POM activity in high-, middle-, and low-income countries. For example, the Perioperative Surgical Home (PSH), "a patient-centered, team-based model, modifying healthcare economics, policy, and organization, to enhance quality and patient safety, decrease costs, augment value, and do away with fragmented and variable care" has been adopted by the American Society of Anesthesiologists.[18,19] Enhanced Recovery after Surgery (ERAS) principles have been widely adopted throughout the world, and there are now numerous societies and published guidelines (e.g., the ERAS society[20] and the Enhanced Recovery After Cardiac Surgery society[21]). Although labeled differently, these endeavors are all versions of POM.[22]

The annual meeting of the Chinese Society of Anesthesiology in 2016 was "from anesthesiology to perioperative medicine," which officially launched the new journey of Chinese anesthesiology.[23] Many hospitals in China have changed the name of their anesthesiology departments to "Department of Anesthesiology and Perioperative Medicine" as proposed by Calvert et al. in the 1990s.

Writing in the *Indian Journal of Anaesthesia* in 2019, Shah et al. articulate some of the India-specific hurdles to adoption of POM, including lack of awareness and reluctance/partial acceptance because of clashes with personal beliefs and traditional teaching but predominantly resource limitations such as "a poor doctor–patient ratio in India."[24] More recently there has been greater recognition of the healthcare burden of postoperative mortality (covered elsewhere in this text) and the massive overlap with population health and that a multidisciplinary integrated program to support POM services are integral to a comprehensive population health strategy.[25,26]

Standards for POM are largely from professional bodies (e.g., Colleges/Associations) and build on existing standards. They are being extended and complemented by younger POM-focused organizations (e.g. the UK Centre for Perioperative Care[14]; the Perioperative Quality Initiative[27]) that publish best evidence-based guidelines using consensus statements and the GRADE methodology. Nevertheless, much of the available evidence that supports recommendations is "weak," underlining the importance of ongoing research to better inform practice. To enable further research to inform standards, as patient-centered outcomes are increasingly used in perioperative clinical trials, the Standardised Endpoints in Perioperative Medicine (StEP) initiative has defined "…which measures should be used in future research to facilitate comparison between studies and to enable robust evidence synthesis."[28]

References

1. Alpert CC, Conroy JM, Roy RC. Anesthesia and perioperative medicine: a department of anesthesiology changes its name. *Anesthesiology.* 1996;84:712–715.
2. Rosenthal MH. Critical care medicine: At the crossroads. *Anesth Analg.* 1995;81:439–440.

3. Evidence Based Perioperative Medicine (EBPOM). https://ebpom.org/about-us/. Accessed June 12, 2021.
4. *University College London. Perioperative Medicine Fellowship*; 2021. https://www.ucl.ac.uk/surgery/research/research-department-targeted-intervention/centre-perioperative-medicine-cpom/perioperative. Accessed August 18.
5. Perioperative Medicine; 2021. https://perioperativemedicinejournal.biomedcentral.com. Accessed August 18th.
6. Monash and UCL Perioperative Medicine Short Course; 2021. https://www.periopmedicine.org.uk. Accessed August 18.
7. *The Royal College of Anaesthetists. Perioperative Medicine—The Pathway to Better Care*; 2021. https://rcoa.ac.uk/sites/default/files/documents/2019-08/Perioperative%20Medicine%20-%20The%20Pathway%20to%20Better%20Care.pdf. Accessed August 18.
8. Royal College of Anaesthetists. Curriculum learning syllabus—stage 3 special interest areas. https://rcoa.ac.uk/documents/perioperative-medicine. Accessed August 18, 2021.
9. Dahl JB, Kehlet H. Perioperative medicine—a new sub-speciality, or a multi-disciplinary strategy to improve perioperative management and outcome? *Acta Anaesthesiol Scand.* 2002;46:121–122.
10. Pausjenssen L, Ward HA, Card SE. An internist's role in perioperative medicine: a survey of surgeons' opinions. *BMC Fam Pract.* 2008;9:4.
11. Levett DZ, Edwards M, Grocott M, Mythen M. Preparing the patient for surgery to improve outcomes. *Best Pract Res Clin Anaesthesiol.* 2016;30:145–157.
12. Fecher-Jones I, Grimmett C, Carter FJ, Conway DH, Levett DZH, Moore JA. Surgery school-who, what, when, and how: results of a national survey of multidisciplinary teams delivering group preoperative education. *Perioper Med (Lond).* 2021;10:20.
13. Rogerson A, Partridge JS, Dhesi JK. Perioperative medicine for older people. *Ann Acad Med Singap.* 2019;48:376–381.
14. *The Centre for Perioperative Care*; 2021. https://cpoc.org.uk. Accessed August 18.
15. Beutler S, McEvoy MD, Ferrari L, Vetter TR, Bader AM. The future of anesthesia education: developing frameworks for perioperative medicine and population health. *Anesth Analg.* 2020;130:1103–1108.
16. Trainees in Perioperative Medicine (TRIPOM). Fellowships in perioperative medicine. https://tripom.org/fellowships/. Accessed August 18, 2021.
17. *The International Board of Perioperative Medicine*; 2021. https://www.internationalboardpom.org. Accessed August 18.
18. King AB, Alvis BD, McEvoy MD. Enhanced recovery after surgery, perioperative medicine, and the perioperative surgical home: current state and future implications for education and training. *Curr Opin Anaesthesiol.* 2016;29:727–732.
19. Kain ZN, Fitch JC, Kirsch JR, et al. Future of anesthesiology is perioperative medicine: a call for action. *Anesthesiology.* 2015;122:1192–1195.
20. *The ERAS Society*; 2021. https://erassociety.org. Accessed August 17.
21. *Enhanced Recovery After Cardiac Surgery Society*; 2021. https://www.erascardiac.org. Accessed August 17.
22. Cannesson M, Ani F, Mythen M, Kain Z. Anaesthesiology and perioperative medicine around the world: different names, same goals. *Br J Anaesth.* 2015;114:8–9.
23. Wang T, Deng X, Huang Y, Fleisher LA, Xiong L. Road to perioperative medicine: a perspective from China. *Anesth Analg.* 2019;129:905–907.
24. Shah SB, Hariharan U, Chawla R. Integrating perioperative medicine with anaesthesia in India: can the best be achieved? *Indian J Anaesth.* 2019;63:338–349.
25. Aronson S, Westover J, Guinn N, et al. A perioperative medicine model for population health: an integrated approach for an evolving clinical science. *Anesth Analg.* 2018;126:682–690.
26. Beutler S, McEvoy MD, Ferrari L, et al. The future of anesthesia education: developing frameworks for perioperative medicine and population health. *Anesth Analg.* 2020;130:1103–1108.
27. Miller TE, Shaw AD, Mythen MG, et al. Evidence-based perioperative medicine comes of age: the Perioperative Quality Initiative (POQI). *Perioper Med (Lond).* 2016;5:26.
28. Moonesinghe SR, Jackson AIR, Boney O, et al. Systematic review and consensus definitions for the Standardised Endpoints in Perioperative Medicine initiative: patient-centred outcomes. *Br J Anaesth.* 2019;123:664–670.

Putting It All Together— Clinical Quality Improvement Examples

Implementation of Enhanced Recovery for Colorectal Surgery: A Real-World Example of Quality Improvement

Alexander Booth, MD ■ Mark Lockett, MD

KEY POINTS

- Enhanced recovery protocols for colorectal surgery have been widely adopted because of their success in reducing length of hospital stay and complications.
- Quality improvement efforts, including enhanced recovery, face significant barriers requiring persistence and redirection to achieve desired outcomes.

Introduction

In contrast to the methodological rigor of randomized trials targeting a specific question, quality improvement (QI) efforts are more complex and nebulous. They often involve many changes at once and rely on coordination between multiple disciplines. Results can be hard to measure and slow to manifest, and outcomes are not always as expected. Whereas scientific trials address a specific question with precision, QI efforts tend to achieve goals through changes to systems and culture. Moreover, the targets, strategies, and agents involved in project implementation must evolve as new knowledge and barriers arise. Lastly, the appetite for change waxes and wanes among stakeholders, requiring frequent stoking of the QI fire.

We present here our journey to improve outcomes in colon surgery. We chose this as a QI project because the case volume is high, and morbidity is significant both in frequency and severity. Length of stay (LOS) can be long, infection rates can be high, and the likelihood of patients returning to the emergency department (ED) or needing readmission is significant.

A number of reports indicate enhanced recovery (ER) programs in colorectal surgery can provide dramatic improvements in LOS, surgical site infection (SSI), and readmission.[1–5] One group suggested the process was easy, noting significantly improved outcomes "*immediately* after implementing enhanced recovery" (emphasis ours).[2] Although adopting the concept of ER was easy, we did not find the actual implementation to be simple, nor did we see immediate improvement in outcomes. In our experience, QI initiatives rarely "flip a switch" or produce rapid and continuous linear improvement. Some process measures change rapidly, but others require more effort and understanding of underlying obstacles before improvement occurs. Some QI literature presents results in an Instagram-like manner, leaving out much of the struggle involved in the journey.

We highlight here some of the successes of our efforts but also point out some of the delays and obstacles we encountered launching a QI program in colorectal surgery (Box 42.1). Specifically, we explore how we instituted process changes such as early feeding and opioid minimization, established acceptance, built momentum, and eventually adopted new processes of care.

Methods

An ER committee was established at our institution in 2016. A multidisciplinary team including surgery, anesthesia, nursing, and administrative staff adopted a charter, approved a series of perioperative order sets, and developed a plan for implementation. The team met quarterly to review the baseline data for colectomy outcomes including LOS, readmissions, and SSIs. Initial quality measurement efforts focused on process measures rather than outcomes. These measures included preoperative oral antibiotics, intraoperative fluid minimization, avoiding patient-controlled analgesia (PCA), diet initiation on postoperative day (POD) 1, and ambulation at least twice daily. Before these standards, each surgeon managed patients with individual algorithms, most of which involved prolonged fasting, nasogastric tubes, and PCAs.

Complicating the effort, our facility transitioned to a new electronic health record (EHR) around the time of implementation. Information technology specialists were needed to install order sets but were unavailable because of many competing projects. In addition, multiple committee discussions, negotiations, and approvals were required to allow the ER protocol to be incorporated into the EHR. Nine months passed before the ER protocol went live. Once the first patients were enrolled, monthly committee meetings were used to monitor compliance with process measures, analyze outcomes, and discuss new and ongoing barriers to implementation.

Multiple data sources were used to track outcomes including coding data, ER-champion chart abstraction data, and data from our facility's membership in the South Carolina Surgical Quality Collaborative (SCSQC).[6] Each data source provided slightly different results as the definitions and accuracy of data capture vary across these sources.

Results

Compliance with ER components is shown in Fig. 42.1. Preoperative oral antibiotics were already standard of care with near 100% compliance (see Fig. 42.1A), but we saw a drop off in compliance over time. Early ambulation remained well below the target goal during the initial year (see Fig. 42.1B). PCA utilization remained high for a full year (see Fig. 42.1C). Compliance with early feeding steadily improved (see Fig. 42.1D). Intraoperative fluid restriction was slower to change but

---

BOX 42.1 ■ Summary of Takeaway Points

Takeaway Points

- Even well-designed and externally valid quality improvement (QI) initiatives take time to initiate and are not immune to challenges in implementation.
- Unanticipated downstream effects are common and may result in unintended consequences.
- Selecting relevant metrics and gathering reliable data are important, but providers must recognize improving care is the goal, not just improving metrics.
- Fostering a culture of improvement requires buy-in at all levels.
- Setbacks are common, should be expected, and should not be allowed to derail the effort.

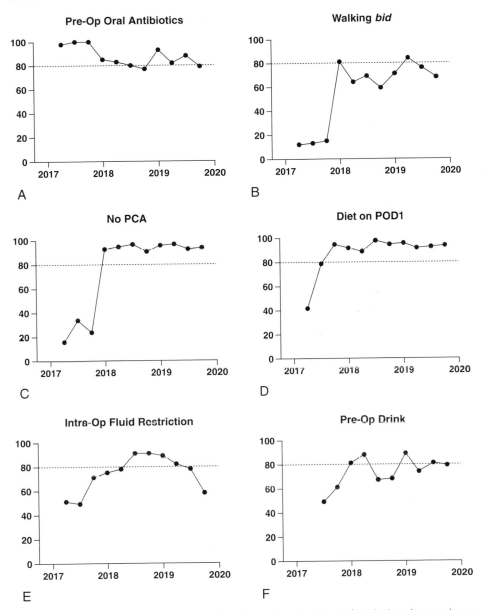

Fig. 42.1 Percentage of process measure compliance for elective colectomy and proctectomy by annual quarter from enhanced recovery implementation. *PCA*, Patient-controlled analgesia; *POD*, postoperative day.

did become standard for an increasing number of anesthesia providers (see Fig. 42.1E). Each component of the ER protocol was adopted but at different rates and with varying impact on outcomes.

Data abstracted by the ER coordinator showed that the rate of SSI increased in the initial period (Table 42.1). This is a common occurrence in QI efforts. Things may get worse before they get better. This is commonly associated with more accurate data being captured compared with baseline rates. For example, the rate of SSI in our baseline period was unusually low and was followed by a

TABLE 42.1 ■ Comparison of Outcomes Before and After Initial ER Protocol Implementation Based on Data Collected by the ER Coordinator

	Pre-Implementation	Post-Implementation
Total Cases	183	97
Mean LOS	6.9	5.85
Median LOS	5	4
Mode LOS	4	4
Readmissions	14 (8.0%)	9 (9.3%)
SSI	12 (6.6%)	11 (13.6%)
Ileus	28 (15.3%)	4 (4.1%)

ER, Enhanced recovery; *LOS*, length of stay; *SSI*, surgical site infection.

spike immediately after ER initiation, potentially because of more awareness of metrics and better overall documentation. Mean and median LOS decreased by 1 day, whereas readmissions were relatively unchanged. These mixed results are common early in QI projects, should be anticipated, and should not discourage the effort.

Analysis of long-term sampled data from the SCSQC (which uses many data elements and well-defined criteria for SSIs, readmissions, etc.) showed decreasing rates of SSI, 30-day readmission, and postoperative ED visits between 2015 and 2020 (Fig. 42.2).

Discussion

Our data shows the ER project improved outcomes but not in a linear fashion, not without setbacks, and with slower than expected progress at times. There were unanticipated hurdles, problems with chosen metrics, and difficulties with consistent outcomes measurement. The path to improving quality is littered with stumbling blocks, wrong turns, and frequently takes longer than anticipated.[7,8] Nevertheless, better outcomes for patients justify the effort needed to identify and implement best practices.

During this effort, we learned multiple lessons that we applied to expanding ER to other specialties. Champions in each discipline are needed to imbed changes into culture.[9] Data capture is time-consuming but critical for tracking progress; facilities need to provide protected time for staff to be involved in these efforts. Data metrics have limitations, which must be recognized, but limitations should not eliminate the use of a given metric. Unintended consequences are common and frequently require adjustments to the original plan. Patience is needed as improvement in outcomes is rarely linear or continuous.

Process changes and metrics can have unforeseen consequences and may not function as expected, requiring adjustments as QI projects mature.[10] For example, we thought PCA use would be decreased simply by omitting them from the postoperative order set. Unfortunately, PCA use persisted long after ER implementation. When we asked surgeons why PCAs were still being ordered, concerns were voiced that patients were not getting intermittent pain medications in a timely fashion. When we asked nurses about the pain medication delays, problematic nurse staffing was the primary factor. Adding to the complexity, the hospital census was so high that patients were being admitted to any bed available and frequently to nonsurgical floors where nurses were not vested in the ER protocol. A key component to lowering PCA use was not removing PCAs from the order set; it was ensuring colectomy patients were admitted to the same surgical floor every time

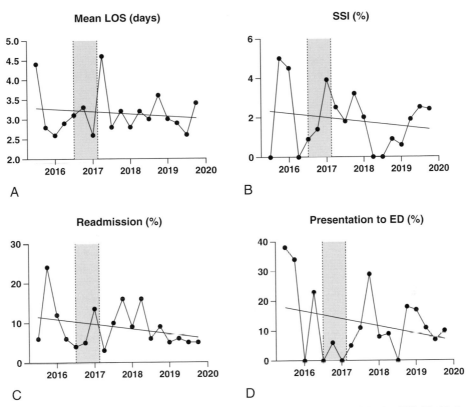

Fig. 42.2 Mean length of stay (*LOS*) (A) and proportion of cases with surgical site infection (*SSI*) (B), 30-day readmission (C), and presentation to emergency department (*ED*) within 30 days (D) by annual quarter, sampled from the South Carolina Surgical Quality Collaborative (SCSQC) database. *Note:* Shaded area represents the baseline period prior to enhanced recovery (ER) implementation.

and making sure nurses were experienced in the ER protocol. This exemplifies how QI efforts need to address root causes, rather than focus solely on a metric. It also demonstrates how systems, not just individuals, are involved in QI efforts because administrative input was required to adjust staffing and bed management processes.

Successful QI efforts in medicine rarely involve making one major fix. The interconnected nature of medical systems guarantee downstream effects will result from any change in input. With the intricacy and complexity in the healthcare environment, it can even be difficult to agree on definitions for measuring high-quality outcomes.[11] Even when providers do agree, the patient, hospital, and funding agencies can define quality with different metrics. When a quality metric is adopted, the ability to measure it in an accurate and meaningful way can still be a challenge. Data definitions, where to find data, how long to track it, who will do the tracking, and how to fund it are only a few of the significant obstacles involved when initiating and maintaining a QI project.

Our struggle to meet the early ambulation metric exemplifies some of the challenges that come with data tracking. Because compliance remained well below the target goal during the initial year (see Fig. 42.1B), the ER committee attributed the deficiency to chart documentation issues rather than a true failure to mobilize patients. Thus data reliability can become a major stumbling block to QI efforts. Much effort was spent on ascertaining whether patients were not ambulating as expected or whether the issue was documenting ambulation in the health record. The reality was both; both ambulation and documentation needed improvement. Dismissing the metric as unreliable was not appropriate but recognizing the metric's limited ability to reflect actual patient care was important to prevent discouraging staff who were trying to improve the metric. Quality reporting systems in health care are fraught with unreliable data and debatable metrics.[10] QI efforts are easily derailed before they even get started if those involved are not willing to accept limitations in data reporting and less-than-ideal outcome measures. If providers feel a chosen metric is not accurate or useful, many other aspects of the project may get disregarded. QI leaders need to become cognizant of this tendency, acknowledge it, and adjust measures and implementation to keep the project on the right path.

To facilitate process improvement, healthcare providers are commonly asked to use QI frameworks that are not ideally suited for use in health care. Most QI structures were developed in industry and may not adequately adjust for the complexities involved in health care. As an example, many hospitals use High Reliability Organization (HRO) principles or Lean as part of their QI efforts.[12] These QI systems were developed by investigating "complex" industries such as nuclear power, manufacturing, and air travel. The complexity of the industries in which these systems were developed pales in comparison to that of managing even a single patient, much less an entire healthcare system. QI platforms developed in industries where foundational facts and linear outcomes are the norm may not translate well to healthcare settings. We know what makes planes fly and land because we built them. We have far less knowledge about how the human body works and responds to various interventions. We do not always know why one patient developed an infection while another did not, even when all correct processes were followed for both patients. Patient-specific factors, social determinants of health, and many yet unknown factors impact outcomes in health care. The complexity of health care exponentially exceeds that of the industries on which many QI improvement platforms were structured. These QI frameworks are still useful, but QI providers need to be cognizant of their limitations and be willing to adapt them to the dynamic and complex world of health care.

Motivation to improve is an often-overlooked prerequisite to QI. People have an inherent desire to improve work quality and efficiency but also tend to overestimate abilities. Over 80% of people believe they are an above-average driver.[13] Most surgeons believe they are above average and have above average outcomes. One of the biggest hurdles at the outset of any QI project is generating the urgency for improvement.[14] We found most providers liked the concept of ER on paper, but motivating them to actively change a practice in the real world was more time consuming and challenging than anticipated. Old habits truly are hard to break. The provision of reliable data was key to getting clinicians engaged and focused on following the process measures.

Another foundational step in any QI initiative is identifying an aim that is both worthy and realistic. Without such a cornerstone, any initiative is bound to fail because of lack of buy-in from those involved. The motivation to improve and momentum toward change flow from the aim. Tracking outcomes and sharing data with stakeholders can help build momentum for projects; successes fuel more effort to improve even further.[15] In addition, care must be taken at the outset to ensure measures are not overly simplified and account for unintended consequences. As an example, efforts to lower patient pain scores, although valid and easily measurable, could lead to worse outcomes vis-à-vis opioid overprescribing. Unintended consequences can discourage providers and negatively impact patients. QI leaders must continually look at the overall outcomes associated with any process changes, not just the chosen metrics.

People who have tried to lose weight or get in shape know the complex interactions involved at a personal level to accomplish a personal QI goal. Institutional QI projects are dependent on the QI efforts of everyone involved. Frequently, individuals do not benefit directly from their contributions toward the project, so motivation can be challenging. Would you go on a diet if someone else lost the weight? The need to create a team-based approach to developing a culture that focuses on getting better is paramount to successful QI implementation. Participants need to have an idea how their contribution affects the overall effort and should be rewarded for their efforts. As in economies outside of health care, incentives affect behavior. Measures and rewards should be structured to support introspective analysis and personal responsibility as components of membership in a team seeking a worthwhile goal of better patient care.

Conclusion

QI in health care is complex and dirty work with nonlinear results and frequent failures. Recognition of the struggles and complexities inherent to the process is paramount to keeping providers engaged and motivated in the effort. Reliable, quantifiable metrics are important but not sufficient to improve outcomes. Care must be taken to ensure efforts are truly helping patients, not just improving a metric. QI efforts should be agile and dynamic to achieve the goal of better patient care.

Acknowledgments

The authors thank Geri Johnston, MSN for her dedication to the ER program as coordinator and for providing data for this chapter.

References

1. Zargar-Shoshtari K, Connolly AB, Israel LH, et al. Fast-track surgery may reduce complications following major colonic surgery. *Dis Colon Rectum.* 2008;51(11):1633–1640.
2. Nygren J, Soop M, Thorell A, et al. An enhanced-recovery protocol improves outcome after colorectal resection already during the first year: a single-center experience in 168 consecutive patients. *Dis Colon Rectum.* 2009;52(5):978–985.
3. Keenan JE, Speicher PJ, Nussbaum DP, et al. Improving outcomes in colorectal surgery by sequential implementation of multiple standardized care programs. *J Am Coll Surg.* 2015;221(2):404–414.e401.
4. Shah PM, Johnston L, Sarosiek B, et al. Reducing readmissions while shortening length of stay: the positive impact of an enhanced recovery protocol in colorectal surgery. *Dis Colon Rectum.* 2017;60(2):219–227.
5. Wick EC, Galante DJ, Hobson DB, et al. Organizational culture changes result in improvement in patient-centered outcomes: implementation of an integrated recovery pathway for surgical patients. *J Am Coll Surg.* 2015;221(3):669–677.
6. Lockett MA, Mauldin PD, Zhang J, et al. Facilitated regional collaboration and in-hospital surgical complication. *J Am Coll Surg.* 2021;232(4):536–543.
7. van Zelm R, Coeckelberghs E, Sermeus W, et al. A mixed methods multiple case study to evaluate the implementation of a care pathway for colorectal cancer surgery using extended normalization process theory. *BMC Health Serv Res.* 2021;21(1).
8. Hull L, Athanasiou T, Russ S. Implementation science: a neglected opportunity to accelerate improvements in the safety and quality of surgical care. *Ann Surg.* 2017;265(6):1104–1112.
9. Bonawitz K, Wetmore M, Heisler M, et al. Champions in context: which attributes matter for change efforts in healthcare? *Implement Sci.* 2020;15(1).
10. Lewis CC, Proctor EK, Brownson RC. Measurement issues in dissemination and implementation research. *Dissemination and Implementation Research in Health: Translating Science to Practice.* 2nd ed. Oxford University Press; 2017.
11. Ornstein JT, Hammond RA, Padek M, et al. Rugged landscapes: complexity and implementation science. *Implement Sci.* 2020;15(1).
12. Polonsky MS. High-reliability organizations: the next frontier in healthcare quality and safety. *J Heathc Manag.* 2019;64(4):213–221.
13. McCormick IA, Walkey FH, Green DE. Comparative perceptions of driver ability—a confirmation and expansion. *Accid Anal Prev.* 1986;18(3):205–208.
14. Desveaux L, Ivers NM, Devotta K, et al. Unpacking the intention to action gap: a qualitative study understanding how physicians engage with audit and feedback. *Implement Sci.* 2021;16(1).
15. Powell BJ, Stanick CF, Halko HM, et al. Toward criteria for pragmatic measurement in implementation research and practice: a stakeholder-driven approach using concept mapping. *Implement Sci.* 2017;12(1).

CHAPTER 43

Quality Improvement Through the Lens of the Multicenter Perioperative Outcomes Group

Nirav Shah, MD ■ Kate Buehler, MS, RN ■ Allison Janda, MD

KEY POINTS

- Anesthesiology Performance Improvement and Reporting Exchange (ASPIRE), the quality improvement (QI) arm of the Multicenter Perioperative Outcomes Group (MPOG) and part of the family of Blue Cross Blue Shield Michigan (BCBSM) Collaborative Quality Initiatives (CQIs), works to overcome barriers to accessing information needed for practice analysis and improvement.
- Mechanisms that ASPIRE uses to promote practice change include participation in unblinded performance review sessions, the sharing of institutional quality initiatives throughout the collaborative, and review of cases flagged as not meeting criteria for successful performance for measures of interest, at both the institutional and provider levels, via dashboards and feedback emails.

Introduction

An early titan in healthcare quality improvement (QI), Avedis Donabedian, once said, "The secret to quality is love."[1] Although it is difficult to disagree with that statement, many would agree that the secret to success additionally includes collaboration, persistence, and high-quality data (Fig. 43.1). The previously described Collaborative Quality Initiatives (CQIs) in Michigan are exemplars of how these factors, supported by financial incentives, have resulted in tremendous improvements in care.[2–5]

In this chapter, we will focus on the process by which the Multicenter Perioperative Outcomes Group (MPOG) conducts its QI efforts to enable anesthesiologists and nurse anesthetists to reduce perioperative complications and improve outcomes.

Specifically, we will describe how MPOG infrastructure overcomes barriers to accessing information needed for practice analysis and reflection. We will demonstrate how tools developed by MPOG can be a catalyst for practice improvement. Finally, we will share examples of QI initiatives and the result of such efforts across participating sites.

Context

Founded in 2008, MPOG (https://mpog.org/) is a consortium of hospitals and healthcare systems focused on improving perioperative care and includes sites from around the United States and the Netherlands. MPOG has developed automated processes to extract and validate hospital data

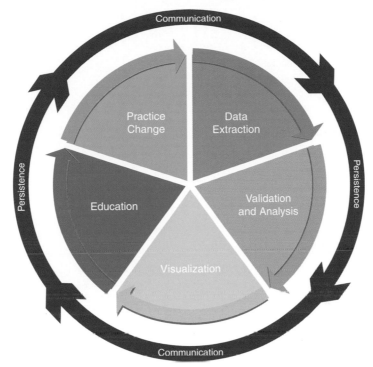

Fig. 43.1 Data extraction, analysis, visualization, education, communication, and persistence, leading to practice improvement.

before submitting the data to its coordinating center at the University of Michigan.[6] In 2014, with funding provided in part from Blue Cross Blue Shield of Michigan's (BCBSM) CQI program, MPOG launched a quality improvement program called the Anesthesiology Performance Improvement and Reporting Exchange (ASPIRE). Over 50 hospitals around the United States participate in ASPIRE, including over 25 hospitals within the state of Michigan.[7]

ASPIRE fulfills its mission to prevent complications and reduce unexplained variation in care by:

1. Using data from the MPOG registry to develop measures based on electronic health records (EHRs) and supplementary data sources.
2. Creating dashboards and visualizations to enable quality champions and practice leaders to view measure performance data, benchmarked with other institutions and filtered down to specific providers and cases (Fig. 43.2).
3. Sending performance feedback emails to providers that enable visualization of measure performance data, including benchmarks and links to specific cases that contributed to the provider's score (Fig. 43.3).
4. Creating supplementary tools, such as QI toolkits. ASPIRE toolkits contain a collection of educational resources, articles, and reference guides. Materials within are intended for use across the collaborative to facilitate the sharing of best practices (https://mpog.org/toolkits/). These toolkits enable local projects to implement practice change and support efforts by anesthesiology departmental quality champions (Fig. 43.4).

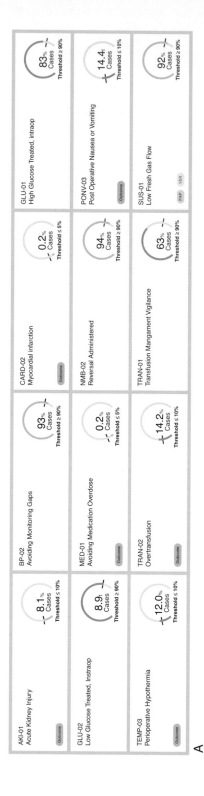

Fig. 43.2 (A–C) Multicenter Perioperative Outcomes Group (MPOG) quality improvement dashboards and measure summaries.

Continued

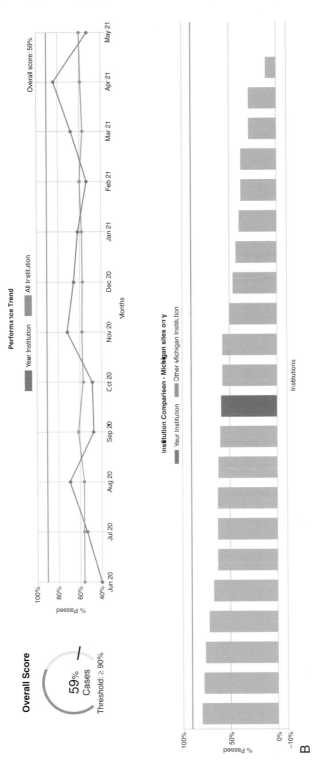

TRAN 01

Performance Trend

Your Institution   All Institution   Overall score: 59%

Overall Score

59% Cases

Threshold: ≥ 90%

Institution Comparison - Michigan sites only

Your Institution   Other Michigan Institution

B

Fig. 43.2, Cont'd

Continued

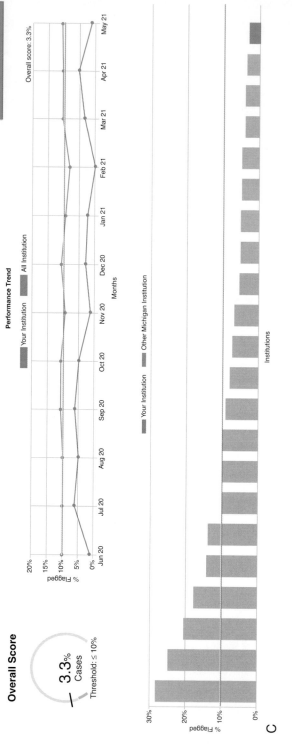

Fig. 43.2, Cont'd

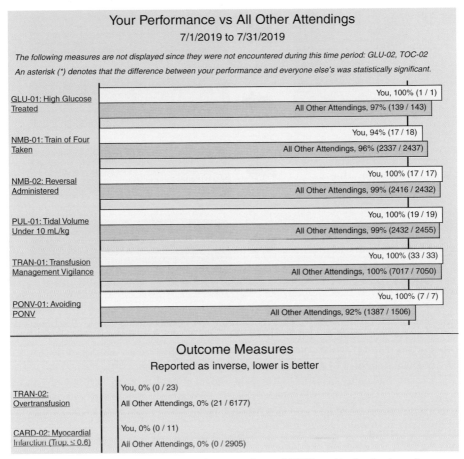

Fig. 43.3 Multicenter Perioperative Outcomes Group (MPOG) provider feedback email.

Importantly, this infrastructure is governed by the ASPIRE Quality Committee, which develops and approves all measure criteria to ensure the appropriate level of evidence or expert consensus is met. In addition, the committee reviews measures at regular intervals to determine whether the measure should be: (1) modified to incorporate recent evidence or (2) retired. The ASPIRE Quality Committee is composed of practice leaders from member institutions and quality champions (a practicing anesthesiologist who has been designated as a quality leader within the department, responsible for communicating measure updates and championing local improvement efforts).

The process by which practice change occurs across ASPIRE sites and providers is varied and tailored to the goal of each institution and individual. Nevertheless, there are several mechanisms that ASPIRE encourages to spark practice change:

1. Attendance and participation in unblinded performance review sessions by quality champions and QI staff
2. Review of cases flagged as not meeting criteria for successful performance for measures of interest (ASPIRE enables this review using software applications developed at the coordinating center at both the institutional and provider levels)

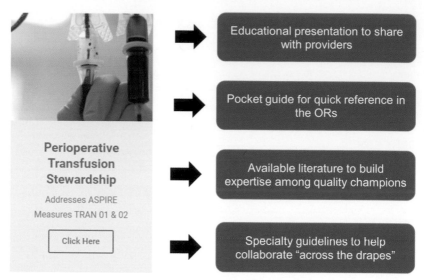

Fig. 43.4 Multicenter Perioperative Outcomes Group (MPOG) quality improvement toolkits.

3. Sharing site QI initiatives or projects with the rest of the collaborative to disseminate best practices and lessons learned
4. Linking these QI efforts with the Maintenance of Certification in Anesthesiology (MOCA) program sponsored by the American Board of Anesthesiology

The factors leading to successful outcomes as a result of implementing a QI initiative include strong evidence to suggest the recommended change in process will improve outcomes, a significant gap between desired and actual behavior, variation in performance across providers and institutions, and the ability to measure change over time.

Example A: Perioperative Transfusion Stewardship

BACKGROUND

Blood product administration in operating rooms can be lifesaving. The risks associated with blood product transfusion—febrile reactions, infectious risks, transfusion-related acute lung injury (TRALI), hemolytic transfusion reaction (HTR), sepsis, anaphylaxis, and more—are uncommon but well known. Transfusions are associated with increased mortality and morbidity and are expensive to administer with estimations of $500 to $1000 per unit.[8–10] Restrictive transfusion triggers (transfusing at relatively low hemoglobin values) have not been shown to increase harm compared with liberal triggers.[11–13]

IMPLEMENTATION

ASPIRE chose transfusion stewardship as a QI initiative because there is ample literature in this area to suggest transfusion should be guided by laboratory tests to avoid unnecessary administration of blood products.[11–13] The collaborative initially created a process measure to assess compliance with monitoring hemoglobin or hematocrit levels before administering any blood product. Exceptions were made for situations of massive hemorrhage, for patients with dangerously low initial hemoglobin or hematocrit levels, and for certain case types (i.e., cesarean deliveries) where specialty guidelines differed from this process.[14,15] The collaborative also developed an outcome measure to assess for "overtransfusion." Specifically, the measure examines hemoglobin and hematocrit values after the final transfusion of a case to determine whether the value is higher than necessary (greater than 10 mg/dL or 30%).[16] Again, exceptions were made for cases with massive blood loss (Fig. 43.5). Initial analysis of performance across ASPIRE sites demonstrated variation in performance across providers and institutions, with opportunities for improvement (Fig. 43.6).

To help sites implement practice change, the ASPIRE coordinating center developed a Transfusion Stewardship Toolkit, which summarized the evidence around transfusion management, procedure-specific guidelines, and ASPIRE process and outcome measure definitions. Financial incentives were provided via the BCBSM Pay for Performance (P4P) program, where performance on this measure was a component of the P4P Index.[17] Site and individual performance was visualized and analyzed through the ASPIRE QI Reporting Tool and sent via email to providers. Finally, education and communication plans were developed, where experts in transfusion management were invited to speak at ASPIRE collaborative meetings and unblinded performance for the transfusion measures was shared and discussed among participating members.

Results

Overall performance for our transfusion process and outcome measures improved over time (Fig. 43.7). Although it is difficult to tease out which intervention led to the most meaningful improvement, we believe that no single intervention is more important and that all are necessary to create the buy-in, motivation, and environment for practice change.

LIMITATIONS

Although data that are automatically extracted and analyzed from the EHR present great opportunities for scale, there are limitations as well. For this initiative, individual case review highlighted several scenarios where the case was flagged by the measure as requiring practice change, but detailed review of the case by a quality champion demonstrated appropriate care was delivered. As an example, blood may be administered by the anesthesiologist and documented in the record. Upon review, however, the quality champion may find the hemoglobin was checked by the perfusion team during cardiopulmonary bypass and was documented outside of the EHR (on paper). The measure algorithm would flag this case, but review would indicate appropriate care was delivered. Additionally, the decision to transfuse blood products is shared among the anesthesia and surgical teams and divergent opinions between those two teams can lead to processes of care not supported by evidence (or the measure algorithms). Nevertheless, these shared decisions should prompt conversations across specialties for optimal care, although such discussions are not easily accounted for in measure algorithms.

This QI initiative also shed light on the differences in resources between institutions. A low-performing institution stated that availability of machines to measure hemoglobin levels intraoperatively was a barrier to practice improvement. In this situation, collective "weight" of a statewide QI initiative, with benchmarking data, and financial incentives provided the necessary evidence and assistance for the quality champion to convince institutional leaders to install the lab machines near the operating rooms.

CONCLUSION

The Perioperative Transfusion Stewardship Initiative within ASPIRE demonstrated processes to achieve success and highlighted limitations associated with blood product management. ASPIRE has built on the successes (and failures) of this initiative as additional opportunities for improvement have arisen.

TRAN 01 (A)

Measure List
Measure Abbreviation
Data Collection Method
Measure Type
Description
Measure Time Period
Inclusions
Exclusions
Success
Other Measure Build Details
Responsible Provider
Threshold
MPOG Concept IDs Required
Data Diagnostics Affected
Rationale
Risk Adjustment
References

TRAN 01

Measure Abbreviation
TRAN-01

Data Collection Method
This measure is calculated based on data extracted from the electronic medical record combined with administrative data sources such as professional fee and discharge diagnoses data. This measure is explicitly not based on provider self-attestation.

Measure Type
Process

Description
Percentage of cases with a blood transfusion that have a hemoglobin or hematocrit value documented prior to transfusion.

Measure Time Period
Up to 36 hours prior to the first transfusion during the case

Inclusions
All surgical patients receiving anesthetics who receive a transfusion of red blood cells.

Exclusions
- Massive Transfusion: Transfusion of 4 or more units of blood; 4 hours before Anesthesia Start to Anesthesia End.
  - Note for sites that document transfusions in ml instead of units: ASPIRE will default to 350ml/unit.
- EBL ≥ 2000 ml
- Patients < 2 years of age
- Patients <12 years old undergoing a cardiac procedure (CPT: 00560, 00561, 00562, 00563, 00567, 00580).
- Patients <12 years old where either transfused PRBC or EBL was greater than 30cc/kb.
- Burn cases (CPT Codes 01951, 01952, 01953)
- ASA 5 & 6
- Labor Epidurals as determined by the MPOG 'Obsteric Anesthesia Type' phenotype results Labor Epidural and 'Conversion (Labor Epidural Portion)'
- Obstetric Non-Operative Procedures - CPT 01958

A

TRAN 02 (B)

Measure List
Measure Abbreviation
Data Collection Method
Measure Type
Description
Measure Time Period
Inclusions
Exclusions
Success
Other Measure Build Details
Responsible Provider
Threshold
MPOG Concept IDs Required
Data Diagnostics Affected
Rationale
Risk Adjustment
References

TRAN 02

Measure Abbreviation
TRAN-02

Data Collection Method
This measure is calculated based on data extracted from the electronic medical record combined with administrative data sources such as professional fee and discharge diagnoses data. This measure is explicitly not based on provider self-attestation.

Measure Type
Outcome

Description
Percentage of cases with a post transfusion hemoglobin or hematocrit value greater than or equal to 10 g/dL or 30%.

Measure Time Period
90 minutes before the last intraoperative transfusion to 18 hours after Anesthesia End

Inclusions
Any patient that receives a red blood cell transfusion, Transfusion is defined as packed red blood cells or whole blood. See MPOG Concept IDs below for complete list.

Exclusions
- Patients < 2 years of age
- Patients <21 years old undergoing a cardiac procedure (CPT: 00560, 00561, 00562, 00563, 00567, 00580)
- Pediatric cases (<12 years old) where either the transfused PRBC or EBL was greater than 30cc/kg.
- ASA 5 & 6
- EBL ≥ 2000ml
- Massive Transfusion: Transfusion of 4 or more units of blood; 4 hours before Anesthesia Start to Anesthesia End
  - Note for sites that document transfusions in ml instead of units: ASPIRE will default to 350ml/unit.
- Labor Epidurals as determined by the MPOG 'Obsteric Anesthesia Type' phenotype results Labor Epidural and 'Conversion (Labor Epidural Portion)'
- Obstetric Non-Operative Procedures – CPT 01958

B

Fig. 43.5 (A–B) Graphic of website screenshot of TRAN 01 and TRAN 02 measures spec.

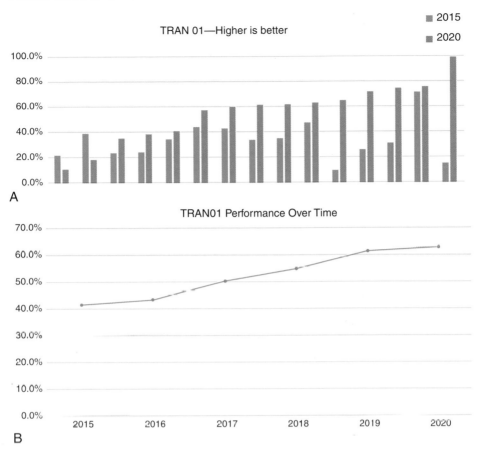

Fig. 43.6 (A) Variation in performance for TRAN 01 across institutions (2015 and 2020 data). (B) Trends in performance across TRAN 01 over time-cumulative cohort 1, 2, 3 institutions.

Example B: Improving Environmental Sustainability in the Operating Room

BACKGROUND

As our society becomes more aware of the effects of climate change and enacts concrete actions to combat it, anesthesia providers are joining these efforts. The healthcare sector provides opportunity for improvement because it accounts for 8% of greenhouse case emissions.[18] Within the operating room, those opportunities include fresh gas flow management and anesthetic agent choice to reduce health care's environmental impact. This type of QI initiative is focused on improving health and wellness at a population level, whereas most initiatives in anesthesiology tend to focus on improving direct patient outcomes. As its first foray into environmental sustainability, ASPIRE selected intraoperative fresh gas flow management.

Halogenated inhalational agents (desflurane, sevoflurane, isoflurane) and nitrous oxide are used to anesthetize patients but are also potent greenhouse gases.[18–20] As these gases undergo minimal metabolism in the body, they are mostly exhaled and then typically vented into the atmosphere

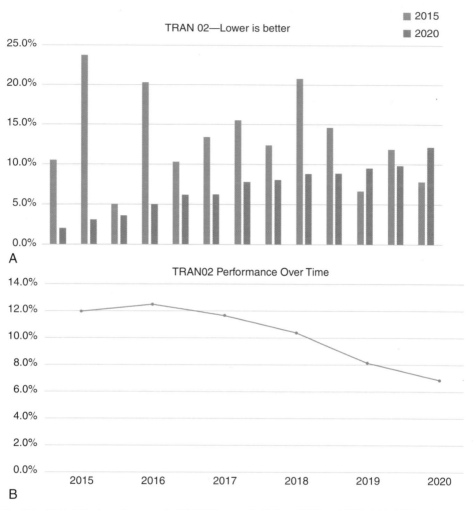

Fig. 43.7 (A) Variation in performance for TRAN 02 across institutions (2015 and 2020 data). (B) Trends in performance across TRAN 02 over time-cumulative cohort 1, 2, 3 institutions.

through scavenger systems. Once in the atmosphere, the effects of gases remain until they are degraded, which can take from 1 to 114 years depending on the agent used (Table 43.1).[21,22] The amount of fresh gas flow is correlated with the amount of agent that is vented into the atmosphere. One method of safely reducing the total amount of vented agent released into the atmosphere is to reduce fresh gas flow while delivering inhaled agent.

IMPLEMENTATION

The QI measure to support this initiative highlights cases where halogenated anesthetic agents and nitrous oxide were administered and fresh gas flow was greater than 3 L per minute,[23] a flow determined to be low enough to be meaningful, but not overly onerous to the provider. We were able to

TABLE 43.1 ■ Greenhouse Gas (GHG) Lifetime and Global Warming Potential (GWP)

1 Minimum Alveolar Concentration (MAC)–Inhaled Agent at Various Fresh Gas Flows (FGF)	Lifetime in Atmosphere (Years)	GWP per kg (100 Year) Compared With CO_2, Where $CO_2 = 1$	Ratio of CO_2/Equivalents Produced	Equivalent Auto Miles Driven per Hour Use of Anesthetic (Miles)
Sevoflurane 2% 2 L FGF	1.1	130	1.0	8
Isoflurane 1.2% 2 L FGF	3.2	510	2.2	18
Desflurane 6% 2 L FGF	14	2540	49.2	400
60% nitrous oxide at 1 L/min with 1 L/min O_2	114	298	7.5	61

Adapted from Axelrod D, Bell C, Feldman J, et al. Greening the operating room and perioperative arena: environmental sustainability for anesthesia practice. Task Force on Environmental Sustainability Committee on Equipment and Facilities. American Society of Anesthesiologists. Revised January 2017. https://www.asahq.org/about-asa/governance-and-committees/asa-committees/committee-on-equipment-and-facilities/environmental-sustainability/greening-the-operating-room.

take advantage of the minute-to-minute granularity of our automated data extract and exclude time periods where high fresh gas flow was necessary (before the endotracheal tube or laryngeal mask airway were placed or when nitric, not nitrous, oxide was administered). Using lessons learned from the Transfusion Stewardship Initiative, ASPIRE asked thought leaders to educate our group and leveraged the BCBSM P4P program to provide financial incentives.

RESULTS

Variation in practice is noticeable across Michigan ASPIRE sites, and there is steady improvement in performance. Although it is difficult to quantify the exact amount of greenhouse gas emissions avoided in the steady improvement demonstrated by providers and sites in this measure, any reduction in greenhouse gas emissions is beneficial (Fig. 43.8).

LIMITATIONS

A major challenge with this sustainability measure is that the ultimate outcome (global reduction of greenhouse gases) relies on the collective efforts of engaged citizens and governments around the world. It can be difficult to link that monumental effort, and the desired outcome, reversal of climate change, to the practice pattern for an individual provider. Technical challenges include the limitations in device integration to the EHR at sites where the gas analyzers that measure inspired and expired concentrations of inhalational agents and the flow sensors that measure fresh gas flow rate are not automatically sending information to the EHR. Without these important device integration capabilities, the measure performance becomes inaccurate and so an early choice was made by ASPIRE to exclude manually entered fresh gas flow data from the EHR from measure calculations. Similar to our transfusion stewardship initiative, we focused efforts on working with institutions to install the appropriate equipment to capture this data automatically, knowing that this effort would lead to more accurate anesthetic records in addition to enabling more accurate measure performance.

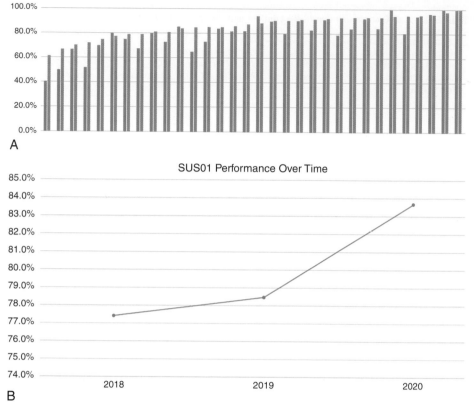

Fig. 43.8 (A) Variation in performance for institutions (all Multicenter Perioperative Outcomes Group [MPOG] sites participating in this measure). (B) Trend in performance for institutions (all MPOG sites participating in this measure).

CONCLUSION

Environmental sustainability is an important yet underrepresented aspect of perioperative care . ASPIRE hopes to build on our initial effort and develop additional measures to help inform providers about how their practice patterns can lead to more efficient use of resources.

Summary

Anesthesiologists have a long history as pioneers in healthcare process improvement. The safety record of anesthesia has sometimes made it an afterthought of the perioperative process. In these two examples provided, however, we see great opportunities for further improvement. The first example (transfusion stewardship) demonstrates how relatively straightforward process changes can lead to a reduction in transfusions administered. The second example highlights the role anesthesia providers can play in one of the most important global health initiatives of our time. Although we continue to face challenges with variation in data quality and resources across our member institutions, we believe that collaborating as a group, instead of working independently, offers the most effective path to addressing those challenges.

Acknowledgments

We acknowledge Mark Dehring for data query and analysis; and Rachel Hurwitz for manuscript review and citation management.

References

1. Mullan F. A founder of quality assessment encounters a troubled system firsthand. *Health Aff.* 2001;20 (1):137–141.
2. Dimick JB, Chen SL, Taheri PA, Henderson WG, Khuri SF, Campbell Jr DA. Hospital costs associated with surgical complications: a report from the private-sector National Surgical Quality Improvement Program. *J Am Coll Surg.* 2004;199(4):531–537.
3. Share DA, Campbell DA, Birkmeyer N, et al. How a regional collaborative of hospitals and physicians in Michigan cut costs and improved the quality of care. *Health Aff.* 2011;30(4):636–645.
4. Hemmila MR, Cain-Nielsen AH, Wahl WL, et al. Regional collaborative quality improvement for trauma reduces complications and costs. *J Trauma Acute Care Surg.* 2015;78(1):78–85. discussion 85–87.
5. Hemmila MR, Jakubus JL, Cain-Nielsen AH, et al. The Michigan Trauma Quality Improvement Program: results from a collaborative quality initiative. *J Trauma Acute Care Surg.* 2017;82(5):867–876.
6. Colquhoun DA, Shanks AM, Kapeles SR, et al. Considerations for integration of perioperative electronic health records across institutions for research and quality improvement: the approach taken by the multicenter perioperative outcomes group. *Anesth Analg.* 2020;130(5):1133–1146.
7. Multicenter Perioperative Outcomes Group. Member Hospitals. https://mpog.org/memberhospitals/. Accessed July 2, 2021.
8. Ejaz A, Frank SM, Spolverato G, Kim Y, Pawlik TM. Potential economic impact of using a restrictive transfusion trigger among patients undergoing major abdominal surgery. *JAMA Surg.* 2015,150 (7):625–630.
9. Salpeter SR, Buckley JS, Chatterjee S. Impact of more restrictive blood transfusion strategies on clinical outcomes: a meta-analysis and systematic review. *Am J Med.* 2014;127(2):124–131.e3.
10. Glance LG, Dick AW, Mukamel DB, et al. Association between intraoperative blood transfusion and mortality and morbidity in patients undergoing noncardiac surgery. *Anesthesiology.* 2011;114(2):283–292.
11. Carson JL, Guyatt G, Heddle NM, et al. Clinical Practice Guidelines from the AABB: red blood cell transfusion thresholds and storage. *JAMA.* 2016;316(19):2025–2035.
12. American Society of Anesthesiologists Task Force on Perioperative Blood Management. Practice guidelines for perioperative blood management: an updated report by the American Society of Anesthesiologists Task Force on Perioperative Blood Management. *Anesthesiology.* 2015;122(2):241–275.
13. Carson JL, Terrin ML, Noveck H, et al. Liberal or restrictive transfusion in high-risk patients after hip surgery. *N Engl J Med.* 2011;365(26):2453–2462.
14. MPOG. Measure Specs—TRAN-01. https://spec.mpog.org/Spec/Public/9. Accessed July 2, 2021.
15. CMQCC. Obstetric hemorrhage emergency management plan: table chart. https://www.cmqcc.org/content/obstetric-hemorrhage-emergency-management-plan-table-chart. Accessed July 2, 2021.
16. MPOG. Measure Specs—TRAN-02. https://spec.mpog.org/Spec/Public/10. Accessed July 2, 2021.
17. BCBSM P4P. https://mpog.org/p4p/. Accessed July 2, 2021.
18. Chung JW, Meltzer DO. Estimate of the carbon footprint of the US health care sector. *JAMA.* 2009;302 (18):1970–1972.
19. Finnveden G, Hauschild MZ, Ekvall T, et al. Recent developments in life cycle assessment. *J Environ Manage.* 2009;91(1):1–21.
20. ISO 14000 family. http://www.iso.org/iso/iso14000. Published 2020. Accessed October 2, 2014.
21. Andersen MPS, Nielsen OJ, Wallington TJ, Karpichev B, Sander SP. Assessing the impact on global climate from general anesthetic gases. *Anesthesia & Analgesia.* 2012;114(5):1081.
22. Ryan SM, Nielsen CJ. Global warming potential of inhaled anesthetics: application to clinical use. *Anesth Analg.* 2010;111(1):92-98.
23. MPOG. Measure Specs—SUS-01. https://spec.mpog.org/Spec/Public/32. Accessed July 2, 2021.

CHAPTER 44

The Michigan Urological Surgery Improvement Collaborative (MUSIC) Reducing Operative Complications From Kidney Stones (ROCKS) Quality Initiative

John Michael DiBianco, MD ■ Casey A. Dauw, MD ■
Khurshid R. Ghani, MB ChB, MS, FRCS (Urol)

KEY POINTS

- A significant proportion of unplanned healthcare encounters after stone surgery (ureteroscopy) are avoidable.
- Improvement in patient education decreases the rate of postoperative emergency department visits after ureteroscopy.
- Nonopioid pain pathways in appropriate patients are safe and feasible without increasing the rates of unplanned postoperative healthcare encounters.
- Providing outcomes data to individual physicians and practices can help motivate changes in behavior to align with best practices and improve patient care and experience.

Introduction

Kidney stone disease is a common, recurrent, and often painful condition affecting 11% of the United States (U.S.) population.[1] Ureteroscopy is a minimally invasive endoscopic procedure, performed mainly at ambulatory centers, where a semirigid or flexible scope is inserted into the ureter or kidney via the urethra to treat urinary stones. It is the most common surgical treatment for nephrolithiasis, with over 500,000 procedures performed annually in the U.S.[2,3] After ureteroscopy (URS), a ureteral stent, which is a small flexible hollow tube that sits within the ureter and bladder, permits drainage of urine from the kidney and is commonly placed for a temporary period.

Postoperative complications represent a significant impact on morbidity and cost of care for patients undergoing kidney stone surgery.[4] Unplanned postoperative healthcare encounters, such as emergency department (ED) visits, add to the patient and caregiver burden, and increase the cost of care.[4,5] The rate of postoperative ED visits after treatment of kidney stones with URS can be as high as 15%.[4] Because kidney stone disease is one of the costliest urological conditions to treat, with greater than $2.1 billion annual costs,[6] efforts to reduce unplanned postoperative encounters after URS represent an area for quality improvement (QI).

The Michigan Urological Surgery Improvement Collaborative (MUSIC) Reducing Operative Complications From Kidney Stones (ROCKS) Framework

The Michigan Urological Surgery Improvement Collaborative (MUSIC) is a physician-led collaborative group made up of urology practices throughout the state of Michigan, supported through funding from Blue Cross Blue Shield of Michigan (BCBSM). The collaborative is designed to evaluate and improve the quality and cost efficiency of urological care to benefit patients, providers, and payers. Initially established to improve care for patients with prostate cancer, it has expanded to other conditions including kidney stones and renal masses/cancer. All patients in the state are eligible to be in MUSIC, regardless of insurance status. MUSIC's goal is to improve patient outcomes through continuous data collection, performance feedback, and sharing of best practices. By collecting clinically relevant and actionable data, comparing performance among peers, and implementing changes in clinical behavior, MUSIC is continually identifying efficient ways to use healthcare resources and improve care delivery for patients with urological disease.

The Reducing Operative Complications From Kidney Stones (ROCKS) program is an initiative within MUSIC, begun in 2016, that aims to improve the quality of care for patients with urinary stone disease. MUSIC ROCKS maintains a prospective clinical registry of URS cases that contains patient demographic, clinical, and operative data entered by trained abstractors at each participating practice. Each patient is followed for 60 days postprocedurally, and appropriate variables are recorded according to a manual of operations. Each practice has a physician clinical champion, and QI projects are developed from the ground up, in conjunction with numerous patient advocates. Providers, healthcare team members, and patient advocates meet three times a year, where the data are evaluated, projects are defined, and the success and challenges of ongoing initiatives are discussed. The MUSIC playbook for QI and how ROCKS is structured is shown in Fig. 44.1.

Understanding the Problem

MUSIC ROCKS developed a QI program designed to understand the problem, enact change, and measure the outcomes. The initial early goal of MUSIC ROCKS was to measure the variation in

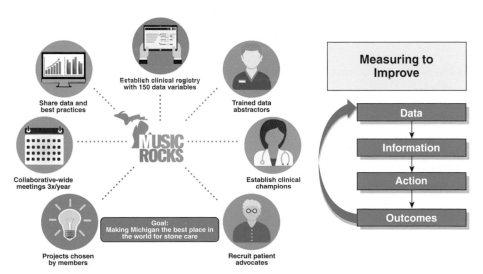

Fig. 44.1 The Michigan Urological Surgery Improvement Collaborative *(MUSIC)* Reducing Operative Complications From Kidney Stones *(ROCKS)* framework.

postoperative ED visits after URS across the state, identify the reasons for these visits, and develop care processes that can reduce unplanned healthcare encounters.

In 2016 a pilot of a limited number of practices within ROCKS was established. The frequency of ED and unscheduled office visits was measured after URS for stones. Patient-, provider-, and practice-level factors were evaluated for predictive factors of an adverse outcome. Additionally, the MUSIC coordinating center performed site visits and structured interviews with the urology care team at ROCKS practices with the lowest rates of postoperative ED visits.

After establishment of the program, ROCKS assessed URS in 21 practices with at least 10 cases per year in the registry and found that the 30-day postoperative ED visit rate was 8.1% but varied from 0% to 14.8% (Fig. 44.2); 70% of these visits occurred within 7 days of surgery. Complaints of pain, hematuria, and urinary symptoms accounted for 36% of these visits. These patients were evaluated in the ED and sent home, indicating that a good proportion of these postoperative ED visits were modifiable and potentially avoidable. Additionally, ureteral stent placement was identified as a predictor of ED visit.[7] A deeper dive into practices with lower rates of these modifiable ED visits showed that they had better efforts at patient education.

Enact Change

As a result of these findings, ROCKS started three initiatives aimed at patient and surgeon education.

PROCEDURE-SPECIFIC EDUCATION

Patient education and health literacy have been recognized to have direct and far-reaching effects on treatment outcomes.[8] Tangible results, as dramatic as reducing hip dislocations threefold after total hip surgery, have been demonstrated.[8,9] In this regard, one study showed that patients who received robust patient education after URS complained of less pain.[10] Therefore MUSIC developed a standardized URS-specific patient education leaflet in conjunction with patient advocates and providers across the state from diverse practices (Fig. 44.3). Particularly because the ureteral stent was the source of great morbidity, a ureteral stent education pamphlet was designed to be given to the patient and caregivers after surgery. This has been disseminated in both a paper format and as an electronic file to incorporate in the patient's electronic health record, as well as a patient educational video.[11]

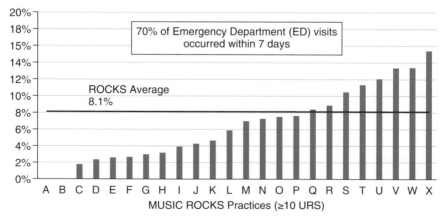

Fig. 44.2   Reducing Operative Complications From Kidney Stones *(ROCKS)* pilot 30-day postoperative ureteroscopy *(URS)* emergency department *(ED)* visit rate in practices with at least 10 cases.

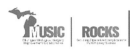 **Managing Pain and Urinary Symptoms after Ureteroscopy**

- You had surgery to remove or fragment your kidney stones, also known as an ureteroscopy.
- After surgery, you may have some degree of pain or discomfort.
- In most patients, these symptoms can be managed with medications.

Common symptoms after kidney stone surgery

 Pain in the bladder, lower abdomen, and/or lower back.

 Urinary frequency and/or urgency

 Burning with urination

 Blood in the urine

 Sensation of incomplete emptying of the bladder

The following recommended medications may be provided by your doctor to reduce symptoms after your kidney stone surgery

Non-Steroidal Anti-Inflammatory Drugs (NSAIDs)	Alpha Blockers
• Best at managing flank and abdominal pain related to kidney stones by reducing inflammation Examples: Toradol, Ibuprofen (Motrin), Naproxen (Aleve), Diclofenac	• Helps with flank pain, abdominal pain, and urinary symptoms after surgery by relaxing bladder and ureter muscles • Helps relieve stent discomfort • May assist kidney stone fragment passage Examples: Tamsulosin (Flomax)
Acetaminophen*	Anticholinergics
• Manages flank and abdominal pain after surgery by blocking pain signals • Very effective when combined with NSAIDs *Do not take more than 3000 mg of acetaminophen in a 24 hour period	• Prevents bladder spasms and bladder pain by preventing involuntary muscle movements • Helps relieve stent discomfort Examples: Oxybutynin (Ditropan) and Tolterodine (Detrol)

You may also be prescribed the following optional medications to help reduce your symptoms

Opiolds**,***	Pyridium
• Manages flank and abdominal pain after surgery by blocking some pain receptors • Can cause nausea, vomiting, constipation Examples: Norco, Vicodin, Oxycodone	• Helps with painful urination by interacting with the bladder surface to provide pain relief • May turn urine orange

**Shorter duration (less than 3 days) is recommended to prevent dependence
***Most patients are able to manage symptoms without these drugs

Fig. 44.3 Surgery-specific patient education material.

ROCKS PAIN CONTROL OPTIMIZATION PATHWAY (POP): IMPROVING PAIN MANAGEMENT AFTER SURGERY

Pain or discomfort is common after URS and was the primary driver of unplanned healthcare encounters in ROCKS. Historically, pain management strategies after URS included oral administration of opiate medication and nonsteroidal anti-inflammatory drugs (NSAIDs). Opiates are well established to effectively manage postoperative pain,[12] but it is estimated that more than 10 million Americans misuse prescription opiates, with an estimated risk of overdose-related death of

4 per 1000 patients.[13,14] New persistent opiate use, defined as use for more than 90 days after surgery in an opiate-naïve patient, occurs in more than 6% of those undergoing URS.[15] Importantly, opiates may not be necessary after URS because opiate-free pathways after URS have been developed.[16]

NSAIDs have been suggested to be superior to opiates in the treatment of renal colic by impeding inflammation and reducing pain.[15] Additionally, NSAIDs play an important role in the multimodal treatment of symptoms after URS, which includes alpha-adrenergic blockers, anticholinergic drugs, and urinary mucosal analgesia. The American Urological Association (AUA) stone management guidelines recommend alpha-adrenergic blockers for reducing stent-related symptoms.[17] Anticholinergic medications are also recommended for symptoms after URS in patients where a ureteral stent is placed.

The ROCKS Pain Control Optimization Pathway (POP) recommends the use of NSAIDs, and narcotic analgesics if the potential patients participating in ROCKS POP screen positive for NSAID allergy, intolerance, and possible contraindications. ROCKS POP recommends that education about the patient's disease process and the expected treatment course occurs. Circumstances giving rise to pain during URS, and a discussion regarding the benefits and potential toxicities of drugs to be considered for use, as they apply to the patient's comorbidities and nonurological drug requirements, should be provided.

ROCKS POP is designed not to alter the intraoperative care of any patient, each of whom will receive standard analgesia as deemed appropriate during the operation by their anesthesiologist and surgeon. ROCKS POP recommends postoperative care includes NSAIDs and acetaminophen, provided these agents are not contraindicated. Anticholinergic agents are recommended in patients receiving a ureteral stent for the duration of the stent dwell time. Other agents, such as Pyridium, which can reduce urinary irritation, are optional medications. Importantly, patients are not given a prescription for opioid medications as routine use after URS. Nonpharmaceutical alternatives to managing pain, such as applying ice or heat, meditating, or walking are also encouraged.

MUSIC ROCKS REPORT CARDS

The Hawthorne effect describes the change in behavior as a result of the subject knowing that they are being observed.[18] Prior work has demonstrated significant change in physician behavior to align with best practices and QI initiatives using "scorecards," leveraging the Hawthorne effect.[19] This was the motivation for MUSIC ROCK to develop practice and physician data summaries, report cards with anonymous peer comparator data, that are shared with urology practices and physicians to inform on their performance and identify variation in the QI activities. Specifically aligning with ROCKS initiatives, practices and physicians receive information on the postoperative ED visit, unplanned hospitalization, and opioid prescription rates (Fig. 44.4).

Measuring the Outcomes

Since its inception in 2016, the ROCKS initiative has understood several key findings from the data collected in its clinical registry. First, a significant proportion of unplanned healthcare encounters after URS for stone treatment are avoidable. Second, improvement in patient education can decrease the rate of modifiable postoperative ED visits related to pain and urinary symptoms. Third, it is safe to implement nonopioid postoperative pain pathways in appropriate patients without increasing the rates of unplanned postoperative healthcare encounters.[20] Lastly, providing physician and practice outcomes data may motivate changes in physician behavior to more effectively align with best practices. The driving force for the substantive improvements witnessed in MUSIC, however, are because of the culture of collaboration in implementing statewide programs that benefit all centers and patients.

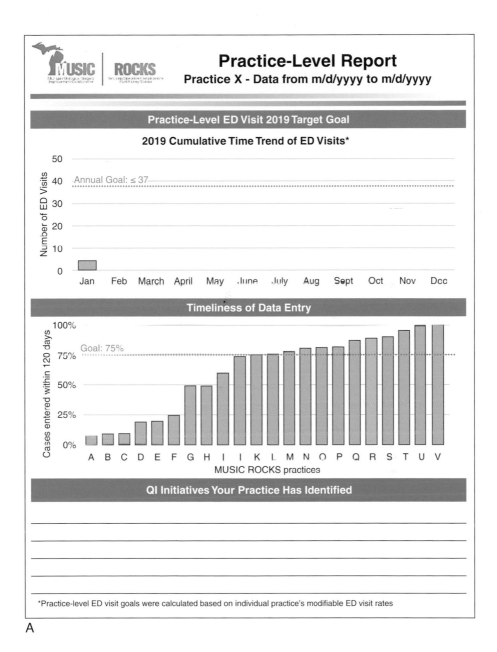

A

Fig. 44.4 (A–B) Michigan Urological Surgery Improvement Collaborative *(MUSIC)* Reducing Operative Complications From Kidney Stones *(ROCKS)* report cards. *ED*, Emergency department; *NSAIDs*, nonsteroidal anti-inflammatory drugs; *QI*, quality improvement.

Continued

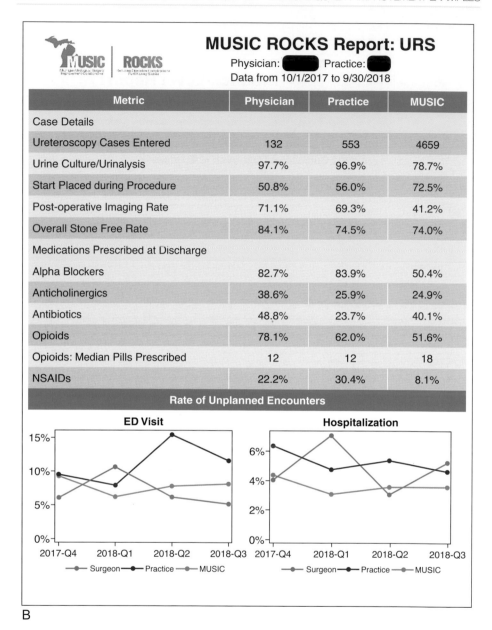

Metric	Physician	Practice	MUSIC
Case Details			
Ureteroscopy Cases Entered	132	553	4659
Urine Culture/Urinalysis	97.7%	96.9%	78.7%
Start Placed during Procedure	50.8%	56.0%	72.5%
Post-operative Imaging Rate	71.1%	69.3%	41.2%
Overall Stone Free Rate	84.1%	74.5%	74.0%
Medications Prescribed at Discharge			
Alpha Blockers	82.7%	83.9%	50.4%
Anticholinergics	38.6%	25.9%	24.9%
Antibiotics	48.8%	23.7%	40.1%
Opioids	78.1%	62.0%	51.6%
Opioids: Median Pills Prescribed	12	12	18
NSAIDs	22.2%	30.4%	8.1%

Fig.44.4, Cont'd

EMERGENCY DEPARTMENT VISITS

Analysis of the MUSIC ROCKS clinical registry revealed an initial postoperative ED visit rate after URS of 10%. After implementation of the strategies previously noted, this has dropped to a current rate of 6% (Fig. 44.5), an approximate 40% decrease in postoperative ED visits after URS ($p < .01$).

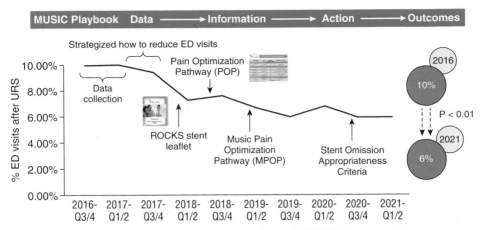

Fig. 44.5   Reducing Operative Complications From Kidney Stones *(ROCKS)* Ureteroscopy 30-day postopera tive ED visit rate. *ED,* Emergency department; *MUSIC,* Michigan Urological Surgery Improvement Collaborative; *URS,* ureteroscopy.

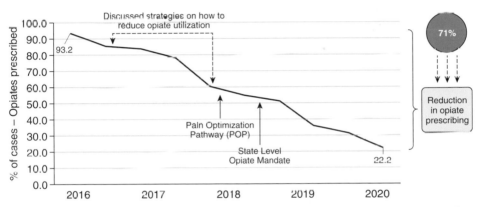

Fig. 44.6   Reducing Operative Complications From Kidney Stones *(ROCKS)* postoperative ureteroscopy opiate prescription rates.

PRESCRIPTION RATES

The rate of postoperative opioid prescriptions after URS at the start of the ROCKS initiative was 93.2% of all URS cases (Fig. 44.6). In 2020 the rate dropped by 71% to an overall rate of 22.2%.

MUSIC ROCKS REPORT CARDS

The report card initiative empowered urologists to measure their own outcomes. Practice and physician data summaries with anonymous peer comparator data allowed surgeons and practices to know where they belonged in the spectrum of performance in the state of Michigan.

Limitations

The ROCKS registry provides clinical information used for QI, where data collection must be manageable, nimble, and actionable. This may have limitations, compared with data collected during prospective clinical trials, which can be very detailed. Confounding can be a factor with QI data. The three initiatives reviewed spanned similar timeframes and evaluating the contribution of each initiative specifically to favorable results cannot be obtained within the observational QI design. Additionally, ROCKS POP was begun during the period in which the State of Michigan instituted regulations aimed at reducing opioid use, which may also have driven physician behavior.

Conclusions

Through modifications in patient education, pain management, and physician empowerment, the MUSIC ROCKS initiative has improved the journey for patients undergoing surgery for kidney stones. By asking the right questions in partnership with patient advocates, a diverse group of practices, and providers, and with trained abstractors inputting high-quality clinical data, ROCKS has been able to understand variations in care and promote best practices. ROCKS is a great example of the power of collaborative QI to improve healthcare delivery in the state and improve the care of patients which can potentially be replicated.

Funding

MUSIC is funded by the Value Partnerships program of BCBSM. Investigations are initiated and conducted by the members and group practices, where data collection, analysis, and resulting actions are independently coordinated under the guidance of the MUSIC Coordinating Center. BCBSM has no access to the data and does not direct the QI activities. The authors acknowledge the significant contributions of the physician clinical champions, urologists, administrators, and data abstractors in each participating MUSIC practice (details around specific participating urologists and practices can be found at www.musicurology.com), as well as members of the MUSIC Coordinating Center, located within the University of Michigan.

References

1. Scales Jr. CD, Smith AC, Hanley JM, et al. Prevalence of kidney stones in the United States. *Eur Urol.* 2012;62:160–165.
2. Saigal CS, Joyce G, Timilsina AR, et al. Direct and indirect costs of nephrolithiasis in an employed population: opportunity for disease management? *Kidney Int.* 2005;68:1808–1814.
3. Geraghty RM, Jones P, Somani BK. Worldwide trends of urinary stone disease treatment over the last two decades: a systematic review. *J Endourol.* 2017;31:547–556.
4. Scales Jr. CD, Saigal CS, Hanley JM, et al. The impact of unplanned postprocedure visits in the management of patients with urinary stones. *Surgery.* 2014;155:769–775.
5. San Juan J, Hou H, Ghani KR, et al. Variation in spending around surgical episodes of urinary stone disease: findings from Michigan. *J Urol.* 2018;199:1277–1282.
6. Tundo G, Vollstedt A, Meeks W, et al. Beyond prevalence: annual cumulative incidence of kidney stones in the United States. *J Urol.* 2021;205:1704–1709.
7. Hiller SC, Daignault-Newton S, Pimentel H, et al. Ureteral stent placement following ureteroscopy increases Emergency Department visits in a Statewide Surgical Collaborative. *J Urol.* 2021;205(6): 1710–1717.
8. Wittink H, Oosterhaven J. Patient education and health literacy. *Musculoskelet Sci Pract.* 2018;38:120–127.
9. Lubbeke A, Suva D, Perneger T, et al. Influence of preoperative patient education on the risk of dislocation after primary total hip arthroplasty. *Arthritis Rheum.* 2009;61:552–558.
10. Abt D, Warzinek E, Schmid HP, et al. Influence of patient education on morbidity caused by ureteral stents. *Int J Urol.* 2015;22:679–683.
11. Ureteral Stents. *What you need to know*; 2021. https://musicurology.com/stent-video/.
12. Cheung CW, Ching Wong SS, Qiu Q, et al. Oral oxycodone for acute postoperative pain: a review of clinical trials. *Pain Physician.* 2017;20:SE33–SE52.

13. Bohnert AS, Valenstein M, Bair MJ, et al. Association between opioid prescribing patterns and opioid overdose-related deaths. *JAMA*. 2011;305:1315–1321.

14. Lee JS, Hu HM, Edelman AL, et al. New persistent opioid use among patients with cancer after curative-intent surgery. *J Clin Oncol*. 2017;35:4042–4049.

15. Tam CA, Dauw CA, Ghani KR, et al. New persistent opioid use after outpatient ureteroscopy for upper tract stone treatment. *Urology*. 2019;134:103–108.

16. Large T, Heiman J, Ross A, et al. Initial experience with narcotic-free ureteroscopy: a feasibility analysis. *J Endourol*. 2018;32:907–911.

17. Assimos D, Krambeck A, Miller NL, et al. Surgical management of stones: American Urological Association/Endourological Society Guideline, Part I. *J Urol*. 2016;196:1153–1160.

18. Sedgwick P, Greenwood N. Understanding the Hawthorne effect. *BMJ*. 2015;351, h4672.

19. Das A, Cohen JE, Ko OS, et al. Surgeon scorecards improve muscle sampling on transurethral resection of bladder tumor and recurrence outcomes in patients with nonmuscle invasive bladder cancer. *J Urol*. 2021;205:693–700.

20. Hawken SR, Hiller SC, Daignault-Newton S, et al. Opioid-free discharge is not associated with increased unplanned healthcare encounters after ureteroscopy: results from a Statewide Quality Improvement Collaborative. *Urology*. 2021;158:57–65.

CHAPTER 45

Enhanced Recovery After Surgery Protocols— Implementation Across a US Health System: System-Level Principles

Michael Scott, MB ChB, FRCP, FRCA, FFICM ▪ Paula Spencer, MSHA, PMP, CPHIMS

KEY POINTS

- Enhanced Recovery After Surgery (ERAS) is a series of evidence-based protocols that improve outcomes after surgery by optimizing patients before surgery, reduce stress and injury during surgery, and promote rapid return of preoperative function.
- ERAS pathways can be used as a framework for all health system surgical perioperative care pathways to reduce length of stay, improve quality, reduce variance, and improve patient satisfaction.
- Executive leadership support is key to implementing an ERAS program across a health system.
- Return on investment is high, meaning ERAS truly offers value-based health care.
- Assembling a dedicated team of a medical director, quality improvement (QI) director, QI managers, and data analysts is likely to be necessary to tackle the enormity of health system transformation.
- Initial outlay of costs is low and return on investment is high.
- Surgical and anesthesia champions are needed with dedicated time.
- Advanced practice providers, nurses, and all bedside providers need to be involved in pathway organization.
- Vertical and horizontal implementation of ERAS principles accelerate the standardization of perioperative pathways across the health system.
- Using the electronic medical record (EMR) can help drive real-time compliance of ERAS elements and produce audits but may require a lot of new resources in current EMR versions.
- Data assessing the compliance of ERAS elements and complications, length of hospital stay, and direct and indirect costs can improve the process and guide ongoing QI projects.

Introduction

Enhanced Recovery After Surgery (ERAS) pathways are multimodal, evidence-based perioperative care protocols designed to improve outcomes after surgery.

The concept was pioneered in the early 2000s by Henrik Kehlet, a Danish colorectal surgeon. In 2005, the ERAS Society was founded and published and formalized key elements of ERAS.[1] The overall principle of ERAS is to optimize the patient's health before surgery, minimize stress to the body, maintain homeostasis, and restore function to normal rapidly.[2] The result of ERAS pathways is a more predictable length of hospital stay (LOS) and reduced complications, without increased readmissions. ERAS principles can be applied to all types of elective surgery and even emergency general surgery.[3] The cost of implementing ERAS is minimal but the challenges to reorganizing the surgical pathway can be significant. In the UK, the Enhanced Recovery Partnership successfully embedded ERAS as a standard of care in at least four specialties over 4 years across all UK hospitals.[4] There have been consistent cost savings and improvements in patient care in other countries where ERAS has been implemented.[5] In health systems where ERAS has been adopted as the standard (e.g., Alberta Health System, Canada), there have been net health system savings per patient ranging from $26.35 to $3606.44 and return on investment (ROI) ranging from 1.05 to 7.31, meaning that every dollar invested in ERAS brought $1.05 to $7.31 in return.[6] The results of improved quality for less cost fits with the value-based proposition for United States (US) health care. Demand for elective surgical services continues to rise and the COVID-19 pandemic has put increased pressure on operating room (OR) utilization as the backlog of surgical cases is addressed. The increased bed capacity ERAS releases is an important aspect to help address this issue. Because the US has been unable to reduce healthcare costs despite attempts, the Centers for Medicaid and Medicare Services (CMS) and private payers are moving from pay per use to episode payment models to control costs with a focus on better outcomes.[7] With the reduction in variance, increase in predictable LOS, and reduction in complications and readmissions as a result of ERAS pathways, ERAS can be a key pillar of delivering health care in the future.

Making ERAS principles the standard of care for all patients is one way to deliver care via reliable processes that afford better predictability of outcomes and costs.

ERAS Implementation Across a US Health System

In 2016, Virginia Commonwealth University (VCU) Health recruited Dr. Michael Scott (coauthor) from the UK (where he had been a National Lead for ERAS) as Lead for ERAS implementation and Medical Director to work in the Department of Clinical Effectiveness alongside the Director, Paula Spencer (coauthor). Reductions in LOS, cost per case, and complications were immediately realized with the first colorectal surgery pathway in 2016. In February of 2017, a system-wide ERAS implementation in all surgical specialties was launched. We found an optimal way to accelerate adoption by creating a vertical and horizontal implementation strategy, which we believe to be unique. By engaging key resources in each vertical care phase to design standard work, ERAS care principles were suddenly available to all elective surgery patients. Our new vertical implementation strategy was launched in early 2018 and was running toward completion by summer of 2021.

The whole of the perioperative process was reset, focusing on three parts of the patient's journey: preoperative, intraoperative, and postoperative, including discharge (Fig. 45.1).

- In the preoperative phase, the patient is prepared physically, socially, and emotionally. Engagement is from the time of being seen in the surgery clinic and involves interaction with a preoperative clinic (the Preoperative Assessment Communication and Education Clinic [PACE]).

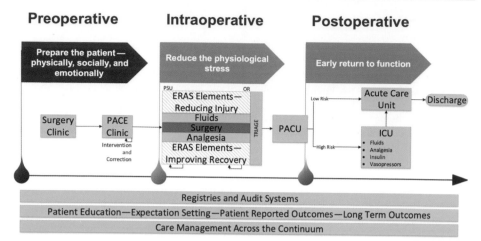

Fig. 45.1   The three phases of the patient's journey: preoperative, intraoperative, and postoperative, including discharge.

■ The aim of the intraoperative phase is to reduce the physiological stress of surgery. The key stakeholders are the surgeon, anesthesia team, and perioperative nursing. The surgeon minimizes injury and blood loss, and the anesthesiology team minimizes pain and stress and optimizes blood flow and perfusion. Many of the ERAS elements during the intraoperative phase are now standards of care (e.g., postoperative nausea and vomiting [PONV] prophylaxis, deep venous thrombosis [DVT] prophylaxis, warming) and as such just need to be done effectively. Nevertheless, opioid-sparing analgesia and fluid and hemodynamic therapy need to be individualized for the patient, type of surgery, and surgical approach. Different pathways were created with standardization of most ERAS elements but with separate analgesia and fluid pathways. At the end of surgery, patients are optimized, reviewed, and triaged in the postanesthesia care unit (PACU) and go to the appropriate postoperative care unit.

■ Postoperatively, a standardized de-escalation of care appropriate to the type of surgery is implemented to restore function and accelerate recovery so that the patient is drinking, eating, mobilizing, and sleeping on postoperative day 1.

It is key to success that the patient is engaged throughout their journey, starting with preoperative education, informed consent, and expectation setting. Registries and audit systems are mandatory to map compliance with processes and provide patient-reported outcomes and long-term outcomes. Planning care management across the pathway ensures appropriate and timely discharge from the hospital.

Organizing Around the Health System Model

Health systems in different countries are funded and function in different ways, but the principles of ERAS apply internationally.

Here we summarize the key steps to effect impactful change in a health organization:
1. Ensuring executive buy-in
2. Ensuring a governance structure for change
3. Creating an effective transformation team
4. Designing process mapping across the patient pathway
5. Designing process mapping for the health system
6. Effecting change management

7. Adopting Lean principles
8. Providing an audit of compliance and outcomes
9. Providing regular feedback to providers with mechanisms for change to continue ongoing quality improvement (QI)

EXECUTIVE BUY-IN

Sponsorship from the executive suite is key to success in any QI project.

It is imperative that a clear vision is created along with a realistic time frame for implementation and visualization of benefits for the organization (Fig. 45.2). An outline business case should be prepared, which should demonstrate costs and ROI. With ERAS releasing bed days, increased capacity can be used for performing further surgical procedures. Reduction of complications will reduce costs, which is mandatory for episode payment bundling. Other downstream benefits such as acute kidney injury (AKI) reduction and reduced episode costs have also been demonstrated.

The importance of developing efficient, standardized processes that integrate the clinical principles of ERAS throughout the patient journey from preoperative to perioperative and postoperative are key to ensuring high-quality, low-variance, and optimal patient experiences.

A GOVERNANCE STRUCTURE FOR CHANGE

We implemented key governance changes with executive support. An ERAS steering committee consisted of key leaders in surgery, anesthesia, nursing, allied health, quality and safety, and operations. The steering committee was cochaired by the quality and safety officer and the vice president of perioperative services. Together, these oversight teams signify the unified, committed sponsorship of ERAS necessary for sustained success (Fig. 45.3).

Two key clinical groups were formed to establish the system-wide program: the ERAS Provider Champions Team and the ERAS Nursing Committee members. The Perioperative Executive Committee (PEC) is the main governing body for perioperative operations, and is composed of

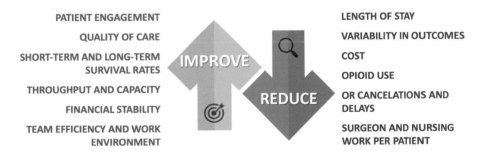

Why IS ERAS Important to VCU Health?

PATIENT ENGAGEMENT

QUALITY OF CARE

SHORT-TERM AND LONG-TERM SURVIVAL RATES

THROUGHPUT AND CAPACITY

FINANCIAL STABILITY

TEAM EFFICIENCY AND WORK ENVIRONMENT

IMPROVE

REDUCE

LENGTH OF STAY

VARIABILITY IN OUTCOMES

COST

OPIOID USE

OR CANCELATIONS AND DELAYS

SURGEON AND NURSING WORK PER PATIENT

American College of Surgeons standard of care
Opportunity for VCU Health to be a U.S. leader
Market demand for value-driven care

Fig. 45.2 Importance of Enhanced Recovery After Surgery (ERAS) to Virginia Commonwealth University (VCU) health.

Governance

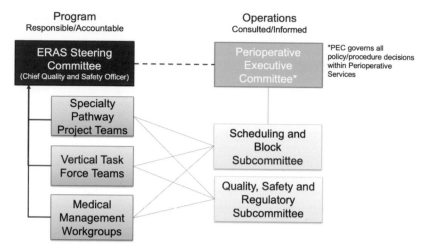

Fig. 45.3   Governance structure.

the chief of operations, the surgical department chairs, the chair of anesthesia, and the vice president of perioperative services. This committee is responsible for:

- Approving policies
- Supporting operational guidelines
- Holding team members accountable

The Quality, Safety, and Regulatory (QSR) subcommittee of PEC was established to monitor and improve patient and staff quality, safety, regulatory guidelines, and compliance. The committee is responsible for:

- Reviewing regulatory issues
- Identifying key performance indicators
- Ensuring compliance with requirements
- Promoting standardization of patient experience
- Monitoring data

THE ERAS TRANSFORMATION TEAM

Implementation of ERAS affects the whole patient pathway and therefore a large proportion of hospital services. It is essential to engage, educate, and involve all stakeholders in the change management process. Clinical sponsors and champions for each surgical pathway and vertical care-phase task force included the department chair, surgical champion, nurse director, nurse champion, and unit leaders. An anesthesiologist champion is also important for each specialty. Key roles for the team and responsibilities were formalized.[8]

CHANGE MANAGEMENT

Despite adoption of ERAS by VCU Health as standard, we encountered pockets of resistance in the form of both active resistors and passive resistors. We used well-documented implementation strategies and ensured providers and clinicians were provided with the opportunity to participate in designing the change. We addressed how ERAS impacted the individual and the team, the effect on daily workflow, and how individuals might benefit. Key messaging on the "why" of the change, how an ERAS program benefits everyone involved and is patient-centered, was circulated. Regular communications with feedback, including positive gains and improvements, were sent by email, and updates were given at grand round presentations.

Vertical and Horizontal Implementation Model

ERAS implementation in many health systems is initially limited to a few specialties and takes several years to implement. At VCU Health, we started our ERAS transformation with a single pathway for colorectal surgery together with a surgical site infection bundle through a rapid improvement cycle to show stakeholders that improvement was possible and to get confidence to engage in the program across the whole health system.

We followed the successful horizontal specialty-based approach and expanded to four more surgery types.[9] As we worked on these separate projects, we recognized inefficiencies in our approach, such as that it stretched the implementation team too thin. Another unintended consequence was the developing perception of an ERAS patient versus a "non-ERAS" patient. This concerned us because we understood the 22 key elements of care for ERAS to be commonly applicable for all patients, therefore making the ERAS/non-ERAS labeling of patients an opportunity for important care elements that may change a patient's surgical outcome to be missed.

Core ERAS elements are common to all surgery types, so by building a foundation of common ERAS elements at every point of interaction, we could rapidly implement ERAS for all patients, a term we called "vertical implementation" (Fig. 45.4). Although the core principles of ERAS apply to all surgical specialties, a key difference in pathways surrounds analgesia and fluid therapy. We therefore worked with the surgeons, anesthesiologists, and pain team to develop standard guidelines for analgesia and fluids for each surgery type. This allowed us to accelerate the deployment of surgical specialty pathways and build reliability to deliver best practice. We grouped the elements by care phase: preoperative, presurgical unit (PSU), OR, PACU, floor, and added task forces to address these vertical cross-sections.

These new vertically aligned teams were given responsibility to:

- Address design and implementation of ERAS key elements applicable to all surgery types
- Optimize workflows and documentation to support consistent delivery of best-practice care using Lean principles
- Produce a framework for all specialty pathways
- Optimize and fortify the system foundation

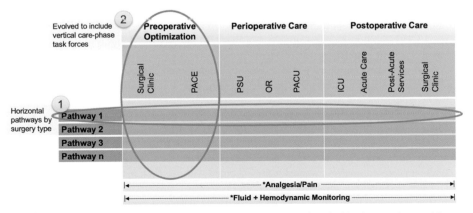

Fig. 45.4 Enhanced Recovery After Surgery (ERAS) horizontal and vertical implementation model.

Our revised methodology, the blending of vertical and horizontal approaches, addressed fundamental change by implementing ERAS principles across surgical specialties as standard work, introducing variation by specialty only where clinically indicated. We took the following steps to stand up our new approach:

- Defined our scope to include all adult patients undergoing inpatient elective procedures that require general anesthesia.
- Developed a single patient-centered pathway that spanned the period from decision for surgery through 90 days after surgery, encompassing all surgical specialties.
- Convened vertical care-phase aligned interprofessional teams with internal consulting resources to develop a systematic framework using Lean thinking.
- Integrated project oversight with perioperative operations governance.
- Formalized an organizational change management strategy.
- Focused on a sustainable infrastructure built around staff and other capabilities, through resource optimization, training and development, analytics, and information technology tools.

CURRENT STATE PROCESS MAPPING AND DESIGNING CHANGE

The first step of designing change is to map the current state workflows with the project team, focusing on what *actually happens,* as opposed to *what is supposed to happen,* and identifying waste. Mapping the current state with all stakeholders is necessary to establish a shared understanding of the surgical pathway, to identify gaps, and to successfully move toward the future state. A process map (see Chapter 27 for more on process maps) allows the team to better identify challenges and opportunities for improvement.

FUTURE STATE PROCESS MAPPING

Processes are often created within silos. Our team focused on a system view of the patient's journey along the surgical continuum to develop more flexible processes. Most importantly, the future state incorporated the new ERAS principles into the process, ensuring that the quality standards of care would be hardwired into the care pathway.

Setting Quality Standards for Perioperative Pathways

The ERAS Society has developed evidence-based pathways for multiple surgical procedures, with recommendations for preoperative, intraoperative, and postoperative elements to improve outcomes. VCU Health used these pathways as a base and individualized pathways to fit our health system and patient population.

A quality standard was developed to represent a fundamental change in clinical practice needed to address ERAS care elements and provide a tool to secure approval and manage expectations regarding consistent care methods rooted in current scientific evidence. These standards act as a guide and reference for all team members involved in the care pathway.

The VCU Health Quality Standards template outlines key information regarding the associated clinical care topic. The format ensures that the governance is maintained and provides staff with information to manage patient care to the quality standard.

1. A surgeon-led interprofessional team is formed with relevant stakeholders.
2. Clinical evidence is reviewed, and a draft document is produced.
3. The document is distributed and reviewed among stakeholders, allowing an opportunity for feedback and refinement.

4. The surgery lead presents the document to the QSR for acceptance and implementation.
5. The document is sent to the PEC for ratification.
6. The quality standard document is published to the intranet and disseminated.
7. The EMR and other system tools are updated to ensure the change in practice.

Formal exceptions to the quality standards can be brought before the QSR for approval provided there is evidence to support the exception and the request is based on patient factors, not individual clinician preferences.

ERAS by Care Phase

To reinforce the importance of the ERAS principles to every phase of patient care, the vertical task force teams identified the top five care points for each and posted them in clinical areas for easy reference. Intraoperative care points were specified for each role.

THE PREOPERATIVE ASSESSMENT COMMUNICATION AND EDUCATION CLINIC

PACE was set up and rapidly expanded to include smaller satellite clinics where surgeons saw patients. The clinic is staffed by advanced practice providers under the supervision of an attending anesthesiologist. This hub-and-spoke model helped all patients listed for surgery get immediate screening, review, and information by a provider and also get immediate input from an attending who would be in the large downtown PACE clinic. This helped identify immediate blood and other tests, which identified any preoperative optimization needed to improve the patient's preoperative status to reduce the risk of complications.[10]

The PACE Clinic had a set of quality standards and algorithms to optimize health status and inform patients of surgery and analgesia options (informed consent). All patients had a screening questionnaire completed based on that published by Vetter's group.[11] All patients received preoperative information and counseling. Other key areas known to reduce postoperative complications were addressed (Fig. 45.5).

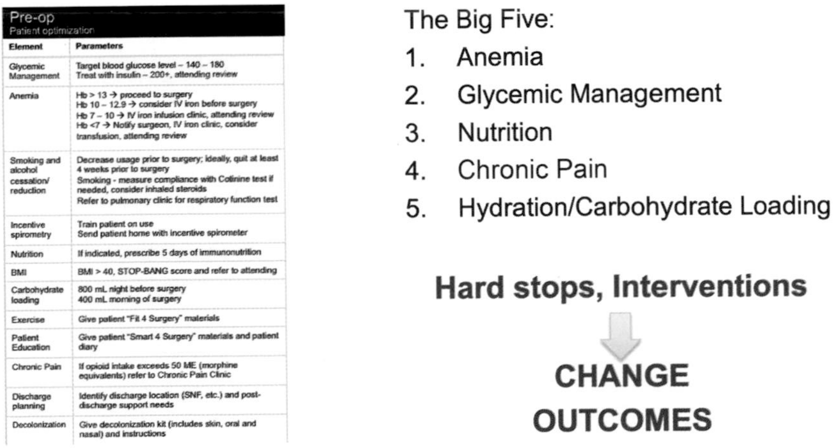

Pre-op Patient optimization	
Element	**Parameters**
Glycemic Management	Target blood glucose level – 140 – 180 Treat with insulin – 200+, attending review
Anemia	Hb > 13 → proceed to surgery Hb 10 – 12.9 → consider IV iron before surgery Hb 7 – 10 → IV iron infusion clinic, attending review Hb <7 → Notify surgeon, IV iron clinic, consider transfusion, attending review
Smoking and alcohol cessation/ reduction	Decrease usage prior to surgery; ideally, quit at least 4 weeks prior to surgery Smoking - measure compliance with Cotinine test if needed, consider inhaled steroids Refer to pulmonary clinic for respiratory function test
Incentive spirometry	Train patient on use Send patient home with incentive spirometer
Nutrition	If indicated, prescribe 5 days of immunonutrition
BMI	BMI > 40, STOP-BANG score and refer to attending
Carbohydrate loading	800 mL night before surgery 400 mL morning of surgery
Exercise	Give patient "Fit 4 Surgery" materials
Patient Education	Give patient "Smart 4 Surgery" materials and patient diary
Chronic Pain	If opioid intake exceeds 50 ME (morphine equivalents) refer to Chronic Pain Clinic
Discharge planning	Identify discharge location (SNF, etc.) and post-discharge support needs
Decolonization	Give decolonization kit (includes skin, oral and nasal) and instructions

The Big Five:

1. Anemia
2. Glycemic Management
3. Nutrition
4. Chronic Pain
5. Hydration/Carbohydrate Loading

Hard stops, Interventions

⬇

CHANGE

OUTCOMES

Fig. 45.5 Preoperative optimization.

INTRAOPERATIVE PATHWAYS

Each specialty service developed an intraoperative pathway for their common procedures. This pathway served as a reference to ensure reproducible care by anesthesia, surgeon, nursing, pharmacy, and availability of appropriate equipment (Fig. 45.6). Most intraoperative elements are now a standard of care and just need to be delivered effectively. We used pop-up reminders in the anesthesia chart if compliance was not achieved as a prompt to action.

PERIOPERATIVE AND POSTOPERATIVE ANALGESIA

Optimal analgesia is key for functional recovery, and it needs to address both visceral pain and wound pain. This obviously depends on the type of surgery, surgical approach, and the patient's own response to pain. We based our plans on the perioperative quality initiative (POQI) papers on analgesia, which address pain to restore function, minimize harm, and ensure comfort.[12,13]

Intraoperative Pathway for Elective Adult X SURGERY
NOTE: PATIENT related factors WILL lead to change from Pathway
This change is an ESSENTIAL part of medical judgement

Element	Pathway	X Surgery	X Surgery
SA-Anes Macro			
Anemia & Blood Utilization	Preoperative Goal For SN-5 Adults		
	Day of Surgery If Hgb @ goal		
Frailty & Geriatric Patients	Preoperative		
	Day of Surgery		
Analgesia (use judgement in elderly, severe Heart/ Liver/, Renal disease)	Preoperative		
	Intraoperative		
PONV Prophylaxis	Risk Factors		
	Age </= 65		
	Age >/= 65		
Antibiotic	Preferred		
	B-lactam Alergy		
Intraop Fluid (use judgement in severe heart & renal disease	Fluid Plan		
	Maintenance Plan		
	Anticipate Vasoactive gtt		
Normothermia	Intraoperative		
DVT Prophylaxis	Intraoperative		
Other Notes			
Equipment			
Position, Rx, or Neuromonitoring			

Fig. 45.6 Intraoperative pathway.

When addressing pain, it is key that:

- Patient expectations for pain management are set before surgery.
- Patients on chronic opioids have a different pathway and their needs are met.
- An opioid-sparing multimodal approach is used with planned de-escalation.
- Opioids are minimized using local anesthetic blocks, regional anesthesia, or adjuncts such as dexmedetomidine or ketamine.
- Oral over intravenous medication routes are chosen when feasible to reduce nursing time and avoid patient-controlled analgesia (PCA), which can lead to decreased mobility.
- Allow intravenous medication for breakthrough pain where oral medications are ineffective.
- Reduce all drug doses according to age and glomerular filtration rate (GFR).
- Take-home opioids should be minimized and not exceed 7 days in duration. Exceptions may be approved by the attending surgeon if extenuating circumstances exist.

We created analgesia pathways with the surgeons and acute pain team to determine optimal multimodal analgesia, decide what type of local anesthetic blocks to use, troubleshoot breakthrough pain for different surgical procedures, and decide which type of surgical approach to use (e.g., laparoscopic versus open; Fig. 45.7).

FLUIDS AND HEMODYNAMICS

Optimal management of fluids and hemodynamics is a key determinant in all-cause outcomes. The combination of cardiac output (flow), blood pressure, and oxygenation are key to supply oxygen and nutrients to cells and remove breakdown products.

Fluid volume ranges are set according to specialty and procedure and provided in the intraoperative pathways; however, timing of fluid administration is just as important. High-risk patients (those with impaired cardiac performance, preexisting renal dysfunction, or who had prolonged surgery and blood loss) will benefit from flow monitoring.[14]

We standardized a goal-directed hemodynamic algorithm, which optimized cardiac output and maintained a mean arterial pressure (MAP) of over 65 mm Hg using low-dose vasopressors (Fig. 45.8). We used a simplified strategy of optimizing stroke volume and cardiac output after induction of anesthesia, maintaining stroke volume and MAP through surgery and then reoptimizing the stroke volume after surgery. Results in colorectal surgery reduced AKI from 15.4% to 7% in 159 patients compared with 162 case controls.

ANESTHESIA ERAS CHECKLIST

A checklist was created and posted on all OR walls and anesthesia machines to constantly remind all anesthesia providers of the key goals of ERAS, culminating in the patient being able to drink, eat a light diet, and mobilize the morning after surgery (Fig. 45.9).

POSTOPERATIVE RECOVERY

Engaged, empowered patients are key to changing outcomes. Setting goals with patients that they can work toward independently and providing tools they can use to track their progress encourages patients to actively participate in their recovery and be better prepared to continue a rapid return to baseline function after discharge.

Patient engagement tools used in the nursing units at VCU Health include:

- Admission (comfort) kits
- Aromatherapy
- Chewing gum
- Patient diaries (Fig. 45.10)
- Unit mobility game boards[15]

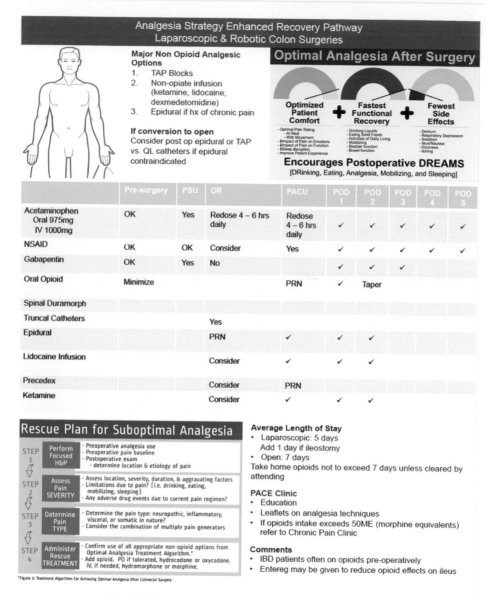

Fig. 45.7 Enhanced Recovery After Surgery (ERAS) anesthesia plan.

- Step tracking apps or devices
- In-room patient communication boards
- Protein drinks
- Progressive care sleep precautions

Electronic Medical Record and Order Sets

EMRs were originally designed as billing tools and despite great improvement in functionality in recent years, they are still not very useful in driving real-time best practice compliance.

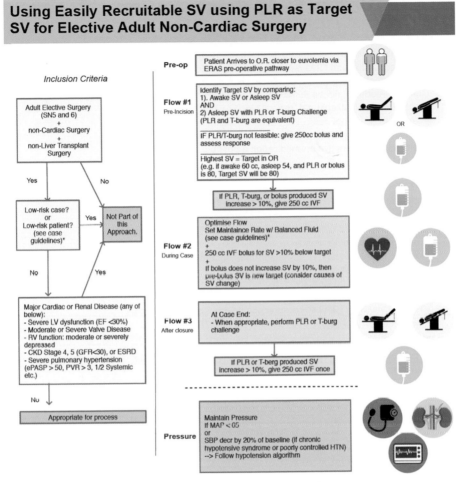

Fig. 45.8 Goal-directed hemodynamic algorithm.

EMR functionality can be used to suggest the most appropriate pathways based on documented results/characteristics, and then flexed to the most appropriate tests, medications, and dosing. To maximize this type of functionality, EMR documentation flows must follow the flow of clinical care and use structured templates to capture data for compliance in a way that can be processed into coded algorithms. The algorithms guide the provider to develop a care plan that reflects the most current evidence, allowing the provider to place their focus on addressing any nonroutine needs of the patient.

Custom views and tracking tools can improve compliance of good practice by serving as an aid for the care team to follow the patient throughout the surgical care journey and intervene as needed to keep the patient on course for the best possible outcome.

Measuring Compliance and Outcomes

As well as contributing to the national Vizient quality data set, we wanted to have a way of being able to collect our own quality data for compliance and outcomes. This ensured we knew the data

Anesthetic Key ERAS Points

Pre-operative

- Patient's health status optimized (anemia, nutrition, diabetes) (PACE)
- Patient education and ERAS pathway planning performed (PACE)
- Oral carbohydrate drink 800 mls evening before, 400 mls early morning of surgery
- Oral multimodal analgesia & s/cut heparin/LMWH* as soon as possible •not if getting neuroaxial block
- Placement of spinal/epidural/truncal block by Acute Pain Service
- Active Warming if needed
- Continue to allow water to drink up to 2 hours before start of surgery
- Avoid/minimize sedative premedication if possible

Intra-operative

- Antibiotic prophylaxis prior to surgery (and re-dose as appropriate)
- Avoid Nasogastric tubes (if needed to decompress stomach remove at end)
- PONV prophylaxis (2 different classes of drugs)
- Short acting anesthetic agents
- Maintenance (if necessary) and monitoring of neuromuscular block
- Depth of anesthesia monitoring where appropriate (elderly/delirium risk)
- Protective ventilation strategy (5–8 mls/kg) with optimal PEEP
- Maintain normoglycemia
- VTE prophylaxis – TEDS, calf compression device, chemoprophylaxis
- Maintenance of normothermia – warming device/fluid warming
- Consider Analgesic technique (neuroaxial block/TEA/TAP/truncal blocks) ketamine/precedex to reduce opioid need postoperatively
- Consider hemodynamic monitoring for patients with comorbidities, blood loss >7mls/kg, high fluid shifts, SIRS, Sepsis, unstable hemodynamics.
- Optimize Stroke Volume, aim for normovolemia, and maintain MAP within 20% of patient's baseline unless there is a clinical indication not to
- Maintain optimal Hemoglobin and oxygen delivery for the patient and procedure

Post-operative

- Rapid awakening from anesthesia
- Controlled extubation to reduce risk of pulmonary microaspiration with full return of neuromuscular and bulbar function
- Optimize analgesia as necessary while minimizing intravenous opioids
- Optimize fluid therapy as necessary during the period of maximal fluid shifts immediately after surgery – monitor/prescribe accordingly
- Intravenous fluids and salt load should be minimized to the amount necessary to maintain normovolemia prior to adequate oral intake
- Start oral feeding and mobilization as soon as feasible
- Maintain normoglycemia
- Ensure multimodal analgesia, antiemetics, & VTE prophylaxis are prescribed

Your patient should be able to drink, eat a light diet and mobilize the morning after surgery

Fig. 45.9   Anesthesia Enhanced Recovery After Surgery (ERAS) checklist.

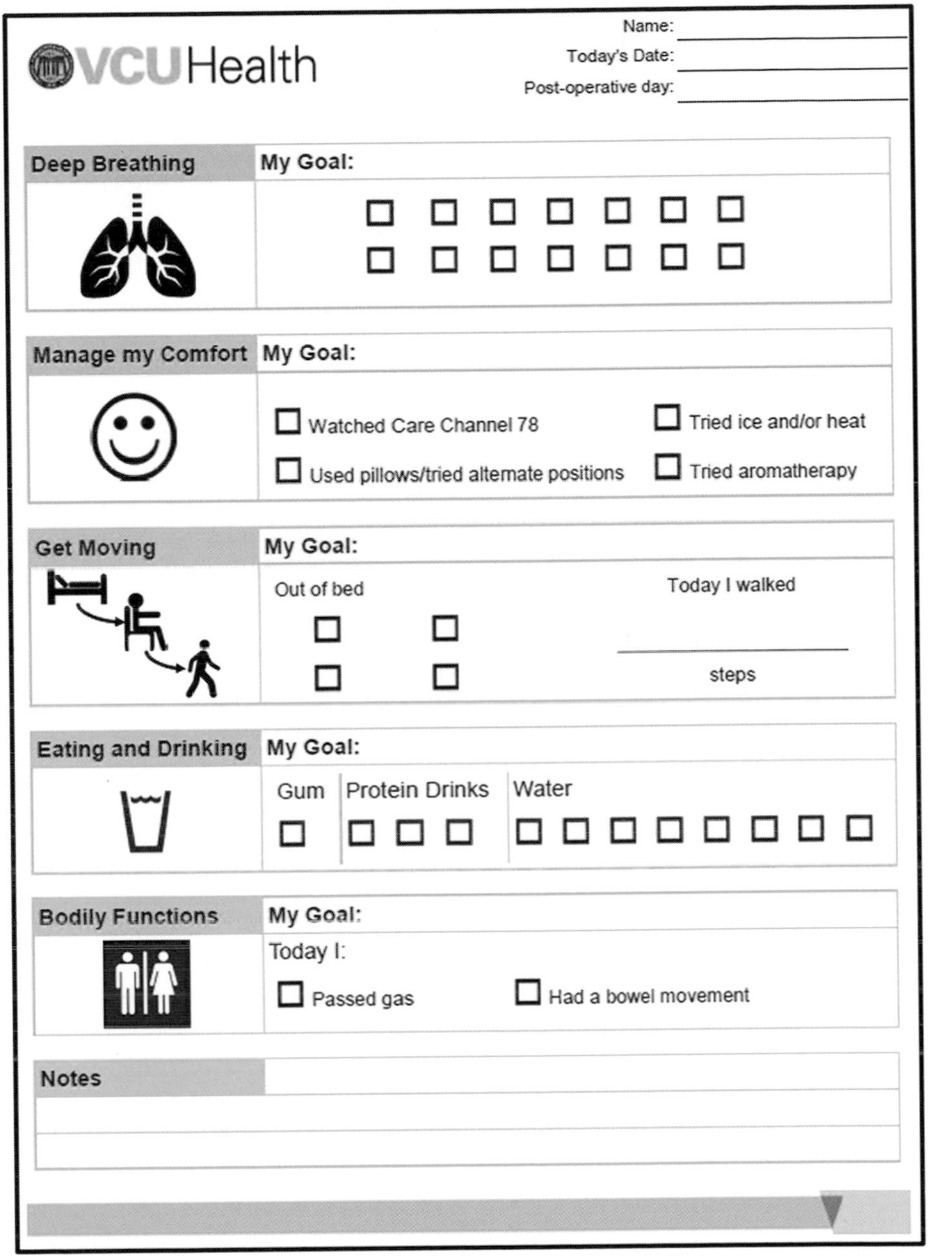
VCU Health

Name:

Today's Date:

Post-operative day:

Deep Breathing My Goal:

☐ ☐ ☐ ☐ ☐ ☐ ☐
☐ ☐ ☐ ☐ ☐ ☐ ☐

Manage my Comfort My Goal:

☐ Watched Care Channel 78
☐ Tried ice and/or heat
☐ Used pillows/tried alternate positions
☐ Tried aromatherapy

Get Moving My Goal:

Out of bed ☐ ☐ ☐ ☐

Today I walked ______ steps

Eating and Drinking My Goal:

Gum ☐ | Protein Drinks ☐ ☐ ☐ | Water ☐ ☐ ☐ ☐ ☐ ☐ ☐ ☐

Bodily Functions My Goal:

Today I:
☐ Passed gas
☐ Had a bowel movement

Notes

Fig. 45.10 Patient diary.

and could feedback in almost real time. We used our analyst to build a data set in Tableau. This required significant funding and time, taking over 9 months to create.

We created run charts to show improvements to maintain buy-in with all stakeholders, showing their work improved patient outcomes. We used dashboards and run charts as a basis to demonstrate sustained improvement.

Summary

VCU Health used ERAS as a backbone to reset the whole of the perioperative space, affecting all patients' surgical pathways. Executive leadership support was vital in the adoption, implementation, and maintenance of momentum of the ERAS program across the health system.

The vertical and horizontal implementation of ERAS principles we used accelerated the standardization of perioperative pathways across the health system. We used the EMR to drive real-time compliance of ERAS elements and produce audits of compliance and outcomes.

Implementing ERAS across surgical specialties fundamentally changed the delivery of care across the entire perioperative pathway and reduced the average LOS, opioid consumption, AKI, all-cause complications, and readmissions. In 2019, the health system had the third lowest colorectal surgical site infection rates in the USA on the Vizient database after ERAS and bundle implementation.[16] The system-wide approach enables the organization to be highly competitive in both local and national markets.

References

1. Fearon KCH, Ljungqvist O, Von Meyenfeldt M, et al. Enhanced recovery after surgery: a consensus review of clinical care for patients undergoing colonic resection. *Clin Nutr.* 2005;24(3). 466–377.
2. Ljungqvist O, Scott M, Fearon KC. Enhanced recovery after surgery: a review. *JAMA Surg.* 2017;152 (3):292–298.
3. Peden CJ, Aggarwal G, Aitken RJ, et al. Guidelines for Perioperative Care for Emergency Laparotomy Enhanced Recovery After Surgery (ERAS) Society recommendations: part 1—preoperative: diagnosis, rapid assessment and optimization. *World J Surg.* 2021;45(5):1272–1290.
4. Mythen MG. Spread and adoption of enhanced recovery from elective surgery in the English National Health Service. *Can J Anaesth.* 2015;62:105–109.
5. Joliat G-R, Ljungqvist O, Wasylak T, Peters O, Demartines N. Beyond surgery: clinical and economic impact of Enhanced Recovery After Surgery programs. *BMC Health Serv Res.* 2018;18:1008.
6. Thanh N, Nelson A, Wang X, et al. Return on investment of the Enhanced Recovery After Surgery (ERAS) multi-guideline, multisite implementation in Alberta, Canada. *Can J Surg.* 2020;63:E542–E550.
7. Burwell SM. Setting value-based payment goals-HHS efforts to improve U.S. health care. *N Engl J Med.* 2015;372:897–899.
8. Spencer P, Scott M. Implementing enhanced recovery after surgery across a United States health system. *Anesthesiol Clin.* 2022;40(1):1–21.
9. Scott MJ, Spencer P, Fain M. Horizontal and vertical implementation strategies for ERAS across a US healthcare system. *Clin Nutr.* 2019;31:133–134.
10. Scott MJ, Spencer P, Fain M, Thakrar S, Fox E, Winborne D. A preoperative ERAS optimization timeline framework to inform surgeons to delay surgery appropriately. *Clin Nutr.* 2019;31:117–118.
11. Vetter TR, Boudreaux AM, Ponce BA, Barman J, Crump SJ. Development of a preoperative patient clearance and consultation screening questionnaire. *Anesth Analg.* 2016;123:1453–1457.
12. McEvoy MD, Scott MJ, Gordon DB, et al. Perioperative Quality Initiative (POQI) I Workgroup. American Society for Enhanced Recovery (ASER) and Perioperative Quality Initiative (POQI) joint consensus statement on optimal analgesia within an enhanced recovery pathway for colorectal surgery: part 1-from the preoperative period to PACU. *Perioper Med (Lond).* 2017;6:8.
13. Scott MJ, McEvoy MD, Gordon DB, et al. American Society for Enhanced Recovery (ASER) and Perioperative Quality Initiative (POQI) joint consensus statement on optimal analgesia within an enhanced recovery pathway for colorectal surgery: part 2-From PACU to the Transition Home. *Perioper Med (Lond).* 2017;6:7.
14. French WB, Scott M. Fluid and hemodynamics. *Anesthesiol Clin.* 2022;40:59–71.
15. Sawyer A, Fox WE, Brown S, Spencer P, Scott MJ. Mobility boards to aid postoperative activity goals. *Clin Nutr.* 2019;31:141.
16. Albert H, Bataller W, Masroor N, et al. Infection prevention and enhanced recovery after surgery: a partnership for implementation of an evidence-based bundle to reduce colorectal surgical site infections. *Am J Infect Control.* 2019;47:718–719.

CHAPTER 46

Pain Care Pathways and Patient Reported Outcomes

Alexander Hallway, BA ■ Michael Englesbe, MD

KEY POINTS

- Overprescribing of opioids and new persistent opioid use after surgery are common problems.
- Granular data involving patient-reported outcomes and clinical behaviors are critical to inform pain care pathways.
- A remarkable number of stakeholders are involved in pain management for even the simplest surgical procedures; all must be included in pathway development.
- Evidence-based and iterative pain care pathways can profoundly reduce the prescription and consumption of opioids.

Introduction

Effective postoperative pain management is critical for successful recovery after surgery, contributing both to positive clinical outcomes and patient satisfaction. Traditional practice has relied on opioid medications as a primary mode of pain management. Although these medications have provided pain control, their role in the escalating opioid use disorder epidemic cannot be ignored. Opioids are overprescribed after surgery, with studies indicating 72% of opioids remain unused.[1] These leftover opioids create opportunities for misuse and diversion into communities. Exposure to opioids may result in new, persistent opioid use for up to 6% of patients after both minor and major surgery.[2]

The reasons for overprescribing opioids after surgery are beyond the scope of this chapter. Nonetheless, right-sizing opioid prescribing is a key priority for both the opioid-naïve and chronic opioid using patient. Creating institutional change for opioid prescribing can best be achieved using various continuous quality improvement frameworks. To do this, patient feedback is critical; thus a system for patient-reported outcomes must be established. We will detail successful opioid prescribing change within a single institution and across a state using the Plan-Do-Check-Act (PDCA) or Plan-Do-Study-Act (PDSA) approach.

Plan — Listen to Operationally Minded Clinical Experts

Efforts to improve opioid prescribing in the state of Michigan began with a review of opioid prescribing practices at one institution. First, the median pill quantity prescribed for postoperative pain management was determined. Each patient undergoing laparoscopic cholecystectomy was surveyed for details regarding their postoperative experience and the quantity of pills they consumed while recovering at home. It was determined that surgeons were prescribing nearly 10 times the number of pills their patients needed for postoperative pain management.[3] In recognition of the fact that surplus pills create opportunities for diversion and misuse, this finding initiated a major change in clinical practice and a mobilization of resources to right-size opioid prescribing after surgery.

A team of clinical stakeholders including nurses, anesthesiologists, surgeons, information technology specialists, and patient advocates assembled to develop best practices and pain-care pathways that reduce excessive opioid prescribing after surgery. These early pathways included simple actions:

- Recommend nonopioid pain medications such as acetaminophen (Tylenol) and ibuprofen (Motrin).
- Counsel patients before surgery about postoperative pain expectations.
- Prescribe evidence-based opioid quantities after surgery, informed by the 90% percentile of patient consumption.

Do—Include As Many Stakeholders As You Can

As clear, actionable pain management pathways emerged, they were vetted with experts and leaders within the institution. Process flow charts, pain management protocol summary documents, and provider training programs were circulated throughout perioperative departments to communicate practice changes and prescribing guidelines for perioperative pain care. Institutional order sets were also revised to streamline medication orders and automate the delivery of better patient instructions. Grand rounds were a high-yield forum to both announce and discuss pain care reform. Visual and verbal communications were used, repeated, and reiterated to emphasize the importance of moving away from the existing model of opioid-centric pain management.

Even for the simplest outpatient procedures, internal process analyses indicated that more than 14 unique stakeholder groups held a role in pain care for surgical patients (Fig. 46.1). These groups extended outside of prescription-writing positions, with surgeons, advanced practice providers, and even surgery schedulers and front desk clerks playing a role in discussing or dictating pain care with patients. It became clear that institutional pain pathways needed to be communicated beyond the people who prescribe the pills.

Check—Most Importantly, With the Patient

Evaluation of perioperative pain management practices requires continuous practice improvement, measured and reported on regular intervals to all stakeholders and leaders. Simple measures in early development of the pathway included type, quantity, and dose of opioid medications prescribed. Additional measures were added to these reports, including nonopioid pain medications prescribed and the existence of institutional pain management instructions in discharge paperwork.

Measuring patient-reported outcomes is essential to checking the progress of clinical change. This is especially important when measuring complex and patient-centered outcomes, such as pain. To ensure patient safety and high-quality care, patient surveys using validated measures were used to assess pain, patient satisfaction, postoperative opioid consumption, recovery time, return to the emergency department, occurrence of pain-related messages, and more. Data collection required a robust patient survey infrastructure, with email, SMS (text messaging), and phone survey distribution capability to collect accurate data and ensure changes to pain management practices created the intended effect (i.e., a reduction in opioid prescribing without compromising patient experience and quality of care). Setting up a robust patient-reported outcomes system was the hardest portion of this early change but ended up being critical for the broad dissemination of this work across the state.

Priority Lap Chole - UM Pain Optimization Pathway Protocol (POPP)

Date:12/20/17

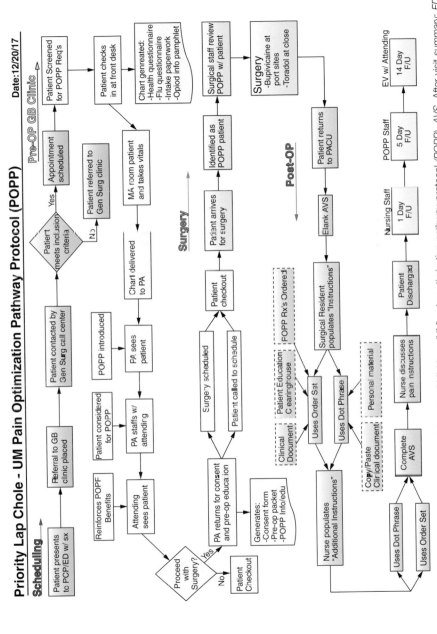

Fig. 46.1 Priority Laparoscopic Cholecystectomy. University of Michigan (UM) pain optimization pathway protocol (POPP). AVS, After visit summary; ED, emergency department; EV, evaluation; F/U, follow-up; GB, gallbladder; PA, physician's assistant; PCP, primary care practitioner; Rx, drugs.

Adjust and Sustain—Informed By Data

Actions and adjustments to the institutional pain management protocol occurred in real time when urgent and in quarterly PDCA cycles. To ensure the maintenance of high-quality care, a multidisciplinary pain committee met on a quarterly basis to review surgical pain management process data, patient-reported outcomes, and provider feedback. Activities of adjustment included revising procedure-specific prescribing recommendations, improving patient education, and adapting medical record documentation processes to improve data visibility. Provider education and the sharing of emerging best practices in surgical pain care became a regular segment of grand rounds discussions.

As practice change took hold, and average discharge prescribing declined to meet average patient consumption, outlier prescribers were targeted by academic detailing sessions in which best practices for postoperative pain management were reviewed with institutional leaders. Detailing sessions also included a review of the outlying prescribers' historical prescription data with comparisons to that of their peers and their patients' measurable needs. These data were a powerful tool for persuasion. Careful, incremental adjustments, backed by high-quality data from both the system and patients, ensured the institution was and is providing the best possible postoperative pain care.

Results

These efforts resulted in a decrease in excessive opioid prescribing for all high-volume procedures. In just 4 years, prescribing after elective laparoscopic cholecystectomy decreased from an average of around 60 Oxycodone 5 mg tablets to just 4. Comparisons of the institution's opioid sparing pathway to a propensity-matched "standard of care" cohort from other hospitals in the state showed that opioid-sparing patients received and consumed 5 times fewer pills than patients receiving nonopioid sparing care. Opioid-spared patients also reported similar satisfaction with their surgical care and lower pain scores; more than 30% of opioid-sparing patients chose to forego an opioid prescription altogether, compared with zero patients in the nonopioid sparing group.[4] We hypothesize this is because of improved preoperative pain discussions, fueled by patient education and informed clinicians. These enhancements may have created opportunities for shared decision making and reduced patient anxiety about pain.

Fortunately, media coverage of the opioid epidemic, and this patient and provider awareness, coincided with the third year of this work. This solidified the efforts and led to broad dissemination and willingness to change.

Change Within the State

As change grew within the institution, the priorities and practices of surgical opioid stewardship were exported to other hospitals across the state. Exchange of these ideas was primarily facilitated by professional organizations, quality collaboratives, and payor-directed financial reimbursement initiatives.[5] Robust patient-reported outcomes data were a critical factor of successful dissemination of opioid-sparing surgical pain management throughout the state. This data infrastructure was created by a strong network of surgical quality data registries and enabled individual hospitals to monitor and maintain high patient satisfaction while iterating a PDCA-based reduction of postoperative opioid prescribing.

With the forces of data, narrative, communications within the lay press, and financial incentive, "rightsizing" opioid prescribing in the state of Michigan was a success. From 2017 to 2018, opioid prescribing in nine common general surgery procedures at 43 Michigan health systems was reduced by a third without any measurable effect on patients' satisfaction with their care.[6] Michigan's efforts to promote evidence-based pain management and opioid prescribing after surgery has made the state a regional leader in postoperative opioid safety. Closing the gap between opioids prescribed and opioids consumed after surgery will reduce excess opioids in the community and hopefully reduce the supply of prescription opioids available for misuse and diversion.

References

1. Hill M, Stucke R, Billmeier S, Kelly J, Barth R. Guideline for discharge opioid prescriptions after inpatient general surgical procedures. *J Am Coll Surg.* 2018;226(6):996–1003.
2. Brummett C, Waljee J, Goesling J, et al. New persistent opioid use sfter minor and major surgical procedures in US adults. *JAMA Surgery.* 2017;152(6):e170504.
3. Howard R, Waljee J, Brummett C, Englesbe M, Lee J. Reduction in opioid prescribing through evidence-based prescribing guidelines. *JAMA Surg.* 2018;153(3):285–287.
4. Anderson M, Hallway A, Brummett C, Waljee J, Englesbe M, Howard R. Patient-reported outcomes after opioid-sparing surgery compared with standard of care. *JAMA Surg.* 2021;156(3):286–287.
5. Howard R, Hallway A, Santos-Parker J, et al. Optimizing postoperative opioid prescribing through quality-based reimbursement. *JAMA Netw Open.* 2019;2(9):e1911619.
6. Vu JV, Howard RA, Gunaseelan V, Brummett CM, Waljee JF, Englesbe MJ. Statewide implementation of postoperative opioid prescribing guidelines. *The New England Journal of Medicine.* 2019;381(7):680–682.

CHAPTER 47

Health Services Research

Jason Tong, MD, MSHP ■ Rachel R. Kelz, MD, MSCE, MBA

KEY POINTS

- The origin of health services research is discussed.
- Quantitative tools, including cross-sectional, cohort, case-control, and difference-in-difference study designs, are briefly reviewed.
- Qualitative tools, such as focus groups, surveys, and interviews, are covered.
- Examples of study designs in perioperative care are used to highlight how health services research can be transformational.

Introduction to Health Services Research

In the wake of World War II and the rapidly evolving landscape of America's identity, the 1946 Hill Burton Act helped to fund the development of hospitals across the country. During the expansion of access to hospital-based services, John Cronin, then chief of the Division of Hospital and Medical Facilities, recognized the need for a new body of research dedicated to better understanding healthcare delivery and access.[1] He not only helped to birth the broad field of health services research but also secured over $10 million in federal funding to jumpstart the field's inception.[1] As health care and its delivery have expanded in complexity over the last several decades, the field of health services research has grown exponentially in response. Now, health services research is defined by the Agency for Healthcare Research and Quality as a "multidisciplinary field of scientific investigation that studies how social factors, financing systems, organizational structures and processes, health technologies, and personal behaviors affect access to health care, the quality and cost of health care, and ultimately our health and well-being."[2]

Health services research is intimately linked to the improvement of healthcare delivery through the concept of transformational research. Transformational research is defined by the National Science Foundation as "research driven by ideas that have the potential to radically change our understanding of an important existing scientific or engineering concept leading to the creation of a new paradigm or field of science or engineering. Such research is also characterized by its challenge to current understanding, or its pathway to new frontiers."[3] As such, transformational research serves as the mechanism through which large advances in care and major paradigm shifts are realized.[4]

In this chapter, we aim to first highlight study designs commonly used in the field of health services research. Subsequently, through the conceptual framework of the five phases of surgical care developed by the American College of Surgeons (ACS), we will provide examples of how these study designs have been successfully implemented as examples of transformational research. Finally, we will summarize the most frequently used standardized reporting guidelines and offer a review of how health services research differs from quality improvement (QI).

Common Study Designs

OBSERVATIONAL STUDY DESIGNS

Before identifying opportunities for improvement and change, researchers must first be equipped with the tools to better understand existing systems in place. Observational studies allow researchers to highlight the existence and magnitude of problems present and see possible correlations between outcomes and exposures.[5] Examples of observational studies include cross-sectional, cohort, and case-control studies. More advanced analytic methods, such as difference-in-difference studies, aid in further exploring correlational relationships.

Cross-sectional studies are a useful descriptive tool to examine relationships between outcomes and exposures within a limited timeframe. They are frequently described as "snapshots" in time.[5,6] These studies may be hypothesis generating for future investigations, providing a powerful tool that can be relatively quick and inexpensive to perform. Given the limited temporal scope of the data, however, cross-sectional studies are most limited by their inability to offer correlational or causal explanations.[6]

Other tools, including cohort and case-control studies, allow for further examinations into the possible correlation between exposures and outcomes of interest. Cohort studies are either retrospective or prospective longitudinal examinations of two study groups. The two study groups consist of one that is associated with a predefined exposure and a second control group that is like the first in most regards except for the exposure variable. The researcher then measures rates of the outcome of interest across the two groups and calculates a relative risk of an outcome associated with that exposure.[5,7] The utility of cohort studies is most limited when examining rare outcomes. Otherwise, cohort studies are subject to the inherent limitations of prospective and retrospective designs. Prospective cohort studies allow for targeted data collection and can examine multiple outcomes from the same exposure, but they are typically costly and may require a lengthy study period depending on the relationship between the study exposure and outcomes. Retrospective studies can be quickly performed using pre-existing data, but their application is limited by the manner and fidelity with which the data was originally collected.[5] Case-control studies are retrospective designs that start with a group containing the outcome of interest and a matched control. The researcher than retrospectively searches and compares the prevalence of an exposure between the case and control groups. They can be relatively quick to perform and are particularly useful in studying relatively rare outcomes. Case-control studies are limited in their ability to study rare exposures and are unable to offer estimates of incidence.[5]

Advanced quasi-experimental study designs exist for specific questions in healthcare delivery. One such design using observational data is the difference-in-difference study. Difference-in-difference studies examine two matched groups over time after an intervention that is limited to only one of the groups. The difference-in-difference analysis then compares the relative difference between respective changes in study outcomes across these two groups over time. In other words, it examines the difference between the respective differences within each study group over time, hence its namesake. Although this can mimic large pseudorandomized retrospective studies examining the isolated effects of individual interventions, difference-in-difference studies are most limited by their internal validity based upon adequate matching between the control and intervention groups.[8] This study design is often used for the evaluation of health policies.

QUALITATIVE STUDIES

Qualitative studies allow for a different approach by recognizing the inherent limitations of objective data to capture the intangible and subjective drivers of complex relationships. Qualitative study designs are typically time-intensive and require specialized training. Given the breadth of qualitative methods, we will only highlight interviews, focus groups, and surveys, which are commonly employed when preparing for the implementation of a quality or safety intervention.

Surveys can be administered through a variety of platforms, including in-person, telephone, video-call, paper-based, and on the Internet. The instrument or questionnaire can be used to obtain information from a broad audience in a standardized fashion. This allows for improved ease of analysis and interpretability. Although often quick to distribute and administer, response rates can be subjective to response bias based on the medium. Additionally, the restrictive format of surveys can prevent subjects from offering clarifying details.

One-to-one interviews can be an immensely powerful tool in exploring intricate details regarding an individual's experience. Themes discovered in these interviews can be hypothesis-generating and lead to future qualitative and quantitative studies. They are limited by their time-intensiveness and their generalizability given the often small sample size. Interviews can be either open-ended or semistructured, allowing for either exploratory discussions or more directed and efficient data collection.[9]

Focus groups allow researchers to not only collect information from numerous individuals but also gain unique insights through group interactions. This additional dimension of complexity can be both beneficial and harmful. Although group interactions may facilitate the discovery of new ideas otherwise not available in one-to-one interviews, focus groups require expertise in navigating and leading a group. Without appropriate guidance, focus groups are subject to dominant opinions and groupthink, which can be counterproductive.[9]

Applications of Study Designs

The 2017 publication of *Optimal Resources for Surgical Quality and Safety* by the ACS outlines five phases of care: surgical preoperative evaluation and preparation, immediate preoperative readiness, and intraoperative, postoperative, and postdischarge phases of care.[10] We will now demonstrate the application of various study designs to these phases of care to demonstrate the breadth and transformative nature of health services research.

SURGICAL PREOPERATIVE EVALUATION AND PREPARATION

The surgical preoperative evaluation and preparation phase is a broad time period leading to the surgeon encounter, which includes issues such as coordinating multidisciplinary resources in anticipation for surgical and postoperative care. In their study, *Impact of Dependent Coverage Provision of the Affordable Care Act on Insurance Continuity for Adolescents and Young Adults With Cancer*, Jeffrey H. Silber, MD, PhD and his coauthors applied a difference-in-difference study design to two matched cohorts with varying degrees of exposure to the policy change.[11] Within the first cohort, they compared two groups of matched patients separated in time such that one group turned 19 years old before the policy change and the other turned 19 years old after the policy change. The second cohort then contained two groups of matched patients similarly separated in time, neither of which experienced the policy change after turning 19 years old. The authors first compared the difference in insurance loss within each cohort. The difference-in-difference study design then offered a method to quantitatively compare the difference between the differences found within each cohort, with control for the other changes to health care that transpired over the study time period, which may have confounded the results.

Ultimately, the study found that the policy change was positively associated with improved insurance retention in young adults with cancer. This offers evidence to both providers and policy makers to suggest that this policy change achieved its intended purpose. Additionally, this work helps to highlight the vulnerable population of young adults with cancer and the need for further attention to help in minimizing coverage loss for these patients.

IMMEDIATE PREOPERATIVE READINESS

The immediate preoperative readiness phase includes care involving the 24 hours immediately preceding the moment the patient arrives in the operating room. To prepare patients mentally and physically for surgery, surgical teams must be able to effectively communicate preoperative instructions to patients. Qualitative tools are an effective means to assess patient expectations and barriers to effective communication.

Gena Dunivan, MD, and her colleagues performed a qualitative study using focus groups to better identify patient priorities in preoperative instructions and education. In their work, *Preferences for Preoperative Education: A Qualitative Study of the Patient Perspective,* they led four focus groups among English- and Spanish-speaking postoperative patients to better understand what elements of the preoperative instructions and education could have been improved. As the authors highlight, "Qualitative research is especially useful when little is known about a particular topic and can aid in hypothesis generation."[12]

They ultimately identified five recurring patient-centered themes to serve as the foundation for future qualitative and quantitative studies. Their work additionally highlights the complex relationship between patient characteristics, such as preferred language, education, medical literacy, and race, and effective patient-surgeon communication.

INTRAOPERATIVE

Within the operating room, surgical safety checklists became increasingly commonplace after the landmark publication of *To Err Is Human: Building a Safer Health System* by the Institute of Medicine.[13] This work prompted a widespread evaluation of the implementation of safety checklists within the surgical field. In Reid B. Adams, MD, and his colleagues' work, *The Surgical Safety Checklist: Lessons Learned During Implementation,* they explored the feasibility of implementing a surgical safety checklist by randomizing a group of surgeons to the use of an intraoperative safety checklist.[14] The study incorporated the use of both postoperative questionnaires and intraoperative video recording to assess the successful use of these checklists.

The authors concluded that the implementation of surgical safety checklists was feasible and, more importantly, could change surgical team behaviors for the better. Additionally, the study's discussion highlighted the tension and discomfort associated with a proposed cultural shift. This identified tension has gone on to inspire numerous subsequent studies exploring the barriers to the successful implementation of surgical safety checklists.

POSTOPERATIVE

In the postoperative space, surgeons have made tremendous strides in streamlining care to reduce inefficiencies and ultimately improve patient care. The concept of "enhanced recovery after surgery" (ERAS) has evolved tremendously and led to major changes in how we think of postoperative care.[15] Simultaneously, it is known that there are racial disparities in postoperative outcomes, potentially because of variations in care. To explore how ERAS has impacted known racial disparities, Daniel I. Chu, MD, and his colleagues published their work, *Enhanced Recovery After Surgery (ERAS) Eliminates Racial Disparities in Postoperative Length of Stay After Colorectal Surgery.*[16]

The authors performed a retrospective matched cohort study to compare postoperative length of stay, mortality, and readmission rates among colorectal surgery patients. Ultimately, they found that the widespread implementation of ERAS protocols was associated with an elimination of preexisting racial disparities in length of stay between White and Black surgical patients. This work's findings helped to point at the potential of protocolized clinical pathways as "a practical approach to achieving health equity in surgery."[16]

POSTDISCHARGE

By streamlining care and increasing the availability of outpatient surgical resources, more and more postsurgical care has shifted into the outpatient domain. With this shift, both patients and providers have encountered novel challenges. To evaluate the barriers and challenges associated with post-discharge care, Phillip M. Dowzicky, MD, MSHP, and his coauthors performed their study, *An Assessment of Patient, Caregiver, and Clinician Perspectives on the Postdischarge Phase of Care.*[17]

Through open-ended interviews employing the free-listing technique with a purposive sample of 40 surgical oncology patients, caregivers, and clinicians, the authors uncovered both overlapping and unique concerns of participants. The findings of this study helped form the basis of future potential investigations investigating a variety of topics including improved preoperative education, standardizing postdischarge engagement by surgical care teams, and improving support systems within patient home environments.

Reporting of Health Services Research

After the successful investigation of a particular research question, it is critical for researchers to follow standardized guidelines for reporting findings. This creates a standardized framework for viewers to digest information and bolsters confidence in the fidelity of research findings. Here, we discuss three commonly cited reporting guidelines for both quantitative and qualitative work.

QUANTITATIVE REPORTING GUIDELINES

The Strengthening the Reporting of Observational Studies in Epidemiology (STROBE) guide-lines offer a 22-item checklist to aid researchers in formatting and presenting their research in an organized and systematic manner consistent with the standards of the epidemiologic commu-nity.[18] This checklist offers items that are both common and specific to cross-sectional, cohort, and case-control study designs.

QUALITATIVE REPORTING GUIDELINES

For qualitative studies, the Standards for Reporting Qualitative Research (SRQR) offers a 21-item checklist that serves to improve transparency in the data collection and content analysis process.[19] Given the complexity in the variety and types of qualitative tools, an alternative reporting guideline known as the Consolidated Criteria for Reporting Qualitative Research (COREQ) offers an alter-native 32-item checklist.[20] The COREQ is a comprehensive tool that is adaptable to a broad array of qualitative study designs.

Differences Between Quality Improvement and Research

Health services research is ultimately dedicated to improving patient and societal well-being through a multidisciplinary exploration into factors surrounding healthcare access and delivery. This concept can sometimes understandably be confused with QI given the commonalities in inves-tigative tools and shared intention of improving patient care. Nevertheless, there are important dis-tinctions between these two fields.

QI is dedicated to improving patient care but is typically rooted in rapid-cycle interventions, such as the Plan-Do-Study-Act framework, to study medical errors and inefficiencies in care deliv-ery.[21] QI projects with the primary intention of improving care. Health services research is similarly directed at improving patient well-being but takes a broader multidisciplinary approach to exploring opportunities for optimizing healthcare organization, delivery, and financing for both individuals and on a societal level.[21] Health services research projects start with the intention of generating new knowledge. The two fields intersect where critical design and appraisal are needed to generate evidence to support practice changes, and when studies are needed to determine best practices for dissemination. Together, quality and safety work alongside health services research to provide the techniques necessary to transform healthcare delivery in surgery.

Summary

In this chapter, we have discussed the definition of health services research and its origin within the US history and highlighted its transformational potential. Subsequently we have discussed quantitative tools available to researchers including cross-sectional, cohort, case-control, and difference-in-difference study designs. Additionally, we have introduced some of the more frequently used qualitative study tools such as interviews, focus groups, and surveys. The included examples of study designs provided highlight the ways in which health services research can be transformative and inspire both immediate action and further research. We also offer three commonly used reporting guidelines to aid in presenting study findings in a standardized and transparent manner. Lastly, this chapter concludes on the distinction between QI and health services research, two closely related, but independent, bodies of work dedicated to advancing patient care.

References

1. McCarthy T, White KL. Origins of health services research. *Health Serv Res.* 2000;35(2):375–387.
2. Agency for Healthcare Research and Quality. An organizational guide to building health services research capacity. Published October 2014. https://www.ahrq.gov/funding/training-grants/hsrguide/hsrguide.html. Accessed October 5, 2021.
3. *Enhancing Support of Transformative Research at the National Science Foundation;* 2007.
4. Dankwa-Mullan I, Rhee KB, Stoff DM, et al. Moving toward paradigm-shifting research in health disparities through translational, transformational, and transdisciplinary approaches. *Am J Pub Health.* 2010;100(suppl 1). https://doi.org/10.2105/AJPH.2009.189167.
5. Rezigalla AA. Observational study designs: synopsis for selecting an appropriate study design. *Cureus.* 2020;12(1). https://doi.org/10.7759/cureus.6692.
6. Wang JJ, Attia J. Study designs in epidemiology and levels of evidence. *Am J Ophthalmol.* 2010;149 (3):367–370. https://doi.org/10.1016/j.ajo.2009.08.001.
7. Setia MS. Methodology series module 1: cohort studies. Ind J Dermatol. 61(1). https://doi.org/10.4103/0019-5154.174011.
8. Dimick JB, Ryan AM. Methods for evaluating changes in health care policy: the difference-in-differences approach. *JAMA.* 2014;312(22):2401–2402. https://doi.org/10.1001/jama.2014.16153.
9. Isaacs A. An overview of qualitative research methodology for public health researchers. *Int J Med Pub Health.* 2014;4(4):318–323. https://doi.org/10.4103/2230-8598.144055.
10. Hoyt DB, Ko CY, Jones RS, Cherry R, Schneidman D, Khalid M. *Optimal Resources for Surgical Quality and Safety;* 2017.
11. Winestone LE, Hochman LL, Sharpe JE, et al. Impact of Dependent Coverage Provision of the Affordable Care Act on insurance continuity for adolescents and young adults with cancer. *JCO Oncol Pract.* 2021;17 (6):882–890. https://doi.org/10.1200/OP.20.00330.
12. Rockefeller NF, Jeppson P, Komesu YM, Meriwether K V, Ninivaggio C, Dunivan G. Preferences for preoperative education: a qualitative study of the patient perspective. *Female Pelvic Med Reconstr Surg.* 2021;27(10):633–636. https://doi.org/10.1097/SPV.0000000000001014.
13. Kohn LT, Corrigan JM, Donaldson MS, eds. *To Err Is Human: Building a Safer Health System.* National Academies Press; 2000.
14. Calland JF, Turrentine FE, Guerlain S, et al. The surgical safety Checklist: lessons learned during implementation. *Am Surg.* 2011;77(9):1131–1137.
15. Ljungqvist O, Scott M, Fearon KC. Enhanced recovery after surgery. A review. *JAMA Surg.* 2017;152 (3):292–298. https://doi.org/10.1001/jamasurg.2016.4952.

16. Wahl TS, Goss LE, Morris MS, et al. Enhanced recovery after surgery (ERAS) eliminates racial disparities in postoperative length of stay after colorectal surgery. *Ann Surg.* 2018;268(6):1026–1035. https://doi.org/10.1097/SLA.0000000000002307.

17. Dowzicky PM, Shah AA, Barg FK, Eriksen WT, McHugh MD, Kelz RR. An assessment of patient, caregiver, and clinician perspectives on the post-discharge phase of care. *Ann Surg.* 2021;273(4):719–724. https://doi.org/10.1097/SLA.0000000000003479.

18. Vandenbroucke JP, von Elm E, Altman DG, et al. Strengthening the Reporting of Observational Studies in Epidemiology (STROBE): explanation and elaboration. *PLoS Med.* 2007;4(10). https://doi.org/10.1371/journal.pmed.0040297.

19. O'Brien BC, Harris IB, Beckman TJ, Reed DA, Cook DA. Standards for reporting qualitative research: a synthesis of recommendations. *Acad Med.* 2014;89(9):1245–1251. https://doi.org/10.1097/ACM.0000000000000388.

20. Tong A, Sainsbury P, Craig J. Consolidated criteria for reporting qualitative research (COREQ): a 32-item checklist for interviews and focus groups. *Int J Qual Health Care.* 2007;19(6):349–357. https://doi.org/10.1093/intqhc/mzm042.

21. Das D, Wilfong L, Enright K, Rocque G. How do we align health services research and quality improvement? *Am Soc Clin Oncol Educ Book.* 2020;40:1–10.

CHAPTER 48

The Perioperative Brain Health Initiative

Alan Tung, MD, FRCPC ■ Jacqueline W. Ragheb, MD ■ Phillip E. Vlisides, MD

KEY POINTS

- Perioperative neurocognitive disorders represent a major public health issue.
- The Perioperative Brain Health Initiative (PBHI) aims to improve brain health in surgical patients through systematic improvements in awareness and clinical practice.
- Preliminary evidence suggests that implementation of perioperative brain health programs optimizes clinical practice for supporting neurocognitive health.

Introduction

The Perioperative Brain Health Initiative (PBHI), first conceived in 2015 by the American Society of Anesthesiologists (ASA), is a patient safety initiative aimed at addressing the growing concern for perioperative neurocognitive disorders in older patients. For example, postoperative delirium occurs in approximately 20% to 50% of older surgical patients[1] and is associated with increased mortality, prolonged hospitalization, and cognitive and functional decline.[2-4] After hospital discharge, cognitive impairment may continue in some patients. Postoperative neurocognitive disorder occurs between 30 days and 12 months after discharge and is defined by a decline in cognitive function identified via standardized neuropsychological tests.[5] Such impairment may occur in up to 40% of older patients after major surgery and is associated with reduced quality of life, depression, and functional impairment.[6] As surgical populations continue to age, neurocognitive complications are expected to persist, and programmatic initiatives are required to mitigate such adverse perioperative outcomes and long-term consequences.

In this context, the mission of the PHBI is to improve brain health in surgical patients through the following aims: (1) Create an accessible program, with supportive tools and resources, to minimize the perioperative impact on cognitive function and trajectory; (2) develop a comprehensive blueprint for anesthesia departments to follow for achieving excellent care; (3) raise awareness for the importance of perioperative brain health among anesthesiologists, perioperative clinicians, and patients; and (4) provide an implementation strategy for the program that can be adopted by various healthcare systems.[7] This chapter will provide an overview of the PBHI, results of implementation strategies to date, and future areas for further development and investigation.

Brain Health Initiative—Actions

In 2018, a panel of experts at the ASA/American Association of Retired Persons (AARP) Perioperative Brain Health Summit discussed strategies for reducing the incidence and burden of perioperative neurocognitive disorders.[8] Important action items identified included the following: raise public awareness, promote adherence to best practices, and provide support to individuals and hospitals for implementing perioperative neurocognitive protection programs.

To raise awareness for perioperative neurocognitive disorders, multiple dissemination strategies have been used. A "Call to Action" arising from the 2018 summit elicited support from various organizations, societies, healthcare systems, and individuals to promote the discussion and management of perioperative brain health on a local and national level.[9] Information, tools, and resources have also been publicly posted to the PBHI website for both patients and providers. Preoperative checklists and tips have been made available for patients, along with definitions of neurocognitive disorders, suggested strategies for reducing confusion after surgery, and key discussion points for perioperative clinic evaluations. For healthcare providers, the PBHI website[a] includes updated definitions and terms, links to clinical guidelines, and a list of key actions for care teams. Representatives from the PBHI have also worked with the AARP Global Council on Brain Health collaborative to further promote perioperative brain health awareness among older patients.

In addition to raising awareness, representatives from the PBHI have also appraised and highlighted best practice recommendations for clinicians. Key actions for care teams have been published on the PBHI website, which summarize clinical recommendations for mitigating perioperative neurocognitive impairment. An expanded appraisal of best practice recommendations, extracted from multiple guidelines, was also recently conducted by an international expert panel.[10] Recommendations were ranked by potential for impact and implementation feasibility, and a summary of these recommendations is outlined in Box 48.1. Important themes include providing preoperative screening for cognitive impairment and risk factors for postoperative delirium, avoiding medications listed by the American Geriatrics Society's Beers Criteria for Potentially Inappropriate Medication Use,[11] considering multimodal analgesia, and conducting a perioperative delirium screening. Resources for supporting these practices have also been made available on the PBHI website.

Lastly, the PBHI has also provided support to physicians and institutions for developing perioperative brain health optimization programs. For example, curated resources for establishing quality improvement (QI) programs have been posted on the PHBI website. Examples include online courses, workshops, books, and links to external organizations (e.g., Agency for Healthcare Research and Quality) with complementary resources. Key recommendations for implementing brain health QI programs are listed in Box 48.2.[12]

BOX 48.1 ■ Best Practice Recommendations—Summary

- Include perioperative neurocognitive disorders as part of the informed consent process
- Conduct baseline cognitive assessment via standardized test
- Perform perioperative delirium screening via standardized assessment tool
- Perioperative medication review
- Avoid deliriogenic medications (e.g., benzodiazepines) and avoid routine use of antipsychotics
- Optimize pain control, particularly with opioid-sparing approaches when possible
- Work to implement multicomponent, nonpharmacological, interdisciplinary delirium prevention programs for high-risk patients
- Educate other healthcare professionals regarding delirium and related neurocognitive disorders
- Help individualize discharge plans for patients experiencing delirium during hospitalization or for those at risk for neurocognitive disorders after discharge

Adapted from Peden CJ, Miller TR, Deiner SG, Eckenhoff RG, Fleisher LA. Improving perioperative brain health: an expert consensus review of key actions for the perioperative care team. *Br J Anaesth.* 2021;126:423–432.

---

[a]https://www.asahq.org/brainhealthinitiative.

BOX 48.2 ■ Key Actions for Quality Improvement Programs

- Collect baseline data—demonstrate need for improvement
- Engage with relevant parties (e.g., hospital staff, patients) to create a platform for change
- Identify issues preventing improvement
- Understand the local system
- Set and communicate achievable goals
- Collaborate to implement the plan
- Build sustainability in the program
- Measure outcomes for ongoing improvement

Adapted from Peden CJ. Ten top tips to make change happen. Perioperative Brain Health Initiative. https://www.asahq.org/brainhealthinitiative/tools/toptips. Accessed May 17, 2021.

Results

Since the launch of the PBHI, there is evidence to suggest that perioperative brain health has gained traction as a major clinical priority. A 2019 survey conducted by the European Society of Anesthesiologists (ESA) reported that 68% of the 566 responses deemed the issue of postoperative delirium to be "very relevant" or "relevant" to daily clinical practice.[13] On an institutional level, several hospitals have pledged support for the campaign and have begun implementation of neurocognitive protection programs.[9,14,15] Some healthcare systems, such as Michigan Medicine, have also launched integrated preoperative evaluation programs that aim to identify older, frail patients at risk for delirium and related geriatric complications.[16] From a research perspective, the US National Institutes of Health funding for projects related to postoperative delirium has also increased, from approximately $4.8 million for 15 projects identified in 2015 to more than $21 million for 54 related projects and subprojects in 2020.[17] Whether this perceived increased prioritization is directly related to the PBHI is unclear; nonetheless, systematic efforts appear to be gaining momentum for improving perioperative brain health.

Although one major aim of the PBHI is to encourage best clinical practices for reducing cognitive risk, adherence to best practice recommendations remains inconsistent among clinicians. An online questionnaire was sent to practicing anesthesiologists in the United States in July 2018 to assess current practices and adherence to available guidelines when caring for older surgical patients.[18] Overall, 81% of survey respondents rarely or never conducted preoperative screening for preexisting cognitive impairment, and 82% rarely or never conducted formal postoperative delirium screening. However, 70% of respondents discussed the risk of developing postoperative delirium or other cognitive disorders. The survey conducted by the ESA mentioned previously, found that 49% of survey participants assessed for postoperative delirium only in select patients, and only 21% used electroencephalogram-based monitoring for depth of anesthesia.[13] As such, adherence to best practice recommendations is not uniform, and reasons for deviation from these recommendations require further analysis.

Lastly, despite implementation of delirium prevention programs, patient outcomes with respect to delirium and related complications have been variable. Some institutions have noted success. For example, with the Tufts Medical Center Total Joint Program, the implementation of delirium prevention protocols has reportedly led to a decreased length of hospitalization, lower proportion of patients requiring discharge to a skilled nursing facility, and reduced healthcare costs.[19] Of note, however, these were preliminary findings that have not yet undergone the peer-review process. Similarly, implementation of a delirium prevention program at the University of California San

Francisco Medical Center led to improved preoperative delirium risk stratification and decreased perioperative administration of deliriogenic medications (as defined by the American Geriatrics Society Beers Criteria for Potentially Inappropriate Medication Use).[11,15] No differences were observed, however, with delirium incidence or length of hospitalization compared with the preimplementation phase. Multiple potential factors may account for the lack of clinical differences observed, including limited detection of delirium, multifactorial delirium etiologies, and preexisting perioperative protocols that may already have independently impacted neurocognitive outcomes. Nonetheless, implementation of neurocognitive protection programs may help optimize care, and further investigation is required to understand (1) barriers to program implementation and (2) why delirium persists in some surgical patients. The PBHI provides a foundation for advancing these clinical/implementation research objectives.

Discussion

The PBHI is an important patient safety initiative that serves to optimize clinical practice for supporting neurocognitive function in surgical patients. The PBHI has led to the creation of new guidelines, resource curation for patients and clinicians, and increased public and professional awareness for perioperative neurocognitive disorders in older surgical patients. There is some evidence to suggest that clinical practice has improved in institutions that have adopted delirium prevention programs; however, the ultimate impact of the PBHI on neurocognitive and clinical outcomes requires additional time and analysis.

At present, success of the PBHI can be evaluated based on progress made with its core missions: increased systematic awareness of perioperative brain health, and the development and implementation of evidence-based programs for optimizing neurocognitive health in surgical patients. Awareness of perioperative brain health has been reflected by recent summits, conferences, practice statements, clinician survey results, and recent increases in postoperative delirium research funding. Whether these results and trends are directly related to the PBHI is unclear, but it is nonetheless encouraging to see that perioperative brain health has been professionally acknowledged via conferences and publications that have arisen. In terms of brain health program implementation, multiple hospital systems have adopted new programs for older surgical patients.[14,15,19] Nevertheless, early adoption of these programs has not yet consistently translated to improved clinical outcomes.[15] Moreover, survey data suggest that clinicians do not consistently adhere to best practice recommendations.[18] Implementation research is required to further understand barriers to clinical guideline adherence and neurocognitive protection program adoption. Ultimately, the success of the PBHI will be judged, in part, by (1) the degree to which practice changes are implemented with respect to neurocognitive care and (2) whether subsequent clinical and neurocognitive outcomes are improved.

The PBHI also imparts several lessons that can be applicable to other, related QI projects. The PBHI raised awareness for perioperative neurocognitive disorders via social media campaigns, publication of guidelines, and meetings at various academic conferences. These strategies can be leveraged for systematic communication to improve public and professional awareness. Additionally, the PBHI developed targeted, accessible tools (e.g., clinical guidelines, online resources) for catalyzing implementation of brain health QI projects. Thereafter, successful initiatives have been publicized on the ASA website and published in high-impact journals, which may encourage others to pursue, and report, similar QIs on perioperative brain health. Importantly, the PBHI also made the issue of perioperative brain health relevant to patients and related organizations, such as the AARP. Hence, an important component of the initiative is the collaboration with other professional organizations and societies aligned with optimizing patient brain health. These elements should be considered for other QI projects.

Important limitations of the PBHI warrant discussion. The pathophysiology of delirium, and related neurocognitive disorders, remains incompletely understood. Without such a thorough neurobiological understanding of these syndromes, the effectiveness of QI programs is likely to be limited. Additionally, like other public health and QI initiatives, the PBHI will be reliant on several factors for sustainability. Such factors include funding, commitment from leaders and stakeholders, and support on the local level from individual clinicians. Implementation of brain health improvement programs will also be predicated on cultural support and acceptance from individual hospital systems. It is encouraging, however, that some institutions have begun implementing perioperative brain health programs with preliminary signs of feasibility, positive shifts in cultural practice,[15] and, possibly, improved clinical outcomes.[19,20] Lastly, a major limitation relates to the COVID-19 pandemic. The pandemic has created conditions that have led to social isolation for hospitalized patients. Additionally, the implementation of preexisting delirium prevention protocols has been limited, given that clinicians spend reduced time at the bedside to limit coronavirus spread.[21] These are challenging conditions for initiatives like the PBHI, and novel strategies—such as virtual neurocognitive assessments and prevention efforts—are being considered and tested.

Conclusions

The PBHI aims to improve perioperative brain health through systematic improvements in awareness and clinical practice. The project has led to the creation of helpful resources, integration of new brain health optimization programs, and new collaborations among professional organizations for improving perioperative brain health. The PBHI will likely continue to advocate for more resources for reducing perioperative neurocognitive impairment and support those working on QI projects for this important patient safety issue.

References

1. Vlisides P, Avidan M. Recent advances in preventing and managing postoperative delirium. *F1000Res.* 2019;8.
2. Witlox J, Eurelings LS, de Jonghe JF, Kalisvaart KJ, Eikelenboom P, van Gool WA. Delirium in elderly patients and the risk of postdischarge mortality, institutionalization, and dementia: a meta-analysis. *JAMA.* 2010;304:443–451.
3. Gleason LJ, Schmitt EM, Kosar CM, et al. Effect of delirium and other major complications on outcomes after elective surgery in older adults. *JAMA Surg.* 2015;150:1134–1140.
4. Hshieh TT, Saczynski J, Gou RY, et al. Trajectory of functional recovery after postoperative delirium in elective surgery. *Ann Surg.* 2017;265:647–653.
5. Evered L, Silbert B, Knopman DS, et al. Recommendations for the nomenclature of cognitive change associated with anaesthesia and surgery—2018. *Anesthesiology.* 2018;129:872–879.
6. Phillips-Bute B, Mathew JP, Blumenthal JA, et al. Association of neurocognitive function and quality of life 1 year after coronary artery bypass graft (CABG) surgery. *Psychosom Med.* 2006;68:369–375.
7. Fleisher LA. Brain health initiative: a new ASA patient safety initiative. *ASA Monitor.* 2016;80:10–11.
8. Mahanna-Gabrielli E, Schenning KJ, Eriksson LI, et al. State of the clinical science of perioperative brain health: report from the American Society of Anesthesiologists Brain Health Initiative Summit 2018. *Br J Anaesth.* 2019;123:464–478.
9. Perioperative Brain Health Initiative. AARP/ASA call to action. https://www.asahq-dev.org/brainhealthinitiative/news/articlesandnews/calltoaction. Accessed May 17, 2021.
10. Peden CJ, Miller TR, Deiner SG, Eckenhoff RG, Fleisher LA. Improving perioperative brain health: an expert consensus review of key actions for the perioperative care team. *Br J Anaesth.* 2021;126:423–432.
11. 2019 American Geriatrics Society Beers Criteria® Update Expert Panel. American Geriatrics Society 2019 Updated AGS Beers Criteria® for potentially inappropriate medication use in older adults. *J Am Geriatr Soc.* 2019;67(4):674–694.
12. Peden CJ. Ten top tips to make change happen. Perioperative Brain Health Initiative. https://www.asahq.org/brainhealthinitiative/tools/toptips. Accessed May 17, 2021.

13. Bilotta F, Weiss B, Neuner B, et al. Routine management of postoperative delirium outside the ICU: results of an international survey among anaesthesiologists. *Acta Anaesthesiol Scand.* 2020;64:494–500.
14. Decker J, Kaloostian CL, Gurvich T, et al. Beyond cognitive screening: establishing an interprofessional perioperative brain health initiative. *J Am Geriatr Soc.* 2020;68:2359–2364.
15. Donovan AL, Braehler MR, Robinowitz DL, et al. An implementation-effectiveness study of a perioperative delirium prevention initiative for older adults. *Anesth Analg.* 2020;131:1911–1922.
16. Min L, Hall K, Finlayson E, et al. Estimating risk of postsurgical general and geriatric complications using the VESPA preoperative tool. *JAMA Surg.* 2017;152:1126–1133.
17. National Institutes of Health. Research Portfolio Online Reporting Tools (RePORT). https://report.nih.gov/. Accessed May 16, 2021.
18. Deiner S, Fleisher LA, Leung JM, Peden C, Miller T, Neuman MD. Adherence to recommended practices for perioperative anesthesia care for older adults among US anesthesiologists: results from the ASA committee on geriatric anesthesia-perioperative brain health initiative ASA member survey. *Perioper Med (Lond).* 2020;9:6.
19. Gordon S. *Spotlight on: Tufts Medical Center's initiatives to prevent postoperative delirium.* American Society of Anesthesiologists: Perioperative Brain Health Initiative; 2018. https://www.asahq.org/brainhealthinitiative/news/articlesandnews/rubenazocarmd.
20. Deeken F, Sánchez A, Rapp MA, et al. Outcomes of a Delirium Prevention Program in older persons after elective surgery: a stepped-wedge cluster randomized clinical trial. *JAMA Surg.* 2021;e216370.
21. Ragheb J, McKinney A, Zierau M, et al. Delirium and neuropsychological outcomes in critically ill patients with COVID-19: an institutional case series. *medRxiv.* 2021. https://doi.org/10.1101/2020.11.03.20225466.

CHAPTER 49

Quality Improvement in Emergency Surgery: Learning From Two Large-Scale Programs to Reduce Mortality After Emergency Laparotomy

Timothy J. Stephens, RGN, BA (Hons), MSc, PhD ■ Carol J. Peden, MB ChB, MD, FRCA, FFICM, MPH

KEY POINTS

- Emergency laparotomy is a common high morbidity and high mortality procedure. Significant efforts have been made within the UK to improve the care of patients needing an emergency laparotomy.
- The EPOCH (Enhanced Perioperative Care for High-Risk Surgical Patients) trial and the Emergency Laparotomy Collaborative (ELC) work offer many important lessons on effective perioperative quality improvement (QI). These include:
  - Keep the improvement intervention simple and focused.
  - Effective QI almost invariably takes much longer than imagined.
  - Ensure sufficient engagement with, and support for, the improvement project, at all levels.
  - Make sure data collection processes are agreed on and in place before starting.

Background

More than 1.53 million adults undergo in-patient surgery in the UK National Health Service (NHS) each year with a 30-day mortality of 1.5%.[1] Patients undergoing emergency laparotomy, however, have a much greater risk of death.[2,3] Emergency laparotomy is a collective term that describes a heterogeneous group of unplanned intra-abdominal surgical procedures that are performed for a variety of indications, including intestinal obstruction, perforation of the bowel, or peritonitis, plus complications of elective surgery.[3] Approximately 30,000 emergency laparotomies are performed annually in England and Wales. Data available before the commencement of the Enhanced Perioperative Care for High-Risk Patients (EPOCH) trial (in 2014) indicated that mortality was high, with a 30-day mortality of between 13.3% and 19%.[2,4,5] A key study in 2012, using data from the Emergency Laparotomy Network, found that there were substantial variations in the way that patients requiring emergency laparotomy were cared for.[2] For example, wide variations were found in the grade of surgeon and anesthetist performing the operation, how long it took to get the patient into the operating room (OR), and whether the patient was admitted to critical care afterward. These variations were found to be associated with differences in mortality rates, and it was hypothesized that standardizing care may lead to improved outcomes.[2] These findings aligned with a report by the Royal College of Surgeons of England, commissioned by the UK Department of Health, which proposed extensive improvements to quality of care for this patient group.[6] Recommendations included interventions across the pre, intra, and postoperative phases, such as consultant-led decision making, cardiac output–guided fluid therapy, and early admission to critical care. A four-center observational study found that implementation of a care bundle to support delivery of some of these key interventions was effective at reducing 30-day mortality.[7,8] This was the background context in the UK NHS that led to the funding, by the National Institute of Health Research, of the EPOCH trial and the Emergency Laparotomy Collaborative (ELC) by the Health Foundation. Concurrently, the Healthcare Quality Improvement Programme (HQIP) funded the National Emergency Laparotomy Audit (NELA), a mandatory national dataset for this patient group.[3]

EPOCH and the ELC: Summary of the Studies and the Main Findings

THE EPOCH TRIAL

The EPOCH trial was a 93-hospital, stepped-wedge cluster randomized trial that ran over 85 weeks, starting in April of 2014.[9–12] Intervention was a quality improvement (QI) program to promote the implementation of a 37-step perioperative care pathway for patients undergoing emergency abdominal surgery (Fig. 49.1). Outcome and process data were acquired through the NELA data set.

The main findings were:

- There was no survival benefit (at 90- or 180-days postsurgery) associated with the national QI program. Furthermore, there was no beneficial effect on hospital length of stay (LOS) or hospital readmission. At a national level, there were only modest improvements among the 10 selected process measures to reflect key processes of care within the pathway. This suggested that implementation failure was the main cause of the lack of effect on patient outcomes.
- Implementation failure likely stemmed from a goal (pathway implementation) that was too ambitious for the time and resources that local QI leads had available to them. There were only 11 clinical processes, which more than half of teams attempted to improve from the clinical pathway (the hard core of the intervention). Ten of the 11 were the same processes as those collected in the NELA dataset, supporting the concept that you cannot improve what you do not measure.
- Ethnographic findings indicated that QI leads predicted, and subsequently experienced, multiple, and often significant, challenges as they attempted to lead change in their hospitals.[11,12] These challenges seemed to shape, to a greater or lesser extent, which components of the pathway they chose to focus on first and how they approached implementation. Major implementation barriers included limited time and scarce resources to support QI leads and, connected to this, an onerous burden of data collection, which limited capacity to subsequently use these data for improvement.
- In particular, the effective use of data for improvement involved a substantial social aspect to help colleagues understand and be motivated by the data, but many QI leads found this aspect challenging and time-consuming.
- Analysis of individual hospital level improvement using run-charts (a form of time-series chart) found that no hospital in the EPOCH trial reliably implemented the care pathway within 6 months of the end of the intervention period. Some areas of improvement were identified, however. In total, 279 (of a possible 800) care processes were improved by hospitals through participation in the EPOCH trial and a small group of hospitals (17.5%, 14/80) were

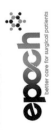

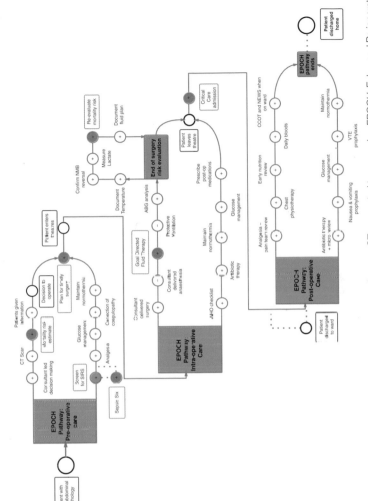

Getting started with the EPOCH Routemap

The EPOCH Intervention Routemap is designed to help you understand the recommendations within the EPOCH Care Pathway.

Users should note the following features in the routemap:

- The positioning of the stations and keys ages gives an indication of the patient journey through the pathway and where the recommended interventions sit within this.
- Within each stage of the pathway there are many interventions and processes that can occur in parallel.
- On the routemap, every station and pathway stage is linked to a page providing more detailed information about it. Simply hover over the item and click to be taken to the relevant page. You can also use the station list (see far left) as links to these pages
- The EPOCH Surgical Survival Six are key areas that we believe teams should focus attention on at the start of pathway implementation. These have been highlighted within the routemap.

Fig. 49.1 The EPOCH trial–recommended care pathway. *ABG,* Arterial blood gas; *CCOT,* critical care outreach team; *CT,* computed tomography; *EPOCH,* Enhanced Perioperative Care for High-Risk Surgical Patients; *NEWS,* National Early Warning Score; *NMB,* neuromuscular blockade; *Sepsis Six,* a protocolized treatment for sepsis; *SIRS,* systemic inflammatory response syndrome; *VTE,* venous thromboembolism; *WHO,* World Health Organization. (From Stephens TJ, Peden CJ, Fearse RM, et al. Improving care at scale: process evaluation of a multicomponent quality improvement intervention to reduce mortality after emergency abdominal surgery [EPOCH trial]. *Implement Sci.* 2018;13:148.)

successful in improving more than six care processes.[10] Effect sizes overall were marginal, but with substantial variance for each process across trial hospitals. The hospital teams that achieved greater care-process improvement also reported using more of the implementation strategies recommended by the QI program, suggesting improvement *may be* possible using a multifaceted approach to improvement.

THE EMERGENCY LAPAROTOMY COLLABORATIVE

The ELC was a 28-hospital QI collaborative that ran for over 24 months, starting in 2015.[13] Intervention was a breakthrough series collaborative (BTS) to promote implementation of a six-step laparotomy care bundle (Fig. 49.2).[14,15] Outcome and process data were acquired through the NELA dataset.

The main findings were:

- The ELC demonstrated an improvement in care-bundle compliance with a concurrent association with decreased 30-day mortality (to 8.3%) during the ELC project. The ELC, however, was designed as a QI project rather than a clinical trial and the observational nature of the study and lack of control group, or a controlled evaluation, means that a causal relationship between the intervention and improved outcomes cannot be confirmed.
- Time series analysis also identified improvements to most of the elements of the care bundle, although more substantial changes in these process measures occurred in the second year of the project, supporting the concept that improvement work takes time to establish.
- Improvements also occurred at different rates. Better attendance by senior clinicians occurred early, as did the measurement of blood lactate levels and admission to the intensive care unit (ICU). Improvement in getting the patient into the OR within the target timeframe was often not maintained, and sustained change occurred late in the project, suggesting that this target was more complex and may first require substantial upgrades to the system at many levels.
- As the ELC started 2 years into NELA data collection, many hospitals had sorted out teething problems with collecting the NELA dataset; for those that had, this was a major burden lifted for the QI leads that enabled them to focus on actually using the data to drive improvements in care. The impact of both NELA and the EPOCH trial on the improvement agenda for this patient group should also be recognized. The issue of poor outcomes was known, and organizations were now being benchmarked on key performance metrics via NELA. As such, organizational leaders became more interested in the ELC as time went on often providing much needed, if sometimes belated, support for local QI leads.

Key Learning From These Studies

What can the frontline clinician learn from these two important studies? Comparing the similarities and differences between EPOCH and the ELC, and drawing on our own experience of being involved in both studies, we suggest these four key points:

1. Keep your improvement intervention simple and focused.
2. Allow enough time for your improvement project.
3. Make sure you have sufficient engagement with and support for your improvement project at all levels.
4. Make sure data collection processes are agreed on and in place before you start.

KEEP YOUR IMPROVEMENT INTERVENTION SIMPLE AND FOCUSED

A key difference between the two studies was the scope and complexity of the intervention (a 37-step pathway vs a six-step care bundle). The EPOCH care pathway represented an ideal gold standard of care but in the context of poor care delivery for this patient group, aiming straight for

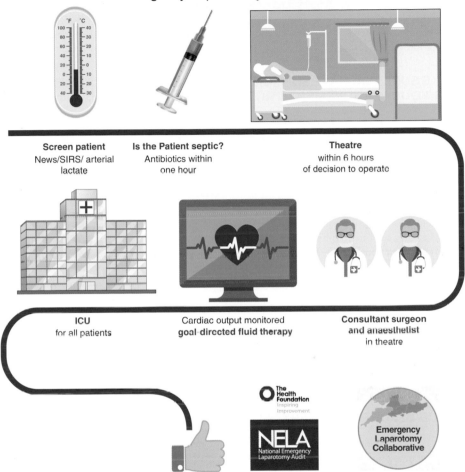

How to save lives in emergency laparotomy

Emergency Laparotomy Collaborative

Screen patient
News/SIRS/ arterial lactate

Is the Patient septic?
Antibiotics within one hour

Theatre
within 6 hours of decision to operate

ICU
for all patients

Cardiac output monitored
goal directed fluid therapy

Consultant surgeon and anaesthetist
in theatre

The Health Foundation
Inspiring Improvement

NELA
National Emergency Laparotomy Audit

Emergency Laparotomy Collaborative

Fig. 49.2 The Emergency Laparotomy Collaborative (ELC) care bundle implemented in 28 hospitals in the South of England. *ICU*, Intensive care unit; *NEWS*, National Early Warning Score; *SIRS*, systemic inflammatory response syndrome. (From Aggarwal G, Broughton KJ, Williams L, Peden CJ. Early postoperative death in patients undergoing emergency high-risk surgery: towards a better understanding of patients for whom surgery may not be beneficial. *J Clin Med.* 2020;9[5]:1288.)

"gold" was perhaps overambitious. Conversely, the ELC care bundle focused on high-impact interventions, all but one of which had strong evidence of benefit (there was still some equipoise around the benefit of cardiac output monitoring–guided fluid therapy for these patients at that time). Also, QI projects should focus on problems in care processes (e.g., screening for sepsis and treating promptly with fluids and antibiotics where identified) and not on structural problems (e.g., increasing the number of available emergency rooms). Structural problems are "money problems"; addressing them may be crucial to improving care delivery but require a different approach than those offered by QI methods, which focus on changing behaviors and care processes.

ALLOW ENOUGH TIME FOR YOUR IMPROVEMENT PROJECT

There is a misperception about QI that it is somehow a quick and easy fix for care delivery problems. This simply is not true. Effective QI almost invariably takes much longer than anyone imagines it will. The healthcare environment is complex and QI methods, as with any behavior change intervention, can be classed as complex interventions. Acknowledge and embrace that complexity and give the desired changes sufficient time at the planning, engagement, and action phases. Be realistic when planning project goals, so that you and your colleagues do not end up disappointed by the lack of rapid progress.

MAKE SURE YOU HAVE SUFFICIENT ENGAGEMENT WITH AND SUPPORT FOR YOUR IMPROVEMENT PROJECT AT ALL LEVELS

QI is essentially a social process and so a large proportion of time for a QI lead will be taken up on activities to engage and influence colleagues and other key stakeholders. This is often a surprise for those who have never led a QI project before! When leading a project, there is a real balance between setting out a strong and clear vision for improvement whilst also allowing colleagues to feel engaged in the process and feeling that their voices are heard and input is valued. Having good-quality data is important to win people over, as is a clear plan of action, but be open to suggestions and advice wherever possible. The complexity of the healthcare context, and the sheer number of people we often work with, means it will take a while for everyone to know what is being improved and what they need to do differently and for them to have their chance to agree/disagree (see also the earlier point about time). Factor this engagement gradient into your project timescales. Also ensure you have engagement from your department and hospital leadership. Wherever possible ensure your QI goals are aligned with organizational ones because this will almost certainly generate senior support for your work.

Beyond engagement, QI is a team sport, and you will need practical support as the QI project leader to optimize your chances of success. Speak to your manager about being allocated time within your job plan and what project support may be available (e.g., for data collection and analysis or for project administrative tasks like posters and other communications). If you try and do everything yourself, you are likely to fail.

MAKE SURE DATA COLLECTION PROCESSES ARE AGREED ON AND IN PLACE BEFORE YOU START

It is very hard (perhaps impossible) to improve what you are not measuring. Concurrently, data collection is almost invariably more challenging than people expect! Because data are crucial, spend time planning this aspect of your project upfront and well before you start the project in earnest. The logistics of data collection (e.g., what exactly is being collected, how often, and by whom) are seemingly simple but often when really considered can present a range of challenges to frontline teams. Ideally you will have started this far enough in advance to generate some baseline data, too. Also consider how often you will analyze your data, the methods you will use, and how you will use these data to inform and motivate your colleagues.

Conclusion

Two major studies provided rich information to highlight themes to facilitate improvement in complex perioperative clinical pathways. Consideration of the key components listed are likely to facilitate success in QI interventions.

References

1. TEF Abbott, Fowler AJ, Dobbs TD, Harrison EM, Gillies MA, Pearse RM. Frequency of surgical treatment and related hospital procedures in the UK: a national ecological study using hospital episode statistics. *Br J Anaesth.* 2017;119(2):249–257.
2. Saunders DI, Murray D, Pichel AC, Varley S, Peden CJ on behalf of UK Emergency Laparotomy Network. Variations in mortality after emergency laparotomy: the first report of the UK Emergency Laparotomy Network. *Br J Anaesth.* 2012;109(3):368–375.
3. NELA Project Team. *First Patient Report of the National Emergency Laparotomy Audit.* London: RCoA; 2015. https://www.nela.org.uk/All-Patient-Reports.
4. Faiz O, Warusavitarne J, Bottle A, et al. Nonelective excisional colorectal surgery in English National Health Service Trusts: a study of outcomes from Hospital Episode Statistics Data between 1996 and 2007. *J Am Coll Surg.* 2010;210(4):390–401.
5. Clarke A, Murdoch H, Thomas MJ, Cook TM, Peden CJ. Mortality and postoperative care after emergency laparotomy. *Eur J Anaesthesiol.* 2011;28(1):16–19.
6. Anderson I, Eddlestone J, Grocott, et al. *The Higher Risk General Surgical Patient—Towards Improved Care for a Forgotten Group.* London: Royal College of Surgeons and Department of Health; 2011.
7. Huddart S, Peden CJ, Swart M, et al. Use of a pathway quality improvement care bundle to reduce mortality after emergency laparotomy. *Br J Surg.* 2015;102(1):57–66.
8. Eveleigh MO, Howes TE, Peden CJ, Cook TM. Estimated costs before, during and after the introduction of the emergency laparotomy pathway quality improvement care (ELPQuIC) bundle. *Anaesthesia.* 2016;71 (11):1291–1295.
9. Peden CJ, Stephens T, Martin G, et al. Effectiveness of a national quality improvement programme to improve survival after emergency abdominal surgery (EPOCH): a stepped-wedge cluster-randomised trial. *Lancet.* 2019;393(10187):2213–2221.
10. Stephens TJ, Peden CJ, Haines R, et al. Hospital-level evaluation of the effect of a national quality improvement programme: time-series analysis of registry data. *BMJ Qual Saf.* 2020;29(8):623–635.
11. Stephens TJ, Peden CJ, Pearse RM, et al. Improving care at scale: process evaluation of a multi-component quality improvement intervention to reduce mortality after emergency abdominal surgery (EPOCH trial). *Implement Sci.* 2018;13(1):142.
12. Martin GP, Kocman D, Stephens T, Peden CJ, Pearse RM. This study was carried out as part of a wider randomised controlled trial EPOC. Pathways to professionalism? Quality improvement, care pathways, and the interplay of standardisation and clinical autonomy. *Sociol Health Illn.* 2017;39(8):1314–1329.
13. Aggarwal G, Peden CJ, Mohammed MA, et al. Evaluation of the collaborative use of an evidence-based care bundle in emergency laparotomy. *JAMA Surg.* 2019;154(5):e190145.
14. Nadeem E, Olin SS, Hill LC, Hoagwood KE, Horwitz SM. Understanding the components of quality improvement collaboratives: a systematic literature review. *Milbank Q.* 2013;91(2):354–394.
15. The Breakthrough Series: IHI's Collaborative Model for Achieving Breakthrough Improvement. In: *IHI Innovation Series White Paper.* Boston: Institute for Healthcare Improvement; 2003.

CHAPTER 50

Perioperative Quality Improvement Programme

Georgina F. Singleton, MB ChB ▪ Kylie-Ellen Edwards, MB ChB ▪
S. Ramani Moonesinghe, OBE, MD(Res), FRCA, FFICM, FRCP

KEY POINTS

- The Perioperative Quality Improvement Programme (PQIP) is a multidisciplinary initiative to evaluate the quality of care and outcomes of patients undergoing surgery in the UK National Health Service (NHS).
- PQIP enrolls patients undergoing major noncardiac surgery and measures complications, failure to rescue, and patient-reported outcomes.
- PQIP aims to develop a high-quality database of perioperative risk and process and outcome data.
- PQIP aims to support local and national quality improvement initiatives focused on the perioperative care of patients.

Why Did We Do This Work?

As surgery and perioperative care have become safer, and mortality after major surgery has declined, we have become more focused on improving outcomes by reducing complications and regaining a good quality of life. Although overall deaths after major surgery have gone down in recent years, postoperative complication rates remain high.[1] Major postoperative morbidity occurs in up to 15% of patients and has consistently been shown to be associated with reduced long-term survival and poor health-related quality of life.[2,3] The impact of postoperative complications on individual patients and the wider healthcare system is therefore clearly evident.

Previous studies from the United States revealed a variation in risk-adjusted postoperative morbidity and mortality between healthcare institutions.[4,5] This variation suggests that structures and processes surrounding perioperative care may have some impact on postoperative outcomes. Therefore there is opportunity to achieve better outcomes by improving the delivery of care.

To address the fact that there was no unified national system for measuring quality of care or outcomes across different types of surgery in the UK National Health Service (NHS), the Perioperative Quality Improvement Programme (PQIP) was created.

PQIP is a multidisciplinary initiative that was established in 2016 by the Health Services Research Centre, working on behalf of the Royal College of Anaesthetists and in collaboration with the Royal Colleges of Surgeons (England), Physicians, and Nursing and the Faculties of Intensive Care Medicine and Pain Medicine. It is a research study that is sponsored by University College London and has had full ethical approval. Patients are required to consent to participation. It has received financial support from the Health Foundation, the Royal College of Anaesthetists, and the National Institute for Health Research's (NIHR) Biomedical Research Centre at University College London Hospital's NHS Foundation Trust.

PQIP has a few aims:

- To support local quality improvement (QI) through feedback of data to clinicians and managers, using near–real-time feedback and regular site-specific reporting
- To develop a high-quality database of perioperative risk and process and outcome data
- To facilitate local and national research into the factors that are associated with clinical outcomes, including objective and patient-reported outcomes

Establishing PQIP

PQIP is a national research study incorporating a theoretically underpinned large-scale improvement intervention. It recruits patients undergoing major and complex surgical procedures in NHS hospitals in the United Kingdom. So far, around 30,000 patients have been recruited in 4 years.

Baseline information and patient questionnaire data are collected preoperatively after written consent has been obtained. On the day of surgery, preoperative, intraoperative, and recovery data are collected. Further inpatient data collection occurs on days 1, 3, and 7 postoperatively and on the date of hospital discharge or death. Long-term data collection occurs at 6 and 12 months after discharge. The data set includes clinical risk factors (for the purpose of descriptive analysis and risk adjustment), process measures, and outcome measures. Process measures are collected prospectively and include the following:

Preoperative Process Measures:

- These include an individualized risk assessment, measurement of HbA_{1c} in patients with diabetes mellitus, detection and management of preoperative anemia, carbohydrate loading, and day of surgery admissions.

Intraoperative Process Measures:

- These include surgical site infection prophylaxis (active warming and appropriate antibiotics), cardiac output monitoring, and use of individualized multimodal analgesia (neuraxial and regional anesthetic techniques).

Postoperative Process Measures:

- These include retention of surgical drains and nasogastric (NG) tubes after leaving the operating room; Drinking, Eating, and Mobilizing (DrEaMing) on postoperative day 1; discontinuation of intravenous fluids; and nutritional support.

Outcome measures were selected based on evidence of previous validation and expert consensus. They include postoperative morbidity and complications, and postoperative patient-reported outcome measures at 6 and 12 months.

All hospitals undertaking PQIP procedures in patients aged over 18 years are invited to participate. The sampling approach varies depending on hospital resources (either all patients within a service or a random sample are approached).

PQIP differs from a purely observational study in that there is provision of almost real-time local process and outcome data to sites as patient recruitment is continuing. There is high-quality regular (quarterly) reporting of local data compared with national data. This feedback loop aims to promote and support local QI processes. The PQIP website (https://pqip.org.uk/content/home) is a central hub for local teams to access process and outcome data for their recruited patients. Dashboards provide site-specific current performance and temporal trends for various PQIP measures (Fig. 50.1). Quarterly and annual reports are individualized to each site and allow sites to compare their performance with averages across all participating hospitals. Underpinning the development of the

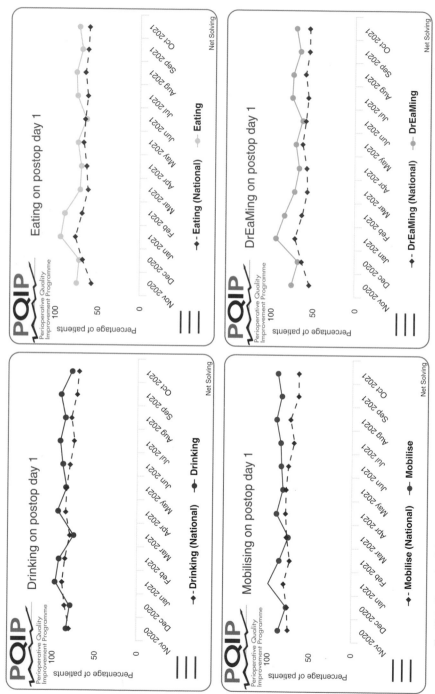

Fig. 50.1 Example of data used for feedback. Run charts with local data shown in blue in comparison with national data, both over time.

PQIP "intervention" was normalization process theory,[6] with the aim of normalizing the use of data for improvement by perioperative teams.

QI tools on the PQIP website provide help local teams to harness their PQIP data to drive improvement. Improvement priorities are set with each annual report cycle (Fig. 50.2). They reflect areas for improvement identified through evaluation of PQIP measures across all sites and incorporate national perioperative improvement targets. Improvement resources include customized support for QI data analysis and process mapping, as well as guidance on the design, implementation, and evaluation of local QI initiatives. Outreach activities by the central PQIP team include newsletters, collaborative events, educational resources, and sharing of successful local PQIP-adjacent QI projects through poster presentations and dissemination of case studies.

The overall effectiveness of PQIP as a tool for improving perioperative outcomes will be evaluated from the comparison of risk-adjusted outcome data from administrative registries (e.g., mortality, length of stay [LOS], and readmission to hospital) between sites participating in PQIP and nonparticipating sites. Temporal trends (for individual sites and the whole cohort) will be analyzed quantitatively and further investigated using qualitative methods. The degree to which PQIP data is being used in local QI initiatives will be assessed by surveys, interviews, and ethnography.

Results

PQIP recruited its first patient in December 2016 and has now recruited more than 31,000 patients; 126 sites have participated across England and Wales, and approval has been gained to involve Northern Irish sites.

To date, PQIP has published three annual reports.[7] Analyses so far reveal that compliance with many key process measures show consistent improvement between the first and third report cycles. These measures include timely measurement of HbA_{1C} for patients with diabetes (69%–82%) and the proportion of patients "DrEaMing" on day 1 postoperatively (54%–66%). Postoperative LOS and unadjusted major morbidity has also reduced consistently over time. Key process measures relating to surgical site infection, including timing of antibiotic prophylaxis and intraoperative warming, appear to be almost universally adhered to (>95% overall compliance).

Despite these improvements and successes, there remain some process measures that do not appear to be as amenable to change; for example, the proportion of colorectal surgical patients who leave the operating room with NG tubes and drains has not changed between report cycles. Furthermore, processes that are still debated in terms of their evidence base (e.g., carbohydrate loading and cardiac output monitoring) have changed little, with some hospitals clearly having adopters and others having very low or zero compliance.

To encourage involvement from local sites and in line with PQIP's ethos of collaborative working and sharing learning experiences, PQIP has held three collaborative events. These bring together collaborators from across the UK with national leads for perioperative care, the presidents of the Royal Colleges of Anaesthesia and Surgery, and the central PQIP project team. The events launch the PQIP annual report and provide panel discussion about improving perioperative care, QI training, and updates on best practice in perioperative care. The events provide a forum for sharing stories of PQIP successes and challenges, learning how to make the most out of PQIP at a local level, and holding specialty-specific discussions. It was evident from these events that PQIP data is facilitating local QI projects.

The annual PQIP poster competition has provided further evidence of site-level QI work, either using PQIP data or PQIP's top five improvement priorities. We have seen high-level QI initiatives relating to numerous topics, including enhanced recovery, individualized risk assessment, and anemia.

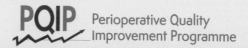

PQIP Perioperative Quality Improvement Programme

Top 5 National Improvement Priorities for 2019-20

1 Preoperative assessment

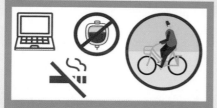

Individualised risk assessment
Anaemia detection & treatment
Lifestyle and comorbidity optimisation

2 Diabetes management

Measure HbA1C
Measure compliance against local pathway
Restore usual nutrition as soon as possible

3 Communication and multidisciplinary working

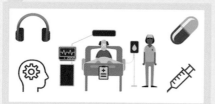

The whole MDT and patients can use PQIP to lead local improvement

Regular, multi-modal communication keeps PQIP in focus for the clinical team

Build discussion into clinical routines - team briefs, staff meetings, MDT meetings

Make your data work for you: use it to build business cases, support local reward systems etc.

4 Individualised pain management

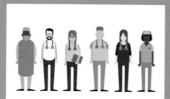

Expectation setting and management
Multimodal analgesia
Local anaesthesia techniques
Distraction therapy
Regular, early post-op review by pain teams

5 Enhanced Recovery

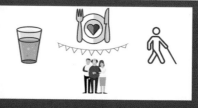

Surgery school or other tailored preparation
Pre-op nutritional assessment, carbohydrate loading and minimising starvation
Drinking, Eating (or nutritional supplementation) & Mobilising within 24h
Minimise tubes, drains and 'institutionalisation'

Read our reports: www.pqip.org.uk   Follow us: @PQIPNews   Join our team: PQIP@rcoa.ac.uk

Fig. 50.2 Infographic about Perioperative Quality Improvement Programme (PQIP) priorities.

Discussion

Although the principles of QI are now well recognized as playing a fundamental role in improving health care, this project has not been without its challenges.

First, as with any project in which local data are fed back to a national team, there were concerns from some clinicians that hospital-level data would be used to generate league table ranking and be used to identify individual clinicians or hospitals. PQIP responded to these anxieties by reassuring hospitals that data would be used to capture and share learning but without hospitals being exposed as poor performers. PQIP also promoted the concept of "positive deviance," highlighting high-performing hospitals in its annual report and not drawing attention to hospitals with less positive results.

Secondly, there is no doubt that any clinical trial or research study is associated with an administrative burden, which can be challenging for any clinical department. To assist local sites with this, PQIP has encouraged sites to apply for funding from the NIHR for research nurse support. This has been made possible by the fact that PQIP has been adopted as a portfolio study. PQIP has welcomed the support that the NIHR has provided to date.

Thirdly, the PQIP project team is aware that supporting local recruitment and engagement requires a focus on avoiding onerous data collection and maintaining a streamlined data set, while ensuring data utility for QI activity. For the most part, this has been achieved without issue and there appears to be meaningful measurement for the vast majority of process and outcome measures. Regular review and interim analysis of the data set has revealed some items that require further refinement and additional data collection to provide meaningful data. An example is the collection of hemoglobin and anemia treatment data. Initially, a single preoperative hemoglobin measurement was collected (the most recent value before surgery). In 2020 an additional item was added to collect treatment for anemia occurring within 3 months of surgery (aligning with national priorities and a Commissioning for Quality and Innovation [CQUIN] project). Subsequent analyses have revealed that these data are insufficient for sites to reliably identify a cohort of patients with preoperative anemia and assess the effect of any intervention. The data successfully identify patients with anemia at the time of surgery and whether they have received treatment. What cannot be identified from the current data set is patients with anemia who have received effective treatment and have a normal hemoglobin level immediately before surgery or any degree of treatment success in patients on anemia treatment who remain anemic at the time of surgery (but may have had a significantly lower hemoglobin at initial preoperative presentation). In response, an additional item has been added to the data set for patients receiving anemia treatment, measuring the lowest hemoglobin value within 3 months of surgery.

It is not immediately clear why PQIP has been effective in facilitating improvement in certain process measures but other measures have remained relatively static. This has occurred despite some of these measures (e.g., individualized risk assessment) being key improvement priorities in annual report cycles. What is evident is that despite relatively poor performance of the overall cohort, there are specialty groups and individual sites that are showing positive deviance in terms of either their baseline rates of compliance with these measures or improvement over time. These sites provide potential for identification of exemplars of good practice, which will be explored using qualitative research methodology. This will facilitate knowledge sharing with other sites through dissemination in annual reports and collaborative event.

The challenges of the sustainability of PQIP can be considered on a macro, meso, and microlevel. At a macrolevel there will be continued requirement for support from PQIP's range of stakeholders and coordination of the project by the PQIP central team. At a meso-level, PQIP relies on its multiple collaborators. PQIP hopes that sites taking part will observe improved healthcare systems and patient outcomes, which, in turn, will facilitate their ongoing involvement. The ability to use PQIP data to meet other healthcare targets such as CQUINs will be a further motivator for local sites. At a microlevel, it is hoped that individuals will benefit from their involvement with PQIP by not only being recognized as collaborators but also taking part in high-quality local QI underpinned by PQIP.

Although still ongoing, we believe that PQIP is having an impact. The growing numbers of hospitals enrolling, attainment of a high-quality and large data set and use of PQIP data to initiate QI at a site-level evidence this. There are several factors that have contributed to PQIP's success, including the regular sharing of hospital level data within the national averages and the ability of participating sites to tailor QI to the local context. In addition, PQIP encourages sharing of best practice and celebrates positive deviance rather than highlighting negative outliers. As stated earlier, the overall aim of the program is not to rank hospitals or to produce league tables but to improve standards of care.

PQIP has already spread from a regional (England) to UK-wide context. The PQIP structure and function provide a model for a large-scale perioperative improvement program that provide support, resources, and data to successfully facilitate local QI and improve care for high-risk surgical patients. The success of PQIP in delivering this without local site financial investment means that it can provide a model for the development of similar programs internationally in comparable health-care settings.

References

1. Abbott TEF, Fowler AJ, Dobbs TD, et al. Frequency of surgical treatment and related hospital procedures in the UK: a national ecological study using hospital episode statistics. *Br J Anaesth.* 2017;119(2):249–257.
2. Moonesinghe SR, Harris S, Mythen MG, et al. Survival after postoperative morbidity: a longitudinal observational study. *Br J Anaesth.* 2014;113:977–984.
3. Manku K, Leung JM. Prognostic significance of postoperative in-hospital complications in elderly patients. II. Long-term quality of life. *Anesth Analg.* 2003;96:590–594.
4. Dimick JB, Pronovost PJ, Cowan JA, Lipsett PA, Stanley JC, Upchurch GR. Variation in postoperative complication rates after high-risk surgery in the United States. *Surgery.* 2003;134:534–540.
5. Ghaferi AA, Birkmeyer JD, Dimick JB. Variation in hospital mortality associated with inpatient surgery. *N Engl J Med.* 2009;361:1368–1375.
6. Murray E, Treweek S, Pope C, et al. Normalisation process theory: a framework for developing, evaluating and implementing complex interventions. *BMC Med.* 2010;8:63.
7. PQIP Project Team. Perioperative Quality Improvement Programme; 2021. Available from: https://pqip. org.uk/Content/home. Accessed April 6, 2021.

CHAPTER 51

Using Real-World Data for Improvement—The Seattle Children's Example

Amber Franz, MD, MEng ■ Daniel Low, BMedSci, BM, BS, MRCPCH, FRCA
■ Lynn D. Martin, MD, MBA

KEY POINTS

- Perioperative opioid-sparing protocols for children are feasible.
- Standardized anesthesia protocols and accessible real-world data displayed as statistical process control charts can inform rapid PDSA (Plan-Do-Study-Act) cycles.
- Challenges to improvement work can be overcome using technology, data, communication, education, time, and a culture that emphasizes willingness to change.

Introduction

Seattle Children's Bellevue Clinic and Surgery Center (Bellevue) is a stand-alone pediatric clinic and ambulatory surgery facility that cares for over 4000 surgical patients annually. Anesthesiologists and nurse anesthetists use standardized anesthesia protocols for the most commonly performed surgical procedures to optimize quality and consistency of patient care. Outcomes are tracked using a software program that can display real-world data from the electronic medical record (EMR) as statistical process control (SPC) charts. These charts are updated daily, allowing for rapid Plan-Do-Study-Act (PDSA) cycles and continuous improvement.[1] One of the outcomes tracked is opioid administration. Data showed that despite using multimodal analgesia, including frequent regional anesthesia, over 70% of surgical patients received intraoperative opioids in 2016 and 2017 (Fig. 51.1).[2]

Starting in July 2018, the Bellevue team began a concerted quality improvement (QI) initiative centered around the removal of intraoperative opioids from standardized anesthesia protocols. The decision to initiate this opioid reduction work was influenced by a series of events that occurred between 2017 and early 2018.

First, a review of 2017 patient outcome data showed that intravenous (IV) acetaminophen was not opioid sparing and was costly. So the team decided to look for a cheaper alternative, identifying dexmedetomidine as a possible replacement. Then in early 2018, the national opioid shortage intensified, leading to a hospital-wide alert to conserve supplies. Finally, opioid use after routine surgery became a recognized gateway to new persistent opioid use.[3,4] In the setting of the national opioid epidemic, concerns began to arise that opioids administered perioperatively could play a role in postoperative opioid consumption through such mechanisms as opioid tolerance and/or opioid-induced hyperalgesia.[5,6]

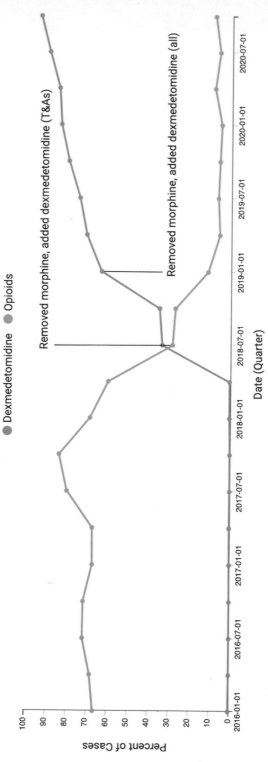

Fig. 51.1 Run chart showing the percent of surgical patients receiving intraoperative dexmedetomidine versus intraoperative opioids at Bellevue. *T&As,* Tonsillectomy and adenoidectomy.

These three events aligned to impel the team to develop a new standardized protocol that eliminated intraoperative opioids for the highest-volume surgery—tonsillectomy and adenoidectomy (T&A)—where opioid-related side effects such as respiratory depression and airway obstruction are not well tolerated.[7,8] Research into dexmedetomidine as an alternative to IV acetaminophen identified several articles evaluating dexmedetomidine in place of morphine for T&As.[8–10] After much discussion, intraoperative morphine and acetaminophen were replaced with dexmedetomidine and ibuprofen. When initial results were not favorable,[11] the team replaced ibuprofen with ketorolac based on (1) evidence of ketorolac's safety for pediatric T&As[12] and (2) similar reoperation rate data in Bellevue's T&A patients receiving ketorolac versus no ketorolac. This protocol change yielded better results, with comparable postanesthesia care unit (PACU) times and maximum pain scores for the dexmedetomidine and ketorolac group versus the morphine-acetaminophen cohort, and no increase in 30-day reoperation rate for tonsillar bleed.[11]

Success with reducing opioid administration for T&As without compromising effective analgesia inspired the team to expand the use of dexmedetomidine (see Fig. 51.1).[13] After multiple PDSA cycles, dexmedetomidine was incorporated into standardized protocols for the most commonly performed procedures, while exploiting opioid-sparing analgesics already popular at Bellevue, such as regional anesthesia and nonsteroidal anti-inflammatory drugs. The results of these interventions were so promising that by January 2019, the team removed intraoperative opioids from all protocols (see Fig. 51.1).[13]

Methods

CONTEXT

At Bellevue, routine ambulatory surgeries are performed on relatively healthy patients. Bellevue's leaders and frontline staff are engaged in and supportive of continuous improvement and meet regularly to update standardized protocols based on best available evidence. Once a new protocol is deployed, it is built into the anesthesia module of the EMR as a case-specific checklist, encouraging protocol compliance. EMR data are stored in the hospital's electronic data warehouse. Selected data can be pulled from the warehouse and displayed as SPC charts by MDmetrix (now known as AdaptX; for more information, go to: https://www.adaptx.com/). Thus clinical teams have immediate access to perioperative data and analytics and can query continuously updated real-world data, create custom patient cohorts, and surface key metrics, allowing for near real-time understanding of how processes are performing and the ability to detect clinical improvement resulting from protocol changes.

INTERVENTIONS

In July 2018, Bellevue's anesthesia team began iterative steps to reduce intraoperative opioid use, with removal of opioids from all protocols by January 2019. Protocol changes for procedures with the greatest monthly surgical volume were prioritized. Table 51.1 summarizes the protocols in place in 2017 and 2020; however, it does not show the PDSA cycles that occurred in the interim. The major changes across all protocols were to substitute intraoperative fentanyl and/or morphine with dexmedetomidine and replace IV acetaminophen with ketorolac.[13]

At Bellevue, most surgical patients receive a mask induction with sevoflurane, a propofol bolus, and lactated ringer solution, plus dexamethasone and ondansetron. Children undergoing myringotomy and tympanostomy tubes are the exception because they undergo surgery without IV access. Premedication with midazolam is rare (<1%); induction rooms allow for parental presence during induction, and a child life specialist is available if needed.[13]

TABLE 51.1 ■ Standardized Intraoperative Anesthesia Protocols for Bellevue's Most
Common Surgeries as of December 2017 (Preintervention) and December 2020
(Postintervention)

	Procedure	Opioid-Inclusive Protocols (2017)	Opioid-Free Protocols (2020)
Otolaryngology	Myringotomy with tympanostomy tubes	Fentanyl 1 mcg/kg intranasal (intraoperatively)	Ibuprofen 10 mg/kg oral (preoperatively)
	Tonsillectomy & adenoidectomy/ tonsillectomy	Morphine 0.1 mg/kg Acetaminophen 15 mg/kg Dexamethasone 0.15 mg/kg (max 4 mg)	Dexmedetomidine 1 mcg/kg[a] Ketorolac 0.5 mg/kg at end of case (max 30 mg) Dexamethasone 0.5 mg/kg (max 8 mg)
	Adenoidectomy	Morphine 0.05 mg/kg Acetaminophen 15 mg/kg	Dexmedetomidine 0.5 mcg/kg[a] Ketorolac 0.5 mg/kg at end of case (max 30 mg)
Urology	Circumcision/buried penis repair/ hypospadias repair	<3 yr: single shot caudal >3 yr: penile block by surgeon Fentanyl 0.5–1 mcg/kg	<15 kg: pudendal block Ropivacaine 0.2% (max 5 mL/side) >15 kg: pudendal block Ropivacaine 0.5% (max 5 mL/side) Dexmedetomidine 0.5–1 mcg/kg[a]
	Orchiopexy/inguinal hernia repair/ hydrocelectomy	<3 yr: single shot caudal >3 yr: ilioinguinal block: Ropivacaine 0.5% 0.1–0.2 mL/kg Fentanyl 1–2 mcg/kg Ketorolac 0.5 mg/kg (max 30 mg)	Ilioinguinal block: Ropivacaine 0.5% 0.1–0.2 mL/kg Dexmedetomidine 0.5–1 mcg/kg[a] Ketorolac 0.5 mg/kg (max 30 mg)
General surgery	Inguinal hernia repair/ hydrocelectomy	<3 yr: single shot caudal >3 yr: ilioinguinal block: Ropivacaine 0.5% 0.1–0.2 mL/kg Fentanyl 1–2 mcg/kg Ketorolac 0.5 mg/kg (max 30 mg)	Ilioinguinal block: Ropivacaine 0.5% 0.1–0.2 mL/kg Dexmedetomidine 0.5–1 mcg/kg[a] Ketorolac 0.5 mg/kg (max 30 mg)
	Umbilical hernia repair/ epigastric hernia repair	Rectus sheath block: Ropivacaine 0.5% 0.2 mL/kg/side Fentanyl 0.5–1 mcg/kg Ketorolac 0.5 mg/kg (max 30 mg)	Rectus sheath block: Ropivacaine 0.5% 0.2 mL/kg/side Dexmedetomidine 0.5–1 mcg/kg[a] Ketorolac 0.5 mg/kg (max 30 mg)
Orthopedics	Knee arthroscopy and meniscus repair	Adductor canal block: Ropivacaine 0.5% 0.1–0.2 mL/kg Fentanyl 0.5–2 mcg/kg	Propofol infusion (TIVA) Adductor canal block: Ropivacaine 0.5% 0.1–0.2 mL/kg

TABLE 51.1 ■ **Standardized Intraoperative Anesthesia Protocols for Bellevue's Most Common Surgeries as of December 2017 (Preintervention) and December 2020 (Postintervention)** (Continued)

	Procedure	Opioid-Inclusive Protocols (2017)	Opioid-Free Protocols (2020)
		Ketorolac 0.5 mg/kg (max 30 mg)	Dexmedetomidine 1 mcg/kg[a] Ketorolac 0.5 mg/kg (max 30 mg)
	Knee arthroscopy and anterior cruciate ligament repair	Adductor canal catheter: Ropivacaine 0.5% 0.1–0.2 mL/kg bolus + 0.2% infusion × 3 days Sciatic nerve block: Ropivacaine 0.5% 0.2 mL/kg Fentanyl 0.5–2 mcg/kg Ketorolac 0.5 mg/kg (max 30 mg)	Propofol infusion (TIVA) Adductor canal catheter: Ropivacaine 0.5% 0.1–0.2 mL/kg bolus + 0.2% infusion × 3 days Sciatic nerve block: Ropivacaine 0.5% 0.2 mL/kg Dexmedetomidine 1 mcg/kg[a] Ketorolac 0.5 mg/kg (max 30 mg)
	Trigger thumb repair	Median nerve block by surgeon Fentanyl 0.5–1 mcg/kg	Median nerve block by surgeon Dexmedetomidine 0.5–1 mcg/kg[a]
Dermatology	Pulse dye laser	Fentanyl 0.5–1 mcg/kg Ketorolac 0.5 mg/kg (max 30 mg)	Propofol infusion (TIVA) Dexmedetomidine 0.5–1 mcg/kg[a] Ketorolac 0.5 mg/kg (max 30 mg)
Ophthalmology	Strabismus repair	Fentanyl 1–2 mcg/kg Ketorolac 0.5 mg/kg (max 30 mg)	Propofol infusion (TIVA) Dexmedetomidine 1 mcg/kg[a] Ketorolac 0.5 mg/kg (max 30 mg)

[a]Maximum bolus dose of dexmedetomidine in 2020 was generally 40 mcg (slow administration reduces the incidence of reflex bradycardia from transient vasoconstriction), although for longer cases it was often redosed every couple of hours, consistent with the pharmacokinetics of the drug.

Dexmedetomidine, fentanyl, ketorolac, dexamethasone, propofol, and acetaminophen were administered intravenously intraoperatively if not otherwise specified. Ropivacaine was administered neuraxially or perineurally after induction and before surgery, with a maximum dose of 3 mg/kg if not otherwise specified.

Max, Maximum; *TIVA*, total intravenous anesthetic.

MEASURES

Morphine rescue rate and maximum pain score in recovery were selected as primary outcome measures to assess analgesic efficacy. Morphine is the primary rescue medication used in PACU. Pain scores were recorded by recovery nurses using either the Faces, Legs, Activity, Cry, Consolability tool; Faces Pain Scale—Revised; or a numerical Visual Analog Scale depending on patient age and developmental maturity.[14,15] Each score was converted to an 11-point (0–10) scale for the maximum pain score SPC charts.

The balancing measures of total anesthesia time and total PACU time were selected because dexmedetomidine has been shown to delay wake-up and discharge, which are undesirable in an ambulatory surgery setting.[16] Standardized discharge criteria based on the modified Aldrete scoring system (or return to patient baseline) were used.[17] Patients' surgical sites must be stable before discharge. Total anesthesia time was defined as time from anesthesia start to end after handoff of an extubated patient.

Postoperative nausea and vomiting (PONV) rescue rate were monitored to assess for change after removing opioids from protocols. Medication was administered according to nurse judgment.

ANALYSES

Data were extracted from Seattle Children's data warehouse for all patients undergoing surgery at Bellevue from January 2016 to December 2020 using MDmetrix OR Advisor (now AdaptX, Seattle, WA). Incomplete data were not imported.

SPC charts were used to visualize data. These charts monitor a process over time and help distinguish changes due to special circumstances (i.e., special cause variation, such as improvement from a protocol change) from random variation inherent in a system.[18] Charts were interpreted using Shewhart's theory of variation, with special cause variation identified using standard SPC rules.[18]

DISCLOSURES AND ETHICAL CONSIDERATIONS

This project was submitted to Seattle Children's internal review board and was not deemed a research study. Daniel Low is the Chief Medical Officer and founder of MDmetrix (AdaptX) and Lynn Martin is a shareholder. Lloyd Provost assisted with SPC chart interpretation and is a shareholder and board advisor to MDmetrix (AdaptX).

Results

Between January 2016 and December 2020, over 20,000 patients underwent surgery at Bellevue, with less than 1% excluded because of missing data. Intraoperative opioid reduction efforts officially started in July 2018 with changes to the T&A protocol. Key protocol changes are annotated on the SPC charts. Because otolaryngology surgeries make up approximately 40% of total case volume, changes to these protocols had a large effect on the measures.

Fig. 51.2A–B show the X-bar and S charts for mean maximum pain score in recovery. For both charts, there is no special cause variation and the process is stable, indicating no change in maximum PACU pain score despite the removal of opioids from all protocols by January 2019.

The P chart in Fig. 51.3 shows the percent of patients that required rescue morphine in recovery. There are several special cause signals suggesting changes that are not because of random variation. In the second and third quarter of 2018, there are two breaches of the upper control limit that are likely related to PACU nurse apprehension about the removal of morphine from the T&A protocol and changes to the T&A protocol (described in the Introduction).[11] Then, there are breaches of the lower control limit in the first two quarters of 2019, when opioids were removed from all protocols, suggesting a possible improvement. This is not sustained, however, into 2020.

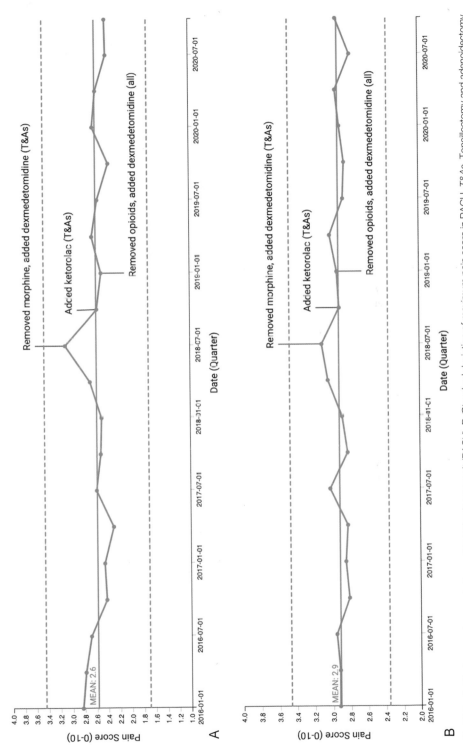

Fig. 51.2 A, Maximum pain score in the postanesthesia care unit (PACU). B, Standard deviation of maximum pain score in PACU. *T&As*, Tonsillectomy and adenoidectomy.

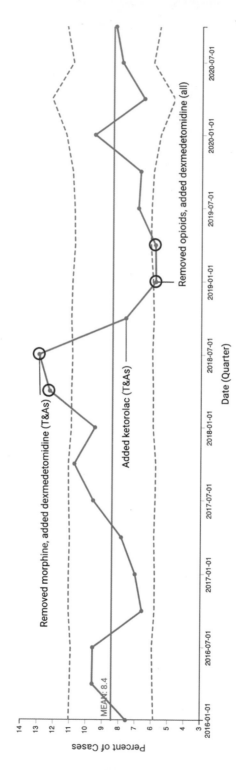

Fig. 51.3 Postanesthesia care unit (PACU) rescue morphine rate. *T&As*, Tonsillectomy and adenoidectomy.

The X-bar and S charts for mean total anesthesia time are shown in Fig. 51.4A–B. In both charts, there is a "shift down" (i.e., lower baseline) that ends in 2019, with several breaches of the upper control limits starting at the end of 2019, consistent with longer anesthesia times. Indeed, a high number of complex cases were diverted to Bellevue because of the closure of multiple Seattle Children's main campus operating rooms starting in May 2019 and then increased operating room availability at Bellevue in the setting of COVID-19. This increase in anesthesia time closely mirrors the increase in surgery time, shown in Fig. 51.5, and is unlikely to be related to the addition of dexmedetomidine to the protocols.

The X-bar and S charts for mean total PACU time are shown in Fig. 51.6A–B. The S chart is stable, indicating no problems with the data. However, there are several special cause signals in the X-bar chart. Although there is a "shift down" that ends when dexmedetomidine was introduced to the T&A protocol, signals near the upper control limit appear only after complex cases started to take place at Bellevue. These PACU time increases coincide with the increased surgery and anesthesia times previously described. In addition, Bellevue also started to accept patients scheduled for admission to the main hospital after surgery in 2019, so the patient population was no longer all outpatients.

There are multiple special cause signals seen in Fig. 51.7, which shows the mean percent of patients requiring rescue medication for PONV (P chart). Several signals near the upper control limit in 2016 suggest an increased PONV rate in 2016 compared with the rest of the cohort. Then, starting in January 2018, there is a downward trend in PONV rate, which may be related to the removal of intranasal fentanyl from the myringotomy with tympanostomy tubes protocol in January; this was done to reduce dosing and administrative burden for anesthesia providers and was not part of a concerted effort to reduce opioids. The downward trend continues as opioids are removed from the T&A protocol and eventually all protocols. There are several signals near the lower control limit in 2019 and 2020, suggesting a reduced PONV rescue rate because of the removal of opioids from all protocols, although this is not sustained throughout the entire 2019 to 2020 time period.

Discussion

Standardized anesthesia protocols and readily accessible real-world data allowed the Bellevue team to perform rapid PDSA cycles, reducing intraoperative opioid administration from 71.7% to 7.6% (see Fig. 51.1) between 2016 and 2020. Maximum PACU pain score remained stable and unchanged during this period. The morphine rescue rate was similar between 2016 and 2017 and 2020. The PONV rescue rate decreased, but improvements were not sustained. Total anesthesia time and PACU time increased in the setting of increased surgery time and case complexity. These results are consistent with the literature, which describes the benefits of opioid-free anesthesia and dexmedetomidine as an analgesic adjunct and opioid-sparing agent.[19,20]

Obstacles to improvement work included team member participation in standardized protocols and recovery nurse apprehension about eliminating intraoperative opioids. These challenges were overcome using technology, data, communication, education, time, and a culture that emphasizes willingness to change. Technology permitted protocols to be embedded into the anesthesia record as customizable checklists and allowed the team to visualize data and track performance over time. Presentations of charts at weekly meetings helped educate and engage team members in thoughtful discussions around improvement. The creation of a workplace culture that supported continuous improvement started from the top down, with recruitment of staff open to change. Over time, the team became used to frequent evidence-based protocol updates, and change became the norm.

Minimizing intraoperative opioids has gained traction outside of Bellevue. At Seattle Children's main hospital, intraoperative opioid use trended down from 2016 to 2020, despite the fact that standardized anesthesia protocols are not the norm, patients are sicker, and the cases are more complex. Fig. 51.8 shows declining intraoperative opioid use (>49,000 cases) and increasing

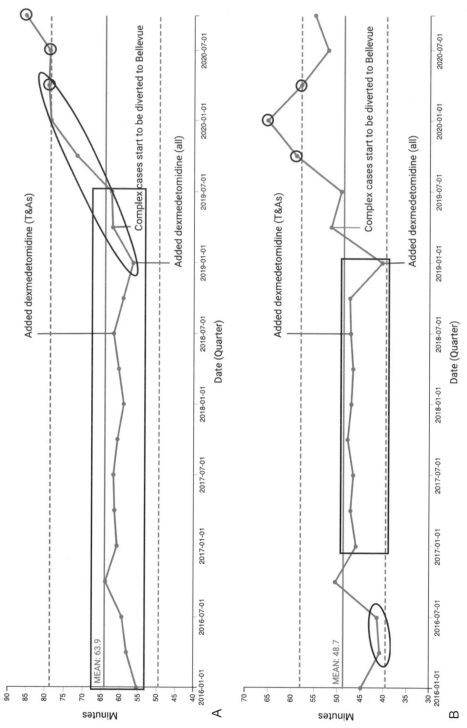

Fig. 51.4 A, Total anesthesia time. B, Standard deviation of total anesthesia time. *T&As*, Tonsillectomy and adenoidectomy.

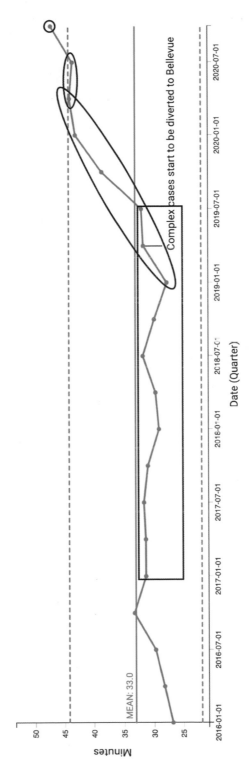

Fig. 51.5 Total surgery time.

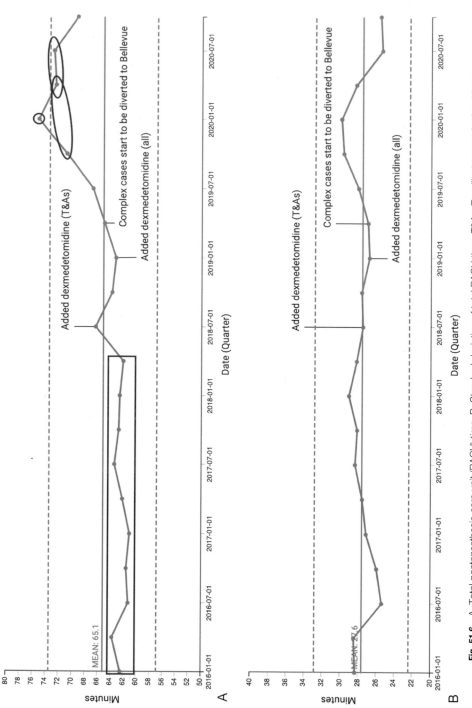

Fig. 51.6 A, Total postanesthesia care unit (PACU) time. B, Standard deviation of total PACU time. *T&As,* Tonsillectomy and adenoidectomy.

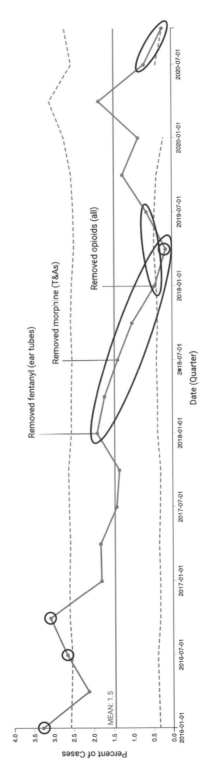

Fig. 51.7 Postoperative nausea and vomiting (PONV) rescue rate. *T&As*, Tonsillectomy and adenoidectomy.

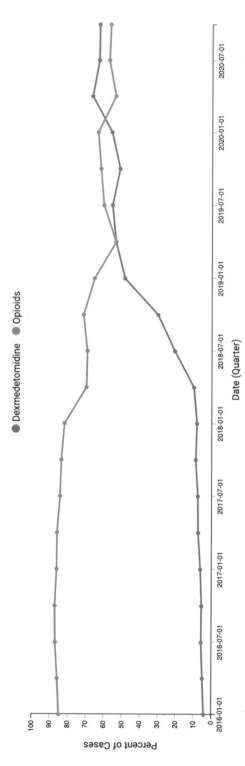

Fig. 51.8 Run chart showing the percent of surgical and procedural patients receiving intraoperative dexmedetomidine versus intraoperative opioids at Seattle Children's main hospital.

dexmedetomidine use (>17,000 patients) in the main operating rooms, gastroenterology suites, cardiac catheterization labs, and interventional radiology suites. This trend is likely due to several factors: the 2018 opioid shortage, vocal advocates of dexmedetomidine, a change in pharmacy practice to make 20 mcg/5 mL dexmedetomidine syringes readily available, awareness of Bellevue's protocols and success at reducing opioids, and presentations to the anesthesia group on dexmedetomidine use and opioid reduction. Importantly, review of 2016 to 2020 main hospital data for over 66,000 cases shows that despite this trend of reduced intraoperative opioids and increased dexmedetomidine, the outcome measures evaluated above have remained stable or improved over time. Taken together, these data suggest that intraoperative opioid reduction is possible at a large academic pediatric hospital.

This QI project has several limitations. First, this project took place at a single outpatient surgery center and findings may not be generalizable to all centers. Second, hemodynamic data were not examined. However, ephedrine and glycopyrrolate administration can be used as proxies for bradycardia and/or hypotension, the most common side effects of dexmedetomidine; in 2016 to 2017 (preintervention), 2018 (intervention), and 2019 to 2020 (postintervention), 5.2%, 5.4%, and 7.0% of patients received ephedrine and/or glycopyrrolate, respectively. Third, three different pain assessment scales were converted into an 11-point (0–10) scale, which is not ideal because pain may be assessed differently depending on who evaluates pain.[21] Finally, and most importantly, there are minimal data on postdischarge pain and opioid use after surgery. Thus it is not known whether there was a change in home opioid administration once intraoperative opioids were replaced with dexmedetomidine.

Readily accessible real-world data allowed the Bellevue team to perform rapid PDSA cycles, leading to the removal of opioids from standardized anesthesia protocols for all the most commonly performed surgeries. By using a combination of dexmedetomidine, nonsteroidal anti-inflammatory drugs, and frequent regional anesthesia, intraoperative opioid use declined by 89% without compromising patient outcomes.

References

1. Toussaint JS, Berry LL. The promise of Lean in health care. *Mayo Clin Proc.* 2013;88(1):74–82.
2. Hollingsworth H, Herndon C. The parenteral opioid shortage: causes and solutions. *J Opioid Manag.* 2018;14(2):81–82.
3. Brummett CM, Waljee JF, Goesling J, et al. New persistent opioid use after minor and major surgical procedures in US adults. *JAMA Surg.* 2017;152(6):e170504.
4. Harbaugh CM, Lee JS, Hu HM, et al. Persistent opioid use among pediatric patients after surgery. *Pediatrics.* 2018;141(1):e20172439.
5. Hayhurst CJ, Durieux ME. Differential opioid tolerance and opioid-induced hyperalgesia: a clinical reality. *Anesthesiology.* 2016;124(2):483–488.
6. Koepke EJ, Manning EL, Miller TE, et al. The rising tide of opioid use and abuse: the role of the anesthesiologist. *Perioper Med.* 2018;7(1):16.
7. McColley SA, April MM, Carroll JL, et al. Respiratory compromise after adenotonsillectomy in children with obstructive sleep apnea. *Arch Otolaryngol Head Neck Surg.* 1992;118:940–943.
8. Olutoye OA, Glover CD, Diefenderfer JW, et al. The effect of intraoperative dexmedetomidine on postoperative analgesia and sedation in pediatric patients undergoing tonsillectomy and adenoidectomy. *Anesth Analg.* 2010;111(2):490–495.
9. Patel A, Davidson M, Tran MCJ, et al. Dexmedetomidine infusion for analgesia and prevention of emergence agitation in children with obstructive sleep apnea syndrome undergoing Tonsillectomy and adenoidectomy. *Anesth Analg.* 2010;11(4):1004–1010.
10. Zhuang PJ, Wang X, Zhang XF, et al. Postoperative respiratory and analgesic effects of dexmedetomidine or morphine for adenotonsillectomy in children with obstructive sleep apnoea. *Anaesthesia.* 2011;66:989–993.

11. Franz AM, Dahl JP, Huang H, et al. The development of an opioid sparing anesthesia protocol for pediatric ambulatory tonsillectomy and adenotonsillectomy surgery—a quality improvement project. *Pediatr Anaesth.* 2019;29(7):682–689.

12. Chan DK, Parikh SR. Perioperative ketorolac increases post-tonsillectomy hemorrhage in adults but not children. *Laryngoscope.* 2014;124:1789–1793.

13. Franz AM, Martin LD, Liston DE, et al. In Pursuit of an opioid-free pediatric ambulatory surgery center—a quality improvement initiative. *Anesth Analg.* 2020;132(3):788–797.

14. Merkel S, Voepel-Lewis T, Shayevitz JR, et al. The FLACC: a behavioral scale for scoring postoperative pain in young children. *Pediatr Nurs.* 1997;23(3):293–297.

15. Wong DL, Baker CM. Pain in children: comparison of assessment scales. *Pediatr Nurs.* 1988;14(1):9–17.

16. Phelps JR, Russell A, Lupa MC, et al. High-dose dexmedetomidine for noninvasive pediatric procedural sedation and discharge readiness. *Paediatr Anaesth.* 2015;25(9):877–882.

17. Aldrete JA. The post-anesthesia recovery score revisited. *J Clin Anesth.* 1995;7(1):89–91.

18. Provost LP, Murray S. *The Health Care Data Guide: Learning From Data for Improvement.* John Wiley & Sons; 2011.

19. Frauenknecht J, Kirkham KR, Jacot-Guillarmod A, et al. Analgesic impact of intra-operative opioids vs. opioid-free anaesthesia: a systematic review and meta-analysis. *Anaesthesia.* 2019;74(5):651–662.

20. Blaudszun G, Lysakowski C, Elia N, et al. Effect of perioperative systemic α2 agonists on postoperative morphine consumption and pain intensity: systematic review and meta-analysis of randomized controlled trials. *Anesthesiology.* 2012;116(6):1312–1322.

21. Manne SL, Jacobsen PB, Redd WH. Assessment of acute pediatric pain: do child self report, parent ratings, and nurse ratings measure the same phenomenon? *Pain.* 1992;48(1):45–52.

CHAPTER 52

Optimizing Value in Perioperative Medicine and the High Value Practice Academic Alliance: A Case-Based Study on Preoperative Assessment

Venkata Andukuri, MD, MPH ■ Christopher J. King, MD ■
Robert L. Fogerty, MD, MPH, SFHM

KEY POINTS

- Perioperative care provides opportunities for the reduction of low-value testing and treatment, in line with evidence-based guidelines.
- Quality improvement (QI) projects focused on perioperative care can have a significant impact on patient outcomes and health system performance.
- There are particular considerations that can arise in designing and implementing a perioperative medicine QI project, such as the need for multidisciplinary engagement across different specialty areas.
- Organizations such as the High Value Practice Academic Alliance (HVPAA) have demonstrated a role in training future physicians in high-value care with QI methodology.

Clinical Case Example

Mrs. Reyes is a 51-year-old woman, who is admitted to a hospital with abdominal pain. She is diagnosed, after her initial laboratory evaluation and imaging findings return, with acute cholecystitis. She has a 5-pack per year history of cigarette use; however, she quit 25 years ago. She has hyperlipidemia and well-controlled essential hypertension. She can walk up two flights of stairs and exercises daily, walking 3 miles per day without chest pain. Her only medication is a high potency statin. Her vital signs are within normal limits. On examination, her respiratory and cardiovascular system are normal. She is managed conservatively with intravenous (IV) fluid hydration and parenteral antibiotics and does well. A surgical consultation is obtained, and she is scheduled for a cholecystectomy once she has fully recovered from the acute episode. The surgical consultant writes in the consult note, "Obtain preop labs and studies, clearance for surgery per medicine."

Using the admission ECG and labs, you perform a revised risk cardiac index (RCRI) risk stratification (https://www.mdcalc.com/revised-cardiac-risk-index-pre-operative-risk) and the patient scores 0 points, which places her in the lowest risk category with a 3.9% risk of perioperative major adverse cardiac events (MACE). She is now eating and drinking normally.

On the day of surgery, the case is cancelled, and the patient is sent back to the floor. You are called by the anesthesiologist who informs you that the case was cancelled because the patient needs to have a preoperative chest radiograph.

You order a two-view chest radiograph, which shows no cardiopulmonary abnormalities.

The patient was able to have a successful laparoscopic cholecystectomy on the next day and was discharged.

Case Review

In the aforementioned case, we see an example of preoperative testing that did not follow evidence-based guidelines and current recommendations from professional societies.

According to the Choosing Wisely® guidelines, it is recommended to avoid routine preoperative testing for low-risk surgeries without a clinical indication.[1] Most preoperative tests, like a complete blood count, prothrombin time and partial thromboplastin time, basic metabolic profile, and urine analysis, are typically normal in an elective preoperative patient. The findings of these tests usually influence less than 3% of management in these patients.[2]

Similarly, the Choosing Wisely® guidelines do not recommend chest x-rays to be routinely performed at admission or preoperatively for ambulatory patients with an unremarkable history and physical examination.[3] Only 2% of images obtained lead to a change in management.[4]

However, it is reasonable to obtain a chest x-ray if acute cardiopulmonary disease is suspected or if there is a history of chronic stable cardiopulmonary disease in a patient older than 70 years who has not had a chest x-ray within 6 months.[4]

Discussion

The case example demonstrates the need for the use of evidence in preoperative management and the need for value-based protocols. Value is defined as quality over cost. The delay to surgery and the extended length of stay and radiograph were likely unnecessary. The appropriate use of preoperative assessment provides opportunities for quality improvement (QI) projects to improve the value of care. A good understanding of QI methodology is required but not sufficient on its own.

A stepwise approach to such a project is helpful for both the novice and experienced professional:

- First, perform a process mapping exercise to understand and document workflows and key decision points.
- Next, obtain data to understand and define the problem. Using data and the process map, the deviation from high-value care can begin to be uncovered via root cause analysis.[4]
- An understanding of the root cause is essential to scope the project, to focus on the use of evidence-based guidelines, and to understand the waste that occurs when guidelines are not applied.
- After this systematic investigation into the problem, a SMART goal[5] is defined, which is **S**pecific, **M**easurable, **A**ttainable, **R**ealistic and defined by a timeline. The SMART goal is used to focus a team effort on an implementation strategy based on an implementation science framework.[6]
- A good QI project may need multiple cycles of Plan-Do-Study-Act (PDSA) tests of change (see the Model for Improvement chapter) to test ideas and achieve the desired changes, consistent with the PDSA approach.[6-9]
- Lastly, a good project should also have a sustainability plan to establish the new process and have an ongoing way to monitor and maintain the changes achieved.

The stepwise process previously defined will be familiar to those who have previously engaged in a QI project in any setting, be it health care or nonclinical. However, there is an aspect to improving preoperative testing, which is about reducing what is done, or "de-implementation" and "doing less." The concept that sometimes it is beneficial for the patient, and to society as a whole, to "do less" can be uncomfortable. Understanding that the approach is supported by high-quality science and an evidence base requires awareness of current guidelines, knowledge of change management, QI, clinical acumen, and an understanding of high-value principles.

Training for "Value" in the High Value Practice Academic Alliance

The High Value Practice Academic Alliance identified the shortage of highly trained physicians able to understand and perform healthcare QI in high-value care. To meet the need of health systems and training programs, the Future Leaders Program (FLP) was created to achieve four main goals for residents and fellow physicians:

1. To develop the knowledge, skills, and attitudes necessary to lead healthcare value QI projects at a local level
2. To develop the knowledge, skills, and attitudes necessary to improve bedside delivery of high value health care
3. To explore the qualities necessary to be an effective healthcare value leader.
4. To connect to national and international organizations focused on healthcare value.

Learners from any medical specialty were encouraged to apply and were accepted into the program after a competitive application review. The application required that candidates propose a healthcare value QI project that they aimed to undertake at their institution over the coming academic year. The selected applicants represented a diverse array of specialties and geographical location, which created challenges. Addressing this cohort of learners required different approaches to curriculum design that used different modalities and tools within the knowledge, skills, and attitudes arenas:

- Knowledge: Given the busy schedules of Graduate Medical Education (GME) learners, the curriculum used asynchronous online learning modules and videos focused on healthcare value concepts, QI strategies, and effective leadership qualities.
- Skills: Learners carried out their proposed healthcare value QI project during the 12 months of the program. Learners were supported through a tiered mentorship model in which day-to-day issues were addressed with the help of a local mentor, and larger topics or those needing an outside lens were discussed with a national mentor (one of the Program Directors).
- Attitudes: Learners were expected to develop an improvement in attitudes to healthcare value through the implementation of their projects, completion of knowledge-focused online modules, and interaction with Program Directors and the national HVPAA organization throughout the year.

Assessment of learner's projects occurred at a local level through discussion with their mentorship team on the appropriate measures for each project. Educational outcomes were measured using a presurvey/postsurvey strategy.

Over the years there have been several projects performed by residents in the FLP in various GME programs across the country to improve preoperative management. The training provided guidance and mentorship, with the help of the combined experience and expertise of the faculty. Implementation science methods were applied and education and training provided for just-in-time issues such as project dissemination, culture change, finances, motivation, buy-in from both front-line colleagues and the C-suite, piloting the project, issues of data gathering within each system's unique medical record, surveys, and finally for analyzing the data.

The FLP provides a roadmap for how to engage physicians-in-training from multiple specialties, and in multiple locations, to improve the value of care that a healthcare system provides, through experiential learning, coupled with asynchronous knowledge acquisition. A tiered mentorship model ensures a robust support team for learners. The goals of the program are broad enough that the underlying learning objectives can be tailored to align with the needs of a healthcare system or GME program. Finally, using an experiential learning system that incorporates resident- and fellow-driven project ideas generates buy-in for action readily and elevates those learners that are enthusiastic about becoming healthcare value leaders.

References

1. Choosing Wisely, ABIM Foundation. *ASCP—Pre-op testing for low-risk surgery*; October 30, 2018. https://www.choosingwisely.org/clinician-lists/american-society-clinical-pathology-routine-preop-testing-for-low-risk-surgeries-without-indication/.
2. Benarroch-Gampel J, Sheffield KM, Duncan CB, et al. Preoperative laboratory testing in patients undergoing elective, low-risk ambulatory surgery. *Ann Surg.* 2012;256(3):518–528. https://doi.org/10.1097/SLA.0b013e318265bcdb.
3. Choosing Wisely, ABIM Foundation. *ACR—Avoid admission or pre-op chest x-rays*; May 2, 2019. https://www.choosingwisely.org/clinician-lists/american-college-radiology-admission-preop-chest-x-rays/.
4. Munro J, Booth A, Nicholl J. Routine preoperative testing: a systematic review of the evidence. *Health Technol Assess.* 1997;1(12):i–iv. 1–62.
5. Joo HS, Wong J, Naik VN, Savoldelli GL. The value of screening preoperative chest x-rays: a systematic review. *Can J Anaesth.* 2005;52(6):568–574.
6. Damschroder LJ, Aron DC, Keith RE, et al. Fostering implementation of health services research findings into practice: a consolidated framework for advancing implementation science. *Implementation Sci.* 2009;4:50. https://doi.org/10.1186/1748-5908-4-50.
7. Heher YK. A brief guide to root cause analysis. *Cancer Cytopathol.* 2017;125(2):79–82. https://doi.org/10.1002/cncy.21819.
8. Aghera A, Emery M, Bounds R, et al. A randomized trial of SMART goal enhanced debriefing after simulation to promote educational actions. *West J Emerg Med.* 2018;19(1):112–120. https://doi.org/10.5811/westjem.2017.11.36524.
9. Christoff P. Running PDSA cycles. *Curr Probl Pediatr Adolesc Health Care.* 2018;48(8):198–201. https://doi.org/10.1016/j.cppeds.2018.08.006.

Further Reading and Resources

Porter ME. What is value in health care? *N Engl J Med.* 2010;363(26):2477–2481. https://doi.org/10.1056/NEJMp1011024.
Smith CD, Alliance for Academic Internal Medicine–American College of Physicians High Value, Cost-Conscious Care Curriculum Development Committee. Teaching high-value, cost-conscious care to residents: the Alliance for Academic Internal Medicine–American College of Physicians Curriculum. *Ann Intern Med.* 2012;157(4):284–286. https://doi.org/10.7326/0003-4819-157-4-201208210-00496.
The High Value Practice Academic Alliance. https://hvpaa.org Accessed November 23,2021.
Health Affairs. Diffusion of innovation to improve health care value: physician-led care redesign. March 14, 2019. https://www.healthaffairs.org/do/10.1377/forefront.20190308.817613.
Guidelines. papers on Pre-operative assessment: Practice Advisory for Preanesthesia Evaluation: an updated report by the American Society of Anesthesiologists Task Force on Preanesthesia Evaluation. *Anesthesiology.* 2012;116:522–538. https://doi.org/10.1097/ALN.0b013e31823c1067.
Fleisher LA, Fleischmann KE, Auerbach AD, et al. 2014 ACC/AHA guideline on perioperative cardiovascular evaluation and management of patients undergoing noncardiac surgery: a report of the American College of Cardiology/American Heart Association Task Force on practice guidelines. *J Am Coll Cardiol.* 2014;64(22): e77–137. https://doi.org/10.1016/j.jacc.2014.07.944.
National Institute for Clinical Excellence (NICE) UK. Routine preoperative tests for elective surgery; 2016. https://www.nice.org.uk/guidance/ng45. Accessed November 23, 2021.
Onuoha OC, Hatch MB, Miano TA, Fleisher LA. The incidence of un-indicated preoperative testing in a tertiary academic ambulatory center: a retrospective cohort study. *Perioper Med (Lond).* 2015;15(4):14. https://doi.org/10.1186/s13741-015-0023-y.
Feely MA, Collins CS, Daniels PR, Kebede EB, Jatoi A, Mauck KF. Preoperative testing before noncardiac surgery: guidelines and recommendations. *Am Fam Physician.* 2013;87(6):414–418.

CHAPTER 53

Perioperative Medicine for Older People: Translating a Geriatrician-Led Perioperative Care Model From an Inner London Teaching Hospital to a District General Hospital

Jugdeep Dhesi, FRCP, PhD ▪ Andrew Rogerson, MB ChB, MRCP ▪
Judith Partridge, FRCP, PhD

KEY POINTS

- The perioperative medicine for older people (POPS) team at Guy's and St Thomas' National Health Service (NHS) Trust (GSTT) has pioneered an award-winning perioperative medicine service model and informed the development of similar services in the United Kingdom.
- National roll-out of POPS services has been slow, particularly in smaller and more financially challenged hospitals.
- A mixed methods study was used to evaluate the translation of the model from GSTT to Dartford and Gravesham Trust (DGT).
- A "logic model" describing the core components of the GSTT service was devised to enable translation with fidelity to the original model.
- Co-design with stakeholders, including patients and relatives, was a key component in the ultimate success of this project.

Introduction: The Need for Geriatrician-Led Perioperative Services

The global surgical population is aging at a faster rate than the general population.[1] The increasing burden of frailty and comorbidity in older patients is associated with perioperative morbidity and mortality.[2,3] Despite this, there is often a case for proceeding with surgery in older, frailer adults to achieve increased longevity and maintain or improve quality of life. The needs of this population are inadequately met by traditional perioperative care models. International reports and guidelines have called for geriatrician-led, integrated perioperative care pathways to address this problem.[4–7]

The perioperative medicine for older people (POPS) model, originally conceived and developed at Guy's and St Thomas' National Health Service (NHS) Trust (GSTT), London, has served as an exemplar in this field. Since beginning as a pilot project in 2003, POPS has established a UK-wide collaborative driving national and international change.[8] This chapter will describe how implementation science methods were used to develop the POPS model at an inner London academic medical center (GSTT) and translate it to a community district general hospital (Dartford and Gravesham Trust [DGT]) while retaining fidelity to the model's guiding principles.

Context: Establishment of POPS Service, Evidence Base, and Scaling Challenges

The POPS service was initially piloted in 2003[9] in older patients scheduled for elective hip and knee arthroplasty. It was based on Comprehensive Geriatric Assessment (CGA) and optimization, which uses multidisciplinary, holistic assessment toprompt multidomain interventions, and has been shown to improve morbidity and mortality in older patients.[10,11] It was hypothesized that preoperative CGA and optimization would improve access to surgery and reduce postoperative complications and length of stay (LOS). A geriatrician-led care model including preoperative CGA and optimization, and collaborative postoperative ward care was tested.

Trial design was informed by the *Framework for Design and Evaluation of Complex Interventions to Improve Health*,[12] which was produced by the UK Medical Research Council in 2000. A "before and after" exploratory trial compared a cohort of 54 patients receiving standard orthopedic care with a 54-patient cohort receiving POPS care. The intervention reduced postoperative complications (notably, pneumonia incidence was reduced by 80% and delirium by 70%), and LOS was shortened by a median of 4.5 days. This study led to the establishment of a substantively funded POPS service that has grown over the past 19 years. In 2004 the team included a geriatric medicine attending (0.2 FTE), a geriatric medicine trainee (0.8 FTE), and a full-time physiotherapist, occupational therapist, social worker, and clinical nurse specialist. In 2022 the team now includes 4.4 FTE attendings, 5 full-time clinical nurse specialists, 4 full-time senior residents, 11 junior residents, an occupational therapist, and an administrator.

In the intervening period, the POPS team has conducted a series of studies demonstrating the impact of CGA in different surgical subspecialties,[13] including a single-site randomized controlled trial that examined the impact of preoperative CGA and optimization on vascular elective surgery patients.[14] It demonstrated a 40% reduction in LOS in the group receiving CGA (predominantly because of fewer medical complications) and was shown to be cost effective.[15] This evidence has subsequently informed additional single-site service evaluations.[16-18] A systematic review of CGA-based perioperative services for older people has also shown improved outcomes in the emergency setting.[19] In emergency laparotomy, big data studies have confirmed the benefit of geriatrician involvement as part of a collaborative perioperative pathway affecting mortality and LOS.[20,21]

Having established an evidence-based single-site service with sporadic uptake at other similar institutions, the challenge of spread to less well-resourced units remains. This chapter now describes the translation of the POPS model from GSTT (POPS@GSTT) to DGT (POPS@DGT).

Intervention

The POPS@GSTT model was translated to DGT in three phases, as will be described, and outcomes were evaluated using a mixed methods study. DGT is a 463-bed district general hospital in a deprived area of Kent County, 16 miles east of GSTT. The partnership between the two sites was approved as one of 50 programs in NHS England's Acute Care Collaboration Vanguard Scheme in 2015. This secured £25,000 funding for the pilot project, which was used to facilitate 2 days per week of input from senior residents in geriatric medicine. They were supported educationally through personal mentoring and a weekly half-day multidisciplinary team meeting led by senior geriatricians from POPS@GSTT.

PHASE 1—DEFINING THE CORE COMPONENTS OF THE MODEL

To facilitate translation of the POPS@GSTT service to another hospital, a standardized description of the core components was required. A logic model to describe these core components was developed by an expert panel of 13 healthcare professionals and the patient involvement group.[22]

PHASE 2—PILOT SERVICE AT NEW LOCATION

The pilot began in elective vascular surgery, providing outpatient, preoperative CGA-based assessment and optimization before lower limb revascularization or aortic aneurysm surgery. After a year, the service was extended to include elective outpatient general surgical patients and postoperative inpatient care for those undergoing general surgery.

The service was codesigned and co-produced with patients, carers, and professionals from the perioperative pathway. Stakeholder relationships were proactively fostered through informal one-on-one meetings, group meetings, departmental presentations, focus groups, and formal interviews and surveys.

To ensure fidelity to the POPS model, reduce duplication of work, and provide a seamless approach to care between hospitals, POPS@GSTT materials were used in the pilot at DGT after adaptation to the local context. These included clinical resources (e.g., outpatient letter template, delirium guidelines, patient information leaflets), education and training materials (e.g., junior doctor teaching slide sets, curricula, capability framework to support upskilling of clinical nurse specialists), and documents to support management processes (e.g., business plans, job descriptions, job adverts).

PHASE 3—DATA COLLECTION, ITERATIVE REFINEMENT OF SERVICE, AND EVALUATION

A prospective, mixed methods, multi-phased "hybrid clinical-implementation" study (i.e., measuring both implementation and clinical data) was undertaken. This approach allowed for an evaluation of clinical, patient-reported, and implementation outcomes comparing a pre-POPS cohort with a post-POPS cohort.

MEASURES

Key performance indicators were defined a priori and aligned with the logic model (Table 53.1). Real time clinical and implementation data findings were visible to the team and discussed

TABLE 53.1 ■ Key Performance Indicators Aligned to the POPS Logic Model

Clinical Outcomes	Patient-Reported Outcomes	Implementation Outcomes
Length of stay	Satisfaction	Feasibility
Readmissions		Acceptability (including staff satisfaction)
Coding for multimorbidity		Uptake
Coding for postoperative complications		Sustainability

POPS, Perioperative medicine for older people.

regularly at both professional and patient and public involvement (PPI) meetings. Semistructured interviews and electronic surveys were used to gather qualitative data on implementation outcomes from staff members. Service user feedback and codesign was facilitated through focus groups. These data were regularly fed back to all stakeholders allowing discussion and iterative adaptation of the service.

Analysis and Ethics

All quantitative implementation and clinical data were analyzed with descriptive statistics using SPSS v.22. Qualitative data (from interviews and focus groups) were transcribed and analyzed with emergent theme analysis using NVIVO v.12. Ethical aspects were considered through the service user liaison element in the study design. Because this is an implementation study rather than research, formal ethics committee approval was not required.

Results

Before the POPS@DGT pilot, no patients scheduled for elective vascular surgery received preoperative CGA and optimization. After establishment of the POPS@DGT pilot, 166 elective vascular surgical patients were seen preoperatively in the POPS@DGT CGA and optimization clinic from October 2016 to October 2018.

In November 2017, the POPS@DGT service was expanded to include patients undergoing elective and emergency general surgery; 77 elective general surgical patients received preoperative CGA in an outpatient setting compared with none receiving it before the pilot.

With respect to emergency general surgery:

- Before the POPS@DGT pilot, 15% of patients over 70 years received geriatrician review.
- After establishment of POPS@DGT, 763 inpatient CGA reviews were conducted.
- The majority of these inpatient reviews ($n = 669$) were emergency admissions, of which 117 underwent emergency laparotomy. Sixty-two of the patients undergoing emergency laparotomy were aged over 70 years, and all were co-managed by the POPS service (one died early postoperatively in critical care).
- A mean reduction in LOS of 2.6 days was observed after introduction of the POPS@DGT pilot service with a reduction in 30-day readmission rate from 30% to 18%.
- An increase in multimorbidity and postoperative complications was observed over the 12-month period, probably reflecting an increase in recognition and documentation as opposed to an increase in incidence.

At the beginning of the pilot, 10 semi-structured interviews were conducted with a range of clinical stakeholders, examining barriers and enablers. These findings were used in the codesign of the service. Nine months into the pilot, an electronic survey of 28 multidisciplinary clinicians was conducted. This showed that more than 80% of staff described an improvement in the overall care of older surgical patients (n = 28, response rate 71%) after introduction of the POPS@DGT pilot service. In addition, staff reported improved understanding of multidisciplinary working and enhanced educational opportunities. Interviews with stakeholders demonstrated improved satisfaction with discharge letter documentation, noted particularly by general practitioners.

Service-user focus groups, conducted at regular intervals during the pilot, were used to facilitate codesign, resulting in improvements to patient experience, such as timing of clinic appointments, content of letters, patient information leaflets, and a hospital map.

Sustainability

A year after the initial POPS@DGT pilot commenced, a business case containing the aforementioned data was submitted to the hospital board and a substantive service was funded. Initial funding was provided for 1.4 FTE consultant geriatricians, 1.0 FTE senior nurse, 0.1 FTE input from a POPS expert from GSTT, and 0.3 FTE occupational therapist input. Further iterative development of the service has resulted in expansion to cover elective and emergency general, vascular, and orthopedic surgery with staffing now including an additional 2.0 FTE senior nurses and 1.0 FTE clinical fellow.

Discussion

In this chapter, we describe the establishment, evaluation, and expansion of the POPS service at GSTT and the translation of the POPS model of care to a community hospital (POPS@DGT).

The POPS model of care has developed over the past 18 years at the initiating site, with evaluations demonstrating improvements in clinician-reported, patient-reported, and process outcomes and in shared decision making. The service has expanded from elective orthopedic surgery to now include all emergency and elective surgical specialties at this academic hospital.

A survey in 2014 demonstrated only three sites employing the POPS model across the UK, with the main barriers to uptake cited as inadequate funding and workforce at both academic and community hospitals.[23] To develop strategies to address these barriers on a national level, the POPS@GSTT team successfully bid for a small grant to pilot POPS at a less financially robust district general hospital with acknowledged workforce issues. Within 18 months, substantive funding from the district general hospital facilitated the establishment of a full clinical team. Key factors contributing to the success of this pilot included sharing of clinical resources from GSTT, allowing the DGT clinical team to apply the model with fidelity in a timely fashion; codesign and co-production with all stakeholders; iterative use of data visible to all to refine the service using rapid Plan-Do-Study-Act (PDSA) cycles; and mentoring, coaching, and clinical supervision from POPS@GSTT building sustainability.

In parallel with the POPS@DGT pilot, other workstreams have been undertaken in preparation for systematic spread of the POPS model of care both nationally and internationally. First, a toolkit of resources, including clinical materials and guidelines, education, and training resources such as curricula and slide sets, as well as management resources such as business plans and job descriptions, has been developed. Second, a(n) (inter)national POPS program employing implementation scientists, coaches, and mentors working with data analysts has been established to support the development of a POPS network. Preliminary data from a second UK survey in 2019[24] demonstrates the impact of these workstreams together with the effect of national advocacy for the POPS approach.[25] There are now approximately 40 sites in the UK delivering POPS-type services, with funding increasingly provided from surgical directorates. A similar picture is seen internationally, with the establishment of programs like Duke Perioperative Optimization of Senior Health (POSH) in the United States and CGA-based services in Australia and Singapore.[8,26–30]

With the challenge of the increasingly older, multimorbid, frail surgical population, new approaches to perioperative care are necessary. CGA-based perioperative services have been demonstrated to be clinically effective, cost-effective, and (as shown in this chapter) translatable across clinical settings and nations. Widespread scale-up requires fidelity to the evidence base, internationally accepted clinical guidelines and standards, implementation science methodology to underpin service development, and evaluation using big data.

Case Vignette

78M

Known comorbidity: hypertension, macular degeneration

Presented with abdominal pain, found to have a 62-mm abdominal aortic aneurysm. Referred to POPS clinic, scheduled for surgery day after POPS review.

Comprehensive Geriatric Assessment Revealed

- 5 recent syncopal events
- Dyspnea
- Cognitive impairment
- Hyponatremia
- Possible lung mass on chest x-ray
- Ischemic electrocardiogram (ECG) changes
- Obstructive bedside spirometry pattern
- Mild frailty and functional impairment

Surgery was delayed for investigation and optimization.

Investigation and Optimization of Comprehensive Geriatric Assessment Issues

Cardiac: Echo showed septal wall motion abnormality. Cardiac catheterization showed nonocclusive coronary artery disease; this was medically managed.

Syncope: 24-hour ECG recording, tilt table test. Found to have episodes of ventricular tachycardia and orthostatic hypotension. Beta blocked and referred for postoperative implanted cardiac defibrillator.

Dyspnea and chest x-ray changes: Formal pulmonary function tests revealed chronic obstructive airways disease, and patient commenced on appropriate inhaler therapy and referred to smoking cessation services and pulmonary rehabilitation classes. Lung cancer was excluded on computed tomography (CT) thorax.

Cognitive impairment: Magnetic resonance imaging (MRI) brain showed small vessel disease. On cognitive assessment, he was felt to have mild vascular cognitive impairment.

Occupational therapy input to support with social isolation, meal preparation, and falls prevention strategies in view of mild frailty.

Hyponatremia: After paired osmolarities and endocrine testing, patient was diagnosed with drug-induced syndrome of inappropriate ADH secretion. Corrected after cessation of medication.

Outcome

The patient underwent open abdominal aortic arch (AAA) repair. An implantable cardioverter device (ICD) was inserted before hospital discharge. Left hospital within 7 days and was well at 12 months post follow-up.

References

1. Fowler AJ, Abbott TEF, Prowle J, Pearse RM. Age of patients undergoing surgery. *BJS*. 2019.
2. Hamel MB, Henderson WG, Khuri SF, Daley J. Surgical outcomes for patients aged 80 and older: morbidity and mortality from major noncardiac surgery. *J Am Geriatr Soc*. 2005;53(3):424–429.
3. Makary MA, Segev DL, Pronovost PJ, et al. Frailty as a predictor of surgical outcomes in older patients. *J Am Coll Surg*. 2010;210(6):901–908.
4. American College of Surgeons. *Introducing the ACS Geriatric Surgery Verification Program*; 2019. https://www.facs.org/quality-programs/geriatric-surgery. Accessed May 19, 2021.
5. National Confidential Enquiry into Patient Outcome and Death (NCEPOD). *An Age Old Problem: A Review of the Care Received by Elderly Patients Undergoing Surgery*; 2010.
6. Griffiths R, Beech F, Brown A, et al, Association of Anesthetists of Great Britain and Ireland. Perioperative care of the elderly 2014: Association of Anaesthetists of Great Britain and Ireland. *Anaesthesia*. 2014;69(suppl 1):81–98.

7. Chow WB, Rosenthal RA, Merkow RP, et al. Optimal preoperative assessment of the geriatric surgical patient: a best practices guideline from the American College of Surgeons National Surgical Quality Improvement Program and the American Geriatrics Society. *J Am Coll Surg*. 2012;215(4):453–466.

8. Norris CM, Dhesi J, Keogh G, et al. Australian hospital calls in the COPS to improve care of older patients. *ACS Bulletin*. 2021. p. 56.

9. Harari D, Hopper A, Dhesi J, Babic-Illman G, Lockwood L, Martin F. Proactive care of older people undergoing surgery ('POPS'): designing, embedding, evaluating and funding a comprehensive geriatric assessment service for older elective surgical patients. *Age Ageing*. 2007;36(2):190–196. https://doi.org/10.1093/ageing/afl163.

10. Grazioli, et al. Comprehensive geriatric assessment toolkit for primary care practitioners. British Geriatrics Society; 2019. https://www.bgs.org.uk/resources/resource-series/comprehensive-geriatric-assessment-toolkit-for-primary-care-practitioners. Accessed May 28, 2021.

11. Ellis G, Gardner M, Tsiachristas A, et al. Comprehensive geriatric assessment for older adults admitted to hospital. *Cochrane Database Syst Rev*. 2017;9(9):CD006211. https://doi.org/10.1002/14651858.CD006211.pub3.

12. Campbell M, Fitzpatrick R, Haines A, et al. Framework for design and evaluation of complex interventions to improve health. *BMJ*. 2000;321:694.

13. Braude P, Goodman A, Elias T, et al. Evaluation and establishment of a ward-based geriatric liaison service for older urological surgical patients: Proactive care of Older People undergoing Surgery (POPS)-Urology. *BJU Int*. 2017;120(1):123–129.

14. Partridge JS, Harari D, Martin FC, et al. Randomized clinical trial of comprehensive geriatric assessment and optimization in vascular surgery. *Br J Surg*. 2017;104(6):679–687.

15. Partridge JSL, Healey A, Modarai B, Harari D, Martin FC, Dhesi JK. Preoperative comprehensive geriatric assessment and optimisation prior to elective arterial vascular surgery: a health economic analysis. *Age and Ageing*. 2021;50(5):1770–1777.

16. Shipway D, Koizia L, Winterhorn N, Fertleman M, Ziprin P, Moorthy K. Embedded geriatric surgical liaison is associated with reduced inpatient length of stay in older patients admitted for gastrointestinal surgery. *Future Hosp J*. 2018;5:108–116.

17. Thu K, Nguyen HPT, Gogulan T, et al. Care of Older People in Surgery for general surgery: a single centre experience. *ANZ J Surg*. 2021;91·890–895.

18. Vilches-Moraga A, Fox J. Geriatricians and the older emergency general surgical patient: proactive assessment and patient centred interventions. *Salford-POP-GS Aging Clin Exp Res*. 2018;30(3):277–282.

19. Khadaroo RG, Warkentin LM, Wagg AS, et al. Clinical effectiveness of the elder-friendly approaches to the surgical environment initiative in emergency general surgery. *JAMA Surg*. 2020;155(4),e196021.

20. Oliver CM, Bassett MG, Poulton TE, et al. Organisational factors and mortality after an emergency laparotomy: multilevel analysis of 39903 National Emergency Laparotomy Audit patients. *Br J Anaesth*. 2018;121:1346–1356.

21. Rachel MA, Judith SLP, Oliver CM, et al. Older patients undergoing emergency laparotomy: observations from the National Emergency Laparotomy Audit (NELA) years 1–4. *Age Ageing*. 2020;49(4):656–663.

22. Jasper EV, Dhesi JK, Partridge JS, Sevdalis N. Scaling up perioperative medicine for older people undergoing surgery (POPS) services; use of a logic model approach. *Clin Med (Lond)*. 2019;19(6):478–484. https://doi.org/10.7861/clinmed.2019-0223.

23. Partridge JS, Collingridge G, Gordon AL, Martin FC, Harari D, Dhesi JK. Where are we in perioperative medicine for older surgical patients? A UK survey of geriatric medicine delivered services in surgery. *Age Ageing*. 2014;43(5):721–724.

24. Joughin AL, Partridge JSL, O'Halloran T, Dhesi JK. Where are we now in perioperative medicine? Results from a repeated UK survey of geriatric medicine delivered services for older people. *Age Ageing*. 2019. https://doi.org/10.1093/ageing/afy218.

25. Lees N, et al. The high-risk general surgical patient: raising the standard. Updated recommendations on the perioperative care of the high-risk general surgical patient. *Royal College of Surgeons of England*. 2018.

26. Rogerson A, Partridge JS, Dhesi JK. Perioperative medicine for older people. *Ann Acad Med Singap*. 2019;48(11):376–381. PMID: 31960018.

27. McDonald SR, Heflin MT, Whitson HE, et al. Association of Integrated Care Coordination With Postsurgical Outcomes in High-Risk Older Adults: The Perioperative Optimization of Senior Health (POSH) Initiative. *JAMA Surg.* 2018 May 1;153(5):454–462. https://doi.org/10.1001/jamasurg.2017.5513. PMID: 29299599; PMCID: PMC5875304.

28. Thillainadesan J, Hilmer S, Close J, Kearney L, Naganathan V. Geriatric medicine services for older surgical patients in acute hospitals: results from a binational survey. *Australas J Ageing.* 2019;38:278–283. https://doi.org/10.1111/ajag.12675.

29. Partridge JSL, Aitken RM, Dhesi JK. Perioperative medicine for older people: learning across continents. *Australas J Ageing.* 2019;38(4):228–230. https://doi.org/10.1111/ajag.12723.

30. Fullbrook AI, et al. A multidisciplinary perioperative medicine clinic to improve high-risk patient outcomes: a service evaluation audit. *Anaesth Intensive Care.* 2022;50(3):227–233.

Putting It All Together: Clinical Quality Improvement Examples: Agency for Healthcare Research and Quality, Improving Surgical Care and Recovery

Elizabeth C. Wick, MD

KEY POINTS

- The Agency for Healthcare Research and Quality (AHRQ) Safety Program for Improving Surgical Care and Recovery (ISCR) was launched in 2016 and aimed to accelerate adoption of enhanced recovery principles across five surgical areas using the principles of the comprehensive unit-based safety program (CUSP).
- CUSP is an implementation framework that emphasizes leadership support and frontline engagement to support meaningful improvement. It has been effective in reducing catheter-associated bloodstream infections and other healthcare-acquired infections.
- Principles of CUSP are woven throughout the ISCR program, and there is a strong emphasis on teamwork and communication. Ultimately, the impact of the program is being evaluated by 30-day surgical outcomes, with a particular focus on healthcare-acquired infections and healthcare utilization.

Why Did We Do This Work—Clinical Issues and Background

Enhanced recovery after surgery (ERAS) sparked excitement in the surgical community, primarily because it works, but also because it is an innovative approach to delivering standardized, evidence-based care. Adoption of ERAS has been associated with reducing surgical complications, improving patient satisfaction, and decreasing length of stay (LOS) and associated hospital costs, while not increasing readmission rates.[1,2] To successfully implement ERAS and achieve improvements, the entire perioperative team must function as a coordinated and collaborative group, breaking down silos among preoperative, operating room, recovery room, and inpatient units and creating transdisciplinary collaboration across perioperative disciplines (surgery, anesthesiology, nursing, pharmacy, and physical therapy).[3] The Agency for Healthcare Research and Quality (AHRQ) partnered with the Johns Hopkins Armstrong Institute for Quality and Safety and the American College of Surgeons (ACS) to rollout evidence-based ERAS pathways within the framework of a comprehensive unit-based safety program (CUSP) across a broad range of US hospital settings over 5 years (Fig. 54.1).[4,5]

Leveraging evidence, prior AHRQ-funded work, and deep experience at the ACS, ISCR developed a comprehensive program to support hospitals in implementing ERAS. The toolkit with ERAS pathways, or bundles of interventions, integrated the adaptive components that are critical

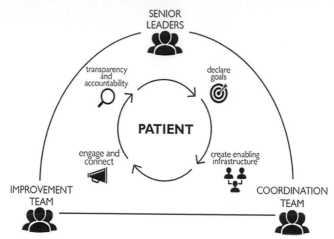

Fig. 54.1   Team dynamics and coordination, with the patient as the focus in the ISCR program. *ISCR,* Improving Surgical Care and Recovery.

to successfully implement, sustain, and seamlessly spread an intervention. Process, outcome, and patient experience are measured to determine the effectiveness of the intervention.[6,7] After implementing ERAS among colorectal surgery patients in cohort 1 (Summer 2017), we applied an iterative and participatory approach to adapt the toolkit to other service lines, such as orthopedics (total hip arthroplasty [THA] and total knee arthroplasty [TKA]) in Spring 2018, gynecology (hysterectomy) in Spring 2019, and emergency general surgery in Fall 2020. Hospitals enroll at set time points in groups or "cohorts" of roughly 100 hospitals and can participate in more than one specialty area. The collaborative is ongoing and will conclude in 2022. Once joining the collaborative, hospitals have access to a variety of resources, including sample pathways, evidence reviews summarizing literature supporting pathway elements, and implementation resources.[4,8] Local hospital teams are encouraged to identify a project team leader (often a clinician) and a data abstractor. Coaching webinars are held monthly to facilitate peer-learning. Participating hospitals also have access to the project team for one-on-one support with implementation and data collection. Participation was open to all US hospitals. Hospitals were recommended to spend 3 months adapting the pathway to their local environment, gathering their team, and ensuring stakeholder buy-in. Participating hospitals have ranged from ERAS novices to those with prior experience who have the desire for further improvement.

All hospitals were required to enter both process measure and 30-day patient outcome measures into a registry. The registry allowed for visualization of performance through data reports and provided benchmarking against other participating hospitals.

Data Sources and Outcomes

The registry was built on the platform of the National Surgical Quality Improvement Program (NSQIP).[9] Trained abstractors extract data from the electronic health record (EHR) using standard data definitions and report both process measure compliance and 30-day outcomes for cases with specific colorectal correct procedural terminology (CPT) codes. The registry variables were parsimonious. Process measures were limited to nine core measures: preoperative bowel preparation, preoperative oral antibiotics, regional analgesia, early mobilization, early liquid intake, early solid intake, early Foley catheter removal, multimodal pain control, and venous thromboembolism (VTE) prophylaxis. Outcomes of interest included 30-day postoperative complications, such as catheter-associated urinary tract infection (CAUTI), VTE, composite of superficial, deep, and organ space surgical site infection (SSI), ileus (defined as return of bowel function >3 days postoperatively), readmission, and prolonged LOS (defined as LOS > 6 days/75th percentile of LOS).

Results

Over 300 hundred hospitals have participated in the program, with many participating in multiple procedure areas. Analysis is underway but preliminary findings exist for hospitals that have participated in colorectal surgery in cohorts 1 and 2. Both LOS and return of bowel function demonstrated substantial improvement over time. Further analyses are needed to understand the association between process measure compliance and outcome improvement. On first pass, there were no common patterns in the characteristics of hospitals who were most likely to succeed in the program. Qualitative analyses have emphasized the complexity of ERAS implementation and the many competing priorities clinicians and hospitals face, as well as limited project management and EHR modifications. Turnover of both the surgical lead and nurse lead, in many instances, prevented a team from remaining in the program.

Discussion

In conclusion, although ERAS and ISCR was timely with regard to the need to drive value in perioperative care, successful implementation, even with the support of a national collaborative and easy-to-use tools, is still challenging and depends heavily on local context, a receptive culture, frontline engagement, and leadership support. In addition to leadership support, it is necessary to have stable and empowered site champions, financial or regulatory incentives, a data platform for monitoring, and expert support to facilitate success. Aligning all of these is hard for most projects; a careful stakeholder assessment is critical before beginning complex quality improvement efforts.

References

1. ERAS Society. http://erassociety.org/.
2. Wind J, Polle SW, Fung Kon Jin PHJ, et al. Systematic review of enhanced recovery programmes in colonic surgery. Br J Surg. 2006;93(7):800–809. https://doi.org/10.1002/bjs.5384.
3. Wick EC, Galante DJ, Hobson DB, et al. Organizational culture changes result in improvement in patient-centered outcomes: implementation of an integrated recovery pathway for surgical patients. J Am Coll Surg. 2015;221(3):669–677. https://doi.org/10.1016/j.jamcollsurg.2015.05.008.
4. Romig M, Goeschel C, Pronovost P, Berenholtz SM. Integrating CUSP and TRIP to improve patient safety. Hosp Pract 1995. 2010;38(4):114 121. https://doi.org/10.3810/hp.2010.11.348.
5. Pronovost P, Needham D, Berenholtz S, et al. An intervention to decrease catheter-related bloodstream infections in the ICU. N Engl J Med. 2006;355(26):2725–2732.
6. Ban KA, Gibbons MM, Ko CY, et al. Evidence review conducted for the Agency for Healthcare Research and Quality safety program for Improving Surgical Care and Recovery: focus on anesthesiology for colorectal surgery. Anesth Analg. 2019;128(5):879–889. https://doi.org/10.1213/ANE.0000000000003366.
7. Ban KA, Gibbons MM, Ko CY, Wick EC. Surgical technical evidence review for colorectal surgery conducted for the AHRQ safety program for Improving Surgical Care and Recovery. J Am Coll Surg. 2017;225 (4):548–557.e3. https://doi.org/10.1016/j.jamcollsurg.2017.06.017.
8. Stone AB, Yuan CT, Rosen MA, et al. Barriers to and facilitators of implementing enhanced recovery pathways using an implementation framework: a systematic review. JAMA Surg. 2018;153(3):270–279. https://doi.org/10.1001/jamasurg.2017.5565.
9. Khuri SF, Daley J, Henderson W, et al. The Department of Veterans Affairs' NSQIP: the first national, validated, outcome-based, risk-adjusted, and peer-controlled program for the measurement and enhancement of the quality of surgical care. National VA Surgical Quality Improvement Program. Ann Surg. 1998;228(4):491–507.

CHAPTER 55

Cardiovascular Disease: Preoperative Testing and Evaluation for Noncardiac Surgery

Michael W. Manning, MD, PhD

KEY POINTS

- More older patients with multiple cardiovascular comorbidities, previous surgery, and other diseases associated with aging are presenting for major surgery.
- Cardiac risk stratification is key to advise the patient on the risks and benefits of surgery and inform discussions with the operative team about the optimal location and timing of surgery or to consider options other than surgery.
- Preoperative electrocardiogram (ECG) is unnecessary for low-risk patients undergoing low-risk procedures.
- Perioperative mortality is rare but approximately 50% of these mortalities are related to cardiac complications; therefore effective identification and management of cardiovascular risk factors is a key component of improving perioperative outcomes.

Introduction

The overall goal of a preoperative cardiovascular evaluation, and the goal of perioperative medicine in general, is to establish the individual's cardiovascular risk.[1-3] Mortality from cardiovascular disease has decreased since the 1970s, most likely from a combination of improved pharmacological management, the development of advanced surgical techniques, and the adoption of healthier lifestyles. Nevertheless, more recently, the rates of cardiovascular disease are increasing and again becoming a key cause-of-death affecting life expectancy in the United States (US) and the United Kingdom (UK).[4]

The mean age of our population is increasing, with "baby boomers" now entering their 70s and 80s. Greater numbers of these patients are now presenting for surgery in advanced age, usually with multiple cardiovascular comorbidities, such as chronic hypertension, renal disease, stroke, pulmonary disease, valvopathies, heart failure, previous surgery, and other diseases associated with aging.[5] We list the conditions that pose the greatest risks in Table 55.1, all of which can have significant implications on surgical risks.[6,7]

Although overall perioperative mortality is only 0.3%, cardiac etiologies account for up to 50% of these perioperative deaths.[8] Myocardial injury, defined as an elevated troponin greater than the 99th percentile, occurs in up to 20% of patients after noncardiac surgery.[9-11] Myocardial infarction (MI) is the most common cardiac complication, occurring within 72 hours postoperatively with the peak incidence at 48 hours. Perioperative MIs have atypical presentations and are almost always non-ST elevation MIs (NSTEMIs). Perioperative evaluation and risk assessment, therefore, becomes a critical step toward the reduction of perioperative morbidity and mortality in this population.

TABLE 55.1 ■ **Cardiovascular Conditions That Increase Perioperative Risk and Negatively Impact Both Short- and Long-Term Outcomes**

High-Risk Cardiac Conditions	Intermediate-Risk Cardiac Conditions	Comorbidities With Cardiac Effects
Recent myocardial infarction (MI; within 12 months)	Remote MI	Diabetes
Decompensated heart failure (HF)	Prior episode(s) of HF	Stroke
Unstable angina	Stable angina	Renal insufficiency
Symptomatic valvular disease	Moderate valvular disease	Pulmonary disease
Symptomatic arrhythmias		

Risk Assessment

One should evaluate perioperative risk within the context of the planned surgical procedure. Low-risk surgeries, in which the risk of MI/death during the perioperative period is less than 1%, include endoscopic and superficial procedures, as well as cataract, breast, or ambulatory surgeries.[2] Several surgeries present with intermediate and/or high risk, adding to the perioperative risk overall. These include carotid endarterectomy and endovascular aneurysm repair, as well as head/neck, intraperitoneal/intrathoracic, orthopedic, prostate, aortic/major vascular, and peripheral vascular surgery (Fig. 55.1).[1]

Besides surgical risk, the timing of surgery should be considered. Surgeries are deemed an *emergency* when life or limb is threatened if not in the operating room within 6 hours or less depending on the underlying condition. Because of such time constraints, there is no or minimal time for optimization and only the most superficial clinical evaluation. *Urgent* procedures are those that threaten life or limb if not in the operating room between 6 and 24 hours. In these instances, there may be slightly more time for a limited or focused clinical evaluation, compared to the *emergency cases*. In contrast with that of a *time-sensitive surgery*, in which a delay of greater than 1–6 weeks to allow for a comprehensive evaluation and significant changes in management could negatively affect outcomes, such as in some aggressive forms of cancer requiring surgery.[12] Most oncological surgeries would fit into this latter category. *Elective surgery* could be delayed for up to 1 year and would include cases like total knee replacement or cataract surgery.[1,2]

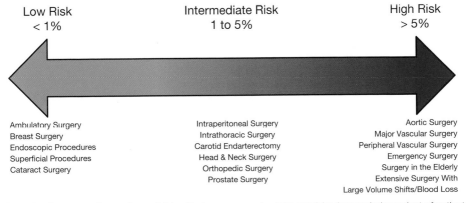

Low Risk < 1%	Intermediate Risk 1 to 5%	High Risk > 5%
Ambulatory Surgery Breast Surgery Endoscopic Procedures Superficial Procedures Cataract Surgery	Intraperitoneal Surgery Intrathoracic Surgery Carotid Endarterectomy Head & Neck Surgery Orthopedic Surgery Prostate Surgery	Aortic Surgery Major Vascular Surgery Peripheral Vascular Surgery Emergency Surgery Surgery in the Elderly Extensive Surgery With Large Volume Shifts/Blood Loss

Fig. 55.1 Spectrum of surgeries and risks. Each surgery carries inherent risks that are independent of patient risk factors or those from anesthesia. Those surgeries that are more invasive or take longer usually carry greater risks.

Perioperative Evaluation

A multidisciplinary, preoperative evaluation of the patient undergoing noncardiac surgery is performed for multiple reasons, including (1) to assess perioperative risks (which can inform the decision to proceed or the choice of surgery), (2) to determine whether addition to or changes in management are needed to minimize risks, and (3) to identify those cardiovascular conditions or risk factors requiring long-term management to help anticipate other postoperative needs (Fig. 55.2). All of these factors must also take into consideration the patient's perspective.

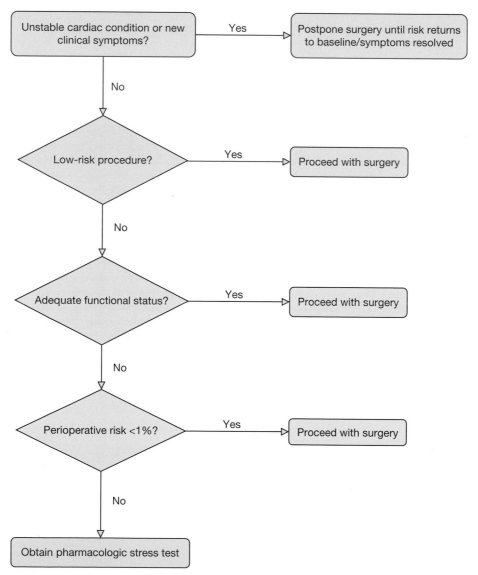

Fig. 55.2 The recommended framework for preoperative evaluation for noncardiac surgery. (Data from Fleisher L.A., Fleischmann K.E., Auerbach A.D., et al. 2014 ACC/AHA guideline on perioperative cardiovascular evaluation and management of patients undergoing noncardiac surgery: executive summary: a report of the American College of Cardiology/American Heart Association Task Force on Practice Guidelines. Circulation. 2014;130(24):2215–2245.)

Although the patient may appear stable and without symptoms at the time of presentation, prior history may be worrisome for intermediate cardiac risks. Although these symptoms may be absent at the time of assessment, they may confer increased morbidity and mortality during times of perioperative stress (see Table 55.1). If present, these symptoms must be evaluated to understand their current status fully and apply best practices for optimization.

As part of the evaluation, a rigorous history and physical examination must be performed to identify the markers of cardiac risk and assess the patient's current cardiac status. Initial evaluation should begin with a good historical overview, which should start as the interview with the patient begins. Observe how they look. Are they calm or restless? Are they short of breath? Do they look fatigued or well rested? Are there obvious signs of labored breathing while speaking? These initial observations are telling and often overlooked, dismissed, or completely ignored by most practitioners today.

As questions of functional status or physiological reserve arise, the determination can then be made as to what, if any, testing is indicated that will better define the risk to the patient. Once this is accomplished, the anesthesia and surgical teams can then best advise the patient on the risks and benefits of surgery and make interventions or modifications as necessary in the allotted time to reduce these risks. Moreover, this may lead to recommendations and discussions with the operative team about the optimal location and timing of surgery (i.e., ambulatory surgery, outpatient hospital, or an inpatient admission) or consideration of other strategies, including avoidance of surgery if that is an option.

PATIENT HISTORY

The perioperative evaluation should follow the framework as outlined by the 2014 American College of Cardiology (ACC)/American Heart Association (AHA) Guideline on Perioperative Cardiovascular Evaluation and Management of Patients Undergoing Noncardiac Surgery.[13] The initial interview should focus on determining the functional status of the patient and understanding their current cardiovascular status.[14] The better approach to achieve this goal begins with asking open-ended questions, such as: *What do you like to do for activity? In which exercises do you like to take part? What keeps you from performing all your desired activities? When do you most get short of breath? How long does it take you to become short of breath? What activities can you do before you get too tired to do more?* Start questions broadly and ensure they are open-ended, then drill down to specifics, trying to avoid asking questions that could be answered with a simple "yes" or "no."[14] Look for and ask about signs or symptoms of other diseases that link to cardiovascular disease, such as kidney disease, diabetes, chronic obstructive pulmonary disorder (COPD), and sleep apnea. Inquire as to the current status of these disease states before testing as well as evaluations that may have been performed and any key findings or current treatments the patient might be receiving. Inquire as to the stability of these symptoms: Have they changed over the past year, 6 months, 3 months, or last month?

Risk calculators, including the metabolic equivalents (METs; Table 55.2),[15] the Revised Cardiac Risk Index (Table 55.3),[16] and the Duke Activity Status Index (DASI)[17] use the patient's history to establish a patient's overall risk for surgery.[7] These scores are used along with findings from the physical examination to provide an overall risk score. This data, taken with the expected surgery, can then help guide conversations/planning with the care team.

PHYSICAL EXAMINATION

Once the comprehensive history is obtained, conduct the most complete physical examination possible with attention given to the subtle findings of heart failure, such as peripheral edema or jugular distention; abnormal heart sounds suggesting valvular disease; or crackles/rales when auscultating the lungs, suggesting fluid overload. If questions arise, having those patients that can physically walk

TABLE 55.2 ■ Metabolic Equivalents (METs) Used to Assess Patients' Physiological and Cardiovascular Status

METs Classification	Common Activities	Surgical Risk
1 MET	Self-Care Eat/Dress/Toilet Walk indoors around house Walk 1–2 blocks on level ground at 2–3 mph Dusting/washing dishes (some classify this as 1–4 METs)	High Risk
≥ 4 METs	Climb 1 flight of stairs -or- walk up a hill Walk on level ground at 4 mph Run a short distance Scrubbing floors/moving heavy furniture Golf, bowling, dance, doubles tennis, throw baseball or football	Intermediate Risk
≥ 10 METs	Participate in strenuous sports such as: Singles tennis Football Baseball Skiing	Low Risk

Adapted from Fleisher LA, Fleischmann KE, Auerbach AD, et al. 2014 ACC/AHA guideline on perioperative cardiovascular evaluation and management of patients undergoing noncardiac surgery: executive summary: a report of the American College of Cardiology/American Heart Association Task Force on Practice Guidelines. *Circulation.* 2014;130[24]:2215–2245.

TABLE 55.3 ■ Cardiovascular Risk Calculator Used to Assign Perioperative Risk to Patients Undergoing Noncardiac Surgery

Risk Factor	Points
Cerebrovascular disease	1
Congestive heart failure	1
Creatinine level > 2.0 mg/dL	1
Diabetes mellitus requiring insulin	1
Ischemic cardiac disease	1
Suprainguinal vascular surgery; intrathoracic surgery; or intra-abdominal surgery	1
Total points	_____

Risk of Major Cardiac Events

Points	Risk % (95% Confidence Interval)
0	0.4 (0.05–1.5)
1	0.9 (0.3–2.1)
2	6.6 (3.9–10.3)
≥3	≥11 (5.8–18.4)

Adapted from Lee TH, Marcantonio ER, Mangione CM, et al. Derivation and prospective validation of a simple index for prediction of cardiac risk of major noncardiac surgery. *Circulation.* 1999;100[10]:1043–1049.

a flight of stairs can be incorporated into the physical examination to better gauge functional capacity.

With data now from both history and physical examination, informed decisions can be made as to the need for additional testing (Fig. 55.3). Patients who are at low risk based on clinical features, functional status, and proposed low-risk surgery rarely require any further evaluation. Those patients who are deemed to be at high risk, however, based on clinical features, poor functional status, and consideration for high-risk surgery, will benefit from further evaluation.

Testing/Evaluation/Management

Individuals with at least three clinical risks factors and extensive myocardial ischemia on preoperative stress testing appear to have high complication rates, even with effective medical therapy. These patients should be considered for invasive evaluation and coronary revascularization after a detailed discussion with the surgeon, cardiologist, and anesthesiologist.

In those patients in whom their functional status is questionable, or for patients with physical disabilities that restrict evaluation of their functional status, more formalized cardiovascular testing may need to be performed. This testing can be chemical stress testing or nuclear perfusion stress testing. For those patients undergoing low-risk surgery or who have minimal cardiac risk factors, stress testing is not indicated.[3]

Preoperative 12-lead electrocardiogram (ECG) is appropriate for those patients with previously known cardiovascular disease, history of significant arrhythmias, cerebrovascular disease, or structural defects of the heart. It is unnecessary for low-risk patients undergoing low-risk procedures.[3]

In patients with known or suspected valvular stenosis or regurgitation that is moderate to severe, a preoperative echocardiogram (Echo) should be considered for evaluation.[13,18] If there is a recent Echo ($\leq$1 year) and the patient reports no worsening of symptoms since their last formal evaluation, an Echo is unnecessary. If, however, during an Echo evaluation, the patient is found to have severe stenosis or regurgitation that warrants an intervention, a discussion between the patient, cardiologist, surgeon, and anesthesiologist is encouraged to weigh the perioperative risks against the need for intervention before moving forward.[12]

It is reasonable to evaluate patients with prior or known left ventricular dysfunction and reduced ejection fraction using Echo before surgery, especially if an Echo has not been performed within the past 12 months or symptoms have worsened. If patients have had a recent ($\leq$12 months) exacerbation of heart failure symptoms or hospitalization because of heart failure and the planned surgery is intermediate or high risk, then repeating the Echo is appropriate.[3]

Management of patients taking cardiovascular medication sometimes presents unique challenges. Patients who are on antiplatelet therapy after percutaneous coronary interventions with stent placement require special consideration. Per ACC/AHA guidelines, patients should delay elective, noncardiac surgery for 14 days after balloon angioplasty, for 30 days after bare metal stent (BMS) placement, and at least 1 year after placement of drug-eluting stents (DES).[13]

In special cases where surgery *must* occur within the first 4 to 6 weeks after either BMS or DES placement, dual antiplatelet therapy with aspirin and clopidogrel should continue throughout the perioperative period without interruption.[13] Discussions between the surgeon, prescribing cardiologist, and anesthesiologist should weigh the risks of the planned procedure in this very high-risk group before proceeding to surgery. In patients in whom $P2Y_{12}$ platelet inhibition cannot continue during the perioperative period because of concerns for excessive bleeding, aspirin should continue throughout at the very least, and again conversations with the patient, surgeon, cardiologist, and anesthesiologist should be focused on reducing risks of in-stent thrombosis.

If at any point in the perioperative course, and most especially during the immediate postoperative period, a patient begins to manifest signs or symptoms of an MI, **immediate** diagnosis is required to direct management.[12] High-sensitivity troponin and 12-lead ECG should be

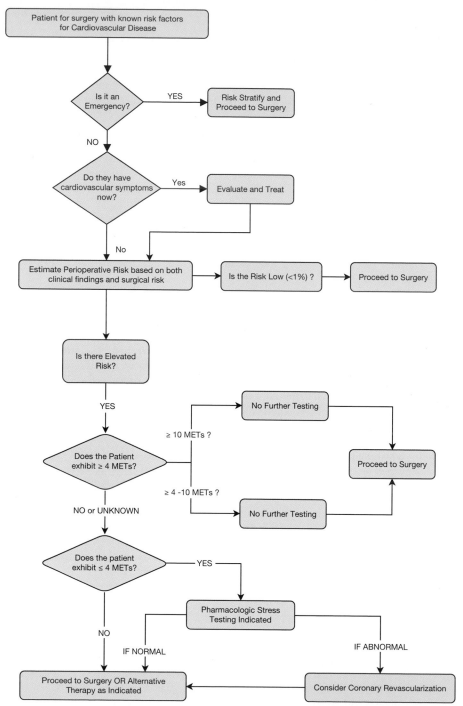

Fig. 55.3 Basic process for contemplating additional cardiovascular testing and evaluation prior to noncardiac surgery. (Adapted from Karnath BM. Preoperative cardiac risk assessment. *Am Fam Physician*. 2002;66 [10]:1889–1896.)

obtained.[9–13] If an ST-elevation MI (STEMI) is diagnosed, immediate intervention in the catheter lab is necessary, whereas an NSTEMI is usually approached with guideline-directed medical management.

Angiotensin-converting enzyme (ACE) inhibitors and angiotensin receptor blockers (ARBs) are generally held within 24 hours of a planned surgery because of the increased risk of hypotension during general anesthesia. Special circumstances, albeit rare, may justify continuation of these medications; however, increased vigilance is necessary by the anesthesia team during surgery to monitor for episodes of hypotension, which may be resistant to catecholamine therapy.[3]

Both beta blockers and statins should be continued during the perioperative period; however, it is widely agreed that beta blockers should not be started the day before major surgery. If medically indicated, beta-blocker therapy should be started a week or more before surgery to allow patients to stabilize on the medication.[3]

Many patients coming for noncardiac surgery have not undergone a recent comprehensive cardiovascular evaluation (or at all). Moreover, a small subset of patients have never had consistent medical care throughout their life. A comprehensive preoperative evaluation with appropriate therapy, therefore, becomes critically important because this may significantly improve both perioperative short-term and long-term outcomes. The use of appropriate risk stratification, perioperative medical management, and proper intraoperative and postoperative surveillance are necessary in these patients and may positively affect long-term outcomes.

References

1. Mukherjee D, Eagle KA. Perioperative cardiac assessment for noncardiac surgery. *Circulation*. 2003;107 (22):2771–2774.
2. Freeman WK, Gibbons RJ. Perioperative cardiovascular assessment of patients undergoing noncardiac surgery. *Mayo Clin Proc*. 2009;84(1):79–90.
3. Fleisher LA, Fleischmann KE, Auerbach AD, et al. 2014 ACC/AHA guideline on perioperative cardiovascular evaluation and management of patients undergoing noncardiac surgery: executive summary: a report of the American College of Cardiology/American Heart Association Task Force on Practice Guidelines. *Circulation*. 2014;130(24):2215–2245.
4. Mehta NK, Abrams LR, Myrskyla M. US life expectancy stalls due to cardiovascular disease, not drug deaths. *Proc Natl Acad Sci U S A*. 2020;117(13):6998–7000.
5. Forman DE, Maurer MS, Boyd C, et al. Multimorbidity in older adults with cardiovascular disease. *J Am Coll Cardiol*. 2018;71(19):2149–2161.
6. Ali MJ, Davison P, Pickett W, Ali NS. ACC/AHA guidelines as predictors of postoperative cardiac outcomes. *Can J Anaesth*. 2000;47(1):10–19.
7. Minto G, Biccard B. Assessment of the high-risk perioperative patient. *Continuing Education in Anaesthesia Critical Care & Pain*. 2014;14(1):12–17.
8. Karnath BM. Preoperative cardiac risk assessment. *Am Fam Physician*. 2002;66(10):1889–1896.
9. Smilowitz NR, Redel-Traub G, Hausvater A, et al. Myocardial injury after noncardiac surgery: a systematic review and meta-analysis. *Cardiol Rev*. 2019;27(6):267–273.
10. Writing Committee for the VISION Study Investigators, Devereaux PJ, Biccard BM, et al. Association of postoperative high-sensitivity troponin levels with myocardial injury and 30-day mortality among patients undergoing noncardiac surgery. *JAMA*. 2017;317(16):1642–1651.
11. Smilowitz NR, Berger JS. Perioperative cardiovascular risk assessment and management for noncardiac surgery: a review. *JAMA*. 2020;324(3):279–290.
12. Mukherjee D, Eagle KA. Perioperative cardiac assessment for noncardiac surgery: eight steps to the best possible outcome. *Circulation*. 2003;107(22):2771–2774.
13. Fleisher LA, Fleischmann KE, Auerbach AD, et al. 2014 ACC/AHA guideline on perioperative cardiovascular evaluation and management of patients undergoing noncardiac surgery: a report of the American College of Cardiology/American Heart Association Task Force on Practice Guidelines. *Circulation*. 2014;130(24):e278–e333.

14. Garcia-Miguel FJ, Serrano-Aguilar PG, Lopez-Bastida J. Preoperative assessment. *Lancet.* 2003;362 (9397):1749–1757.
15. Fleisher LA, Beckman JA, Brown KA, et al. ACC/AHA 2007 Guidelines on perioperative cardiovascular evaluation and care for noncardiac surgery: executive summary: a report of the American College of Cardiology/American Heart Association Task Force on Practice Guidelines (Writing Committee to Revise the 2002 Guidelines on Perioperative Cardiovascular Evaluation for Noncardiac Surgery): developed in collaboration with the American Society of Echocardiography, American Society of Nuclear Cardiology, Heart Rhythm Society, Society of Cardiovascular Anesthesiologists, Society for Cardiovascular Angiography and Interventions, Society for Vascular Medicine and Biology, and Society for Vascular Surgery. *Circulation.* 2007;116(17):1971–1996.
16. Lee TH, Marcantonio ER, Mangione CM, et al. Derivation and prospective validation of a simple index for prediction of cardiac risk of major noncardiac surgery. *Circulation.* 1999;100(10):1043–1049.
17. Hlatky MA, Boineau RE, Higginbotham MB, et al. A brief self-administered questionnaire to determine functional capacity (the Duke Activity Status Index). *Am J Cardiol.* 1989;64(10):651–654.
18. Writing Committee Members, Otto CM, Nishimura RA, et al. 2020 ACC/AHA Guideline for the management of patients with valvular heart disease: executive summary: a report of the American College of Cardiology/American Heart Association Joint Committee on Clinical Practice Guidelines. *J Am Coll Cardiol.* 2021;77(4):450–500.

Further Reading

Duceppe E, Parlow J, MacDonald P, et al. Canadian Cardiovascular Society Guidelines on perioperative cardiac risk assessment and management for patients who undergo noncardiac surgery. *Can J Cardiol.* 2017;33(1):17–32.
Kristensen SD, Knuuti J, Saraste A, et al. 2014 ESC/ESA Guidelines on non-cardiac surgery: cardiovascular assessment and management: the joint task force on non-cardiac surgery: cardiovascular assessment and management of the European Society of Cardiology (ESC) and the European Society of Anaesthesiology (ESA). *Eur Heart J.* 2014;35(35):2383–2431.

CHAPTER 56

Orthopedics and Regional Anesthesia: An Outpatient Total Shoulder Replacement Pathway

Jacques T. YaDeau, MD, PhD ■ Lawrence V. Gulotta, MD ■ Christopher L. Wu, MD

KEY POINTS

- A multidisciplinary group convened to create a standardized protocol for outpatient total shoulder replacement based on available evidence.
- The use of regional anesthesia and analgesia provides superior postoperative analgesia for total shoulder replacement (TSR) compared with general anesthesia and systemic opioids.
- By standardizing preoperative, intraoperative, and postoperative management, we aimed for a reduction in variability in clinical care with an initial goal of 60% to 80% pathway utilization compliance.
- Preliminary results indicate that outpatient TSR in selected patients and with an experienced team is not only feasible but also can be performed successfully with minimal adverse events.

Background

Total shoulder replacement (TSR) is typically performed as a same-day admit/inpatient procedure on approximately 53,000 people in the United States each year.[1] Preliminary small-scale observational studies indicate that outpatient TSR could be a safe and effective alternative to inpatient TSR in appropriately selected patients with no difference in readmission rates and surgical complications.[2,3] However, TSR patients often have severe postoperative pain, which may require an overnight inpatient stay for pain control.

The use of regional anesthesia and analgesia provides superior postoperative analgesia compared with general anesthesia and systemic opioids.[4,5] Peripheral nerve blocks are widely accepted for TSR surgery.[6] An analysis of the National Anesthesia Clinical Outcomes Registry noted that approximately 42% of TSR surgical patients received a peripheral nerve block and that the use of peripheral nerve blocks for this surgery increased over time.[6] Use of a long-acting, single-injection peripheral nerve block along with multimodal analgesia controls postoperative pain after TSR surgery, such that postoperative pain will likely be less than the patient's preoperative pain, few patients require intravenous (IV) opioid analgesia, and, on average, these patients will stop using opioids after 7 days.[7]

With the increasing interest in containing costs of medical care and improving the patient's surgical experience, we created an outpatient TSR pathway for qualified patients.

Creation of the Outpatient Total Shoulder Replacement Pathway

A multidisciplinary group (which included surgery, anesthesiology, nursing, rehabilitation, and case managers) convened to create a standardized protocol for outpatient TSR based on the available evidence. A scoping review of the literature revealed that use of peripheral nerve blocks for TSR improved patient outcomes (e.g., lower pain scores, lower opioid consumption, less postoperative nausea/vomiting).[7,8] The review also clearly noted that the duration of analgesia achieved with the peripheral nerve block could be significantly prolonged with nerve block additives such as dexamethasone, clonidine, or buprenorphine.[9]

Patient selection is important in the success when transitioning from inpatient to outpatient surgery. Certain patient groups or characteristics (e.g., increased comorbidities, morbid obesity) are more likely to have complications and may not be suitable for outpatient surgery. Based on the literature, the multidisciplinary group created a general list of inclusion and exclusion criteria for patient eligibility for outpatient TSR surgery. Inclusion criteria were: age 18 to 75, body mass index (BMI) less than 37.0 and more than 18.5, A1C less than 8.0 for diabetic patients, not currently using warfarin or enoxaparin, and the patient agrees to same-day discharge plan and has a responsible adult to spend the night on the day of discharge (Box 56.1). Exclusion criteria were: contraindication to receiving a peripheral nerve block, active myocardial ischemia, significant valvular disease, significant arrythmias, presence of obstructive sleep apnea, active substance use, chronic pain, no daily use of opioids for more than 3 months, glomerular filtration rate less than 60 mL/min, and the patient lives alone and has no support in the community (Box 56.2).

All operations were performed with the patient in the modified beach chair position (approximately 45 degrees upright) and used a deltopectoral approach. Details of the surgical approach have been described elsewhere.[5] Antibiotic prophylaxis typically was IV cefazolin with vancomycin or

---

BOX 56.1 ■ Inclusion Criteria

- Age 18–75
- Body mass index (BMI) <37.0 and >18.5
- If diabetic, A1C <8.0
- Not currently using warfarin or enoxaparin
- Social support: patient agrees to same day discharge plan and has a responsible adult to spend the night on the day of discharge
- Case should be booked as first or second case
- Low risk patients (see exclusion list [Box 56.2])

BOX 56.2 ■ Exclusion Criteria

- Contraindication to receiving a peripheral nerve block
- Active ischemia
- Significant valvular disease
- Significant arrythmias
- Obstructive sleep apnea
- Active substance use, chronic pain, no daily use of opioids for >3 months
- Glomerular filtration rate <60 mL/min
- Lives alone/no support in the community

clindamycin as substitutes for patients unable to receive cefazolin. For blood conservation, tranexamic acid (1 g) was given IV before surgical incision.

The perioperative anesthetic care was standardized (Table 56.1). Patients received IV sedation of up to 5 mg of midazolam, 20 mg of ketamine, and propofol as determined by the anesthesiologist. Before surgical incision, an ultrasound-guided brachial-plexus peripheral nerve block was performed using approximately 25 mL of 0.5% bupivacaine with adjuncts (e.g., 2 mg preservative-free dexamethasone, 100 mcg clonidine, 150 mcg buprenorphine) to prolong the duration of the peripheral nerve block. Intraoperative sedation/anesthesia was maintained with either IV propofol infusion and additional ketamine (up to a total of 50 mg) or general anesthesia maintained with propofol and sevoflurane. In addition, patients received IV ondansetron (4 mg), famotidine (20 mg), and dexamethasone (4 mg) and ketorolac (15 mg) during surgery. For postoperative analgesia, patients received a multimodal regimen of IV acetaminophen (1000 mg every 6 hours, a total of up to four doses) and IV ketorolac (15 mg every 8 hours, for up to three postoperative doses [fewer doses if shorter stay in hospital] in addition to one dose in the operating room) followed by oral acetaminophen (650 mg every 6 hours for 3 days) and oral meloxicam (7.5–15 mg/day). Oral opioids were

TABLE 56.1 ■ Analgesia for Outpatient Total Shoulder Replacement Pathway

Intraoperative period	Brachial plexus nerve block with additives	0.5% bupivacaine, 25 mL Clonidine, 100 mcg Preservative-free dexamethasone, 2 mg Buprenorphine, 150 mcg
	Intravenous (IV) sedation **OR** General anesthesia	Midazolam, up to 5 mg Propofol, as needed Ketamine, 10–20 mg
		Induction with propofol Insertion of laryngeal mask Airway/ Endotracheal tube Then titrated propofol and sevoflurane
	For **BOTH** IV sedation and general anesthesia	Receive **total** of 50 mg Ketamine Ondansetron 4 mg Famotidine 20 mg Dexamethasone 4 mg Ketorolac 15 mg
Postoperative period	IV acetaminophen, then oral	1000 mg IV × up to 4 doses (adjusted for weight, if needed: If patient is <50 kg; dose is 15 mg/kg every 6 hr) 650 mg by mouth every 6 hr for 3 days
	Low-dose oral opioids (for opioid-naïve patients). Patients with previous exposure to opioids may receive alternative opioid analgesics as clinically indicated.	Mild pain—tramadol 50 mg every 6 hr as needed. Moderate pain—tramadol 100 mg every 6 hr as needed. Severe pain—oxycodone 5 mg every 3 hr as needed. If needed, allow escalation (e.g., oxycodone 5/10/15 mg)
	Ketorolac, then meloxicam	Ketorolac 15 mg every 8 hr, up to 3 more doses. Then meloxicam 7.5–15 mg daily for 2 weeks

available on an as needed basis based on patient's level of pain: 50 mg tramadol for mild pain, 100 mg tramadol for moderate pain, or 5 mg oxycodone for severe pain.

Hospital discharge criteria included a tolerable pain level on oral regimen, no severe nausea, spontaneous voiding, tolerance of regular diet, and temperature less than 39°C without signs of infection. In addition, the patient needed to verbalize understanding of sling management, understanding of home exercise program, understanding of discharge instruction and perform independent ambulation and independent stair climbing. Finally, an adult escort needed to be present before discharge.

After discharge, patients were placed in a shoulder immobilizer for 4 weeks. Patients initiated pendulum exercises and distal range of motion on the first postoperative day. Active range of motion was allowed when the sling was discontinued at 4 weeks. Strengthening was started at 12 weeks with the goal of obtaining a full recovery by 6 months postoperatively.

The objectives for our pathway included reduction of length of stay to 8 hours or less, at least a 75% success rate for discharges on day of surgery, and reduction in the number of surgical complications after TSR surgery. By standardizing preoperative, intraoperative, and postoperative management, we also aimed for a reduction in the variability in clinical care with an initial goal of 60% to 80% pathway utilization compliance.

The metrics we used to assess success included hospital length of stay, 90-day readmission rate, 90-day postoperative revision rate, day of surgery discharge rate, preoperative physical therapy utilization rate, post–acute care service utilization, and PROMIS 10 (Patient-Reported Outcomes Measurement Information System) with comparison of preoperative scores to 6 weeks, 6 months, 1 year, 2 years, and 5 years postoperatively.

Results

Because our outpatient TSR pathway was initiated only in early 2020, our data collection is in progress. Preliminary results indicate that of the 221 TSR procedures scheduled in 2021 by one surgeon (LG), 23 (10%) were performed on an outpatient basis. There were no readmissions and no surgical complications were noted. All patients received a peripheral brachial plexus nerve block that was functioning in the recovery room/postanesthesia care unit (PACU) and provided at least 12 hours of analgesia postoperatively. The vast majority of patients were discharged to home within 4 hours after arrival to the PACU.

Discussion

Our preliminary results indicate that outpatient TSR in selected patients is not only feasible but also can be performed successfully with minimal adverse events. The development of an outpatient TSR protocol was based on the available current literature and standardized perioperative care of these patients. The key component of the intraoperative anesthetic was the peripheral brachial plexus nerve block with adjuvant agents to prolong the duration of the analgesia to approximately 24 hours postoperatively. In addition, a multimodal analgesic regimen using nonopioid analgesic agents on a scheduled basis (acetaminophen and nonsteroidal antiinflammatory drugs) with opioids taken on an as needed basis was standardized.

This project was successful because of many factors. In our opinion, surgeon acceptance of regional anesthesia is critical for the success of an outpatient TSR pathway because uncontrolled postoperative pain is a top reason for need for inpatient admission. In addition, we have a relatively consistent and reliable assignment to these cases of anesthesiologists who are familiar with the TSR pathway. These anesthesiologists have agreed to perform a long-acting (12–24 hours of analgesia) peripheral brachial plexus block on outpatient TRS patients and have an extremely high rate (>95%) of successful nerve blocks, with low complication rates. We have a core group of anesthesiologists working with our shoulder surgeons who perform outpatient TSR procedures, but every anesthesiologist at Hospital for Special Surgery is an expert in regional anesthetic techniques as over 90% of our over 50,000 anesthetic procedures annually incorporate use of regional anesthesia. We have previously documented a high success rate (99.8%) and low complication rate (0% rate of permanent nerve injury) using regional anesthesia for 1169 ambulatory shoulder arthroscopy patients.[10] Our nursing staff was involved with the creation of this pathway and have been instrumental in the smooth discharge of our TSR patients from the PACU.

Our outpatient TSR pathway is sustainable because it is built around a robust clinical framework. In essence, we have modified our previous intraoperative practice to incorporate updated evidence-based practice. Preoperative (e.g., patient education) and postoperative (e.g., nursing discharge direct from PACU) changes are now standardized. We intend to continue to update our pathway based on analysis of the results of our initial cohort or new high-quality evidence as it is published in the literature. Finally, many patients are very happy with the possibility of being discharged to home on the day of surgery.

Other total joint replacement procedures (e.g., total knee and hip replacement) can be done on an outpatient basis. Creation of standardized pathways for these procedures would be similar to what we have undertaken for our outpatient TSR pathway: standardization of patient care based on the best available evidence that can be practically applied to the clinical practice, adequate control of postoperative pain to allow for outpatient discharge, and a multimodal analgesic regimen using primarily nonopioid analgesic agents postdischarge.

There are several implications for outpatient TSR pathways. For these pathways to be successful on a nationwide basis, use of peripheral brachial plexus nerve block for TSR will need to increase dramatically because only 42% of TSR surgical patients currently receive a peripheral nerve block.[6] Transition from inpatient to outpatient TSR would create significant cost savings in our healthcare system. Further study is needed to refine patient selection and determine long-term outcomes. Ideally a randomized controlled trial comparing inpatient to outpatients TSR would be conducted.

In summary, we describe the development of a successful outpatient TSR pathway in selected patients. The pathway standardized care of these patients and was based on the available current literature. The key anesthesia component of outpatient TSR is the use of a long-acting peripheral brachial plexus nerve block, which may provide up to 24 hours of analgesia postoperatively.

Acknowledgments

The HSS outpatient total shoulder pathway development team includes: Brad Crerar, PA (Sports Surgery), Danielle Edwards, PT (Physical Therapy), Wayne Edwards, PA (Sports Surgery), Geri DiLorenzo, RN (Nursing), Lawrence Gulotta, MD (Sports Surgery), Vaughn Hansen, RN (Nursing), Keesha Holmes, RN (Nursing), Kimberly Jean-Louis, RN (Value Management), Eden Kalman (Food and Nutrition), Greg Liguori, MD (Anesthesiology), Linda Russell, MD (Medicine), Rachelle Schwartz, RN (Case Management), Sharlynn Tuohy, PT (Physical Therapy), Peter Vouyoukliotis, Pharm.D. (Pharmacy), and Jacques Yadeau, MD, PhD (Anesthesiology).

References

1. Shoulder Joint Replacement. https://orthoinfo.aaos.org/en/treatment/shoulder-joint-replacement/. Accessed February 22, 2021.
2. Ahmed AF, Hantouly A, Toubasi A, et al. The safety of outpatient total shoulder arthroplasty: a systematic review and meta-analysis. *Int Orthop.* 2021;45:697–710.
3. Harris AB, Best MJ, Weiner S, Gupta HO, Jenkins SG, Srikumaran U. Hospital readmission rates following outpatient versus inpatient shoulder arthroplasty. *Orthopedics.* 2020;1:1–5. https://doi.org/10.3928/01477447-20200925-03.
4. Richman JM, Liu SS, Courpas G, et al. Does continuous peripheral nerve block provide superior pain control to opioids? A meta-analysis. *Anesth Analg.* 2006;102:248–257.
5. Liu SS, Strodtbeck WM, Richman JM, Wu CL. A comparison of regional versus general anesthesia for ambulatory anesthesia: a meta-analysis of randomized controlled trials. *Anesth Analg.* 2005;101:1634–1642.

6. Gabriel RA, Nagrebetsky A, Kaye AD, Dutton RP, Urman RD. The patterns of utilization of interscalene nerve blocks for total shoulder arthroplasty. *Anesth Analg.* 2016;123:758–761.
7. YaDeau JT, Dines DM, Liu SS, et al. What pain levels do TSA patients experience when given a long-acting nerve block and multimodal analgesia? *Clin Orthop Relat Res.* 2019;477:622–632.
8. Chan JJ, Cirino CM, Vargas L, et al. Peripheral nerve block use in inpatient and outpatient shoulder arthroplasty: a population-based study evaluating utilization and outcomes. *Reg Anesth Pain Med.* 2020;45:818–825.
9. Kirksey MA, Haskins SC, Cheng J, Liu SS. Local anesthetic peripheral nerve block adjuvants for prolongation of analgesia: a systematic qualitative review. *PLoS One.* 2015;10:e0137312.
10. Liu SS, Gordon MA, Shaw PM, Wilfred S, Shetty T, YaDeau JT. A prospective clinical registry of ultrasound-guided regional anesthesia for ambulatory shoulder surgery. *Anesth Analg.* 2010;111:617–623.

CHAPTER 57

A Case Study: National Emergency Laparotomy Audit

Emma Stevens, MB BChir, FRCA ■ Carolyn Johnston, BM BCh, MA (Oxon), FRCA ■ Dave Murray, MBBS, BSc, FRCA, MMed

KEY POINTS

- The National Emergency Laparotomy Audit (NELA) collects perioperative data on patients undergoing emergency bowel surgery (emergency laparotomy) from 179 hospitals across England and Wales (2020 figures).
- Data are used nationally, providing real time hospital-level benchmarked performance reports and informing quality improvement programs.
- Outcomes after emergency laparotomy have improved annually since the inception of the audit in 2012.

Introduction

Approximately 30,000 emergency laparotomies are performed annually in England and Wales.[1] In 2012 the UK Emergency Laparotomy Network reported that emergency laparotomies were associated with substantial mortality, and significant variation in outcomes between hospitals and in different patient groups, particularly the elderly or frail. In 2012 the 30-day mortality rate for this procedure in the UK was reported as 14.8%, rising to 24.4% in patients aged 80 or over.[2,3] That mortality rate was very similar to the rate reported in the United States in 2012, using data from the National Surgical Quality Improvement Program.[4]

The National Emergency Laparotomy Audit (NELA) was commissioned by the National Health Service (NHS) Healthcare Quality Improvement Partnership (HQIP) and funded by NHS England and Wales to collect national data with a dual purpose: to benchmark care and risk-adjusted outcomes against published national standards to provide quality assurance and to contribute to quality improvement (QI). NELA facilitates improvements in care by supporting clinicians in using data to reduce variation in processes of care, aid the implementation of best practice, and thus improve outcomes.

Methods

NELA is a continuous audit of prospective patient-level process and outcome measures. Cases are entered by local clinical teams via a dedicated secure website from 179 hospitals across England and Wales (https://data.nela.org.uk/). They are linked to national data sets from Hospital Episode Statistics (HES) and the Office for National Statistics (ONS), adjusted for case-mix, and reported at a named hospital-level. The multidisciplinary Project Team is based at the Royal College of Anaesthetists' Health Services Research Centre, partnered with the Royal College of Surgeons' Clinical

Effectiveness Unit. Stakeholder input is provided by a clinical reference group, including lay representation.

The metrics used for data collection (Tables 57.1 and 57.2) are selected from perioperative best practice recommendations published by the English Royal College of Surgeons, National Institute for Health and Care Excellence, National Confidential Enquiry into Patient Outcome and Death, and the UK and Ireland Association of Surgeons.[5,6]

Comparative information on these process and outcome measures are reported in a variety of publicly available formats and granularity:

- Risk-adjusted outcomes published in annual national report accompanied by a hospital-specific annual report, supported by patient-focused infographics
- Quarterly reports published publicly at provider and regional levels
- These are supplemented by additional dashboards available to healthcare providers behind a firewall to ensure patient confidentiality
- Real-time online dashboard with time series data of key process measures and outcomes, and comparators with regional and national averages, and similar-sized peers (Figs. 57.1 and 57.2). Data can be displayed in a run chart or statistical process control (SPC; I or P chart, depending on the data type) format.

TABLE 57.1 ■ **Examples of Process Measures Relating to Timeliness of Care Throughout the Perioperative Pathway and Delivery of Care Guided by Assessment of Risks of Complications and Death Including Percentages Reported in Year 1 Compared With Year 6**

	Year 1	Year 6
Computed tomography (CT) scans reported by an in-house consultant radiologist before surgery	68%	62%[a]
Access to operating rooms within a time frame appropriate for the urgency of surgery	80%	83%
Documented assessment, before surgery, of the risks of surgery	56%	84%
Presence of consultant surgeon and anesthetist in operating room for high-risk patients	70%	88.5%
Admission to critical care after surgery for high-risk patients	64%	85%
Assessment by a "scare of the older person" specialist for those aged 65+ and frail (or aged 80+)	10%[b]	28.8% (30%)

[a]This metric only includes in-house consultant reporting for Year 6, whereas Year 1 also included outsourced reports.
[b]In Year 1, this was measured for patients aged over 70 years.

TABLE 57.2 ■ **Outcome Measures Published at Hospital Level**

	Year 1	Year 6
Risk-adjusted postoperative 30-day mortality (%)	11.7	9.3
Unplanned return to theatre (%)	10	5
Length of hospital stay (days)	18.1	15.4[a]

[a]Reduction in length of stay representing annual savings estimated at £38,000,000 BP/$51,000,000 USD.

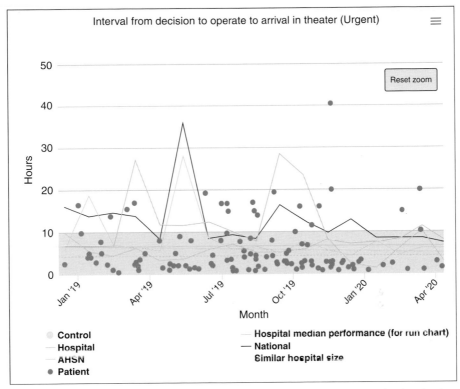

Fig. 57.1 **Example of data output.** This includes patient-level data to track outliers, regional, national, and same size comparators. It also includes control limits and median lines to create a control or run chart. Lines can be toggled on/off for clarity. *AHSN,* Academic Health Service Networks. (From National Emergency Laparotomy Audit Online Dashboard, 2021, with permission from the Healthcare Quality Improvement Partnership, London.)

- Live exponentially weighted moving average (EWMA) charts provide running information on risk-adjusted hospital-level mortality (Fig. 57.3).
- Exception and excellence reporting, detailing the care of high-risk patients, patients who have died in hospital, and patients who have received all the key standards of care

NELA promotes the use of data for QI. Over time, reporting of data has evolved and NELA was one of the first of the NHS National Audit Programme audits to provide real-time data to users. The annual report remains an important tool for quality assurance, interrogation of trends, and national recommendations; however, the recent strategy to supplement this lengthy annual document with more focused, timely outputs has been effective at facilitating data-driven QI.

The NELA website (https://www.nela.org.uk/) hosts a wealth of resources (toolkits, pathway examples, presentations from national conferences) sharing successes from local sites and examples of best practice.

Nationally, NELA has promoted multispecialty involvement from across specialty groups, including emergency medicine and radiology, as well as surgery, anesthetics, and critical care. Importantly, although NELA facilitates improvement initiatives, service improvements are developed, delivered, and funded locally by care providers.

The UK National Clinical Audits (NCAs) have shaped changes in the way clinical care is delivered, but direct measurement of impact remains difficult. The HQIP framework can be applied to look for specific evidence that an audit has effects at national, local, system, and public levels.[7]

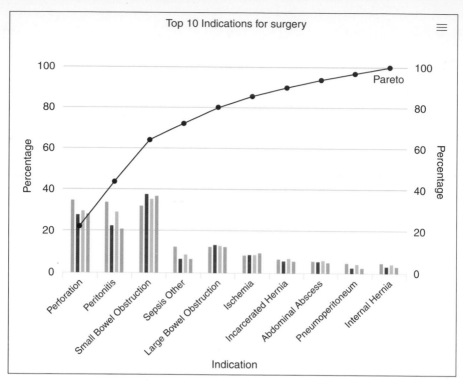

Fig. 57.2 Example of data output. Comparison of indications for surgery, including national, regional, and similar sized trust comparators, and Pareto chart element. (From National Emergency Laparotomy Audit Online Dashboard, 2021, with permission from the Healthcare Quality Improvement Partnership, London.)

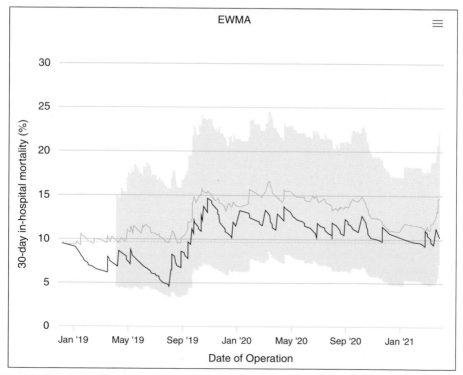

Fig. 57.3 Example of data output. EWMA (exponentially weighted moving average) mortality chart, showing local and national mortality trends, with moving real-time control limits. (From National Emergency Laparotomy Audit Online Dashboard, 2021, with permission from the Healthcare Quality Improvement Partnership, London.)

NATIONAL

Annual reports generated using NELA data describe year-on-year improvements in process and outcome measures. This form of reporting facilitates analysis of national trends and allows the project team to put forward recommendations to help teams improve their outcomes locally.

The generation of peer-reviewed research publications using NELA data and the support of research studies, such as Flo-ela,[8] contributes to the creation of an evidence base for best practice. Using data to produce a risk prediction model specific for patients undergoing emergency laparotomy has enabled the production of accurate risk-adjusted hospital-level postoperative mortality, which can be used to support benchmarking and QI.[9]

In the 6 years of reporting between 2012 and 2020, NELA has collected data on over 140,000 patients. Over the same time, significant improvements have been seen in 30-day mortality (see Table 57.2) and advances have also been seen in other measured processes (see Table 57.1).

LOCAL

The use of an accessible and adaptable platform is crucial to supporting teams to use real-time data to drive change. The NELA dashboard is regularly updated based on user feedback to maximize its use. It is locally adaptable and helps teams benchmark their performance against similar-sized peers and regional and national data.

Sharing of ideas and solutions at a local level is strongly encouraged and facilitated by NELA by promoting examples of good practice within regional collaboratives and on a national level.

Examples of these improvement initiatives include:

1. The creation of an emergency laparotomy operating room "boarding card" to inform the perioperative team about high-risk patients and to ensure that patients have received the recommended treatment before surgery.[10]
2. Using novel mortality review processes to improve learning from deaths in emergency laparotomy patients.[11]
3. Using rectus sheath catheters to manage postoperative pain after emergency laparotomy.[12]

Supporting local delivery of QI goes beyond providing accessible data. The NELA project team has produced a wide variety of educational and training content with a focus on QI skills and tools that can be used to help teams make the most of their data. These resources include short videos outlining relevant core principles, which can help teams plan successful new initiatives (Fig. 57.4); hosting webinars on maximizing the use of the interactive dashboard; hosting topic-specific webinars on topics like sepsis and frailty; and providing workshops, which allow for a more in-depth discussion of QI methodology.

SYSTEM

The use of data to drive improvement is a key feature of national clinical audits, and this goal is often closely aligned with using the data for quality assurance. Reports generated by NELA help highlight deficiencies in the system and help teams recognize positive or negative outlying hospitals. This information is made available to both hospitals and quality regulatory bodies. The NELA project team can provide additional support and advice to hospitals falling outside the expected range of performance.

NELA data-sharing has provided essential support to other NHS-led improvement and innovation programs, such as Getting It Right First Time (GIRFT) and the Academic Health Service Networks (AHSN).

Best practice tariffs (BPTs) are financial incentives for hospitals in England to meet certain quality standards. The introduction of a BPT for emergency laparotomy uses NELA data to establish which providers are meeting the standards.

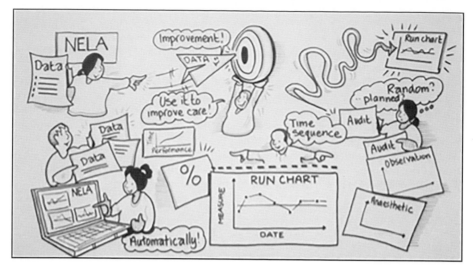

Fig. 57.4 Animations describing how National Emergency Laparotomy Audit (NELA) data can be used to drive local improvement (https://www.nela.org.uk/NELA-QI-Videos#pt).

PUBLIC

Patient involvement in NELA provides unique insights to deliver truly patient-centered care. Some hospitals have created "survivor clubs" to allow patients to share their experiences, which can inform pathway improvements and influence the evolving NELA data set.

The reports compiled by the NELA project team[13] are readily accessible online and publicized by national news outlets.[14,15] Open access publication demonstrates transparency and helps improvements and gaps in patient care, but it can be difficult to distil complex findings in an accessible way for the general population. Careful communication is required to ensure clarity in messaging.

Discussion

Over the last 10 years, data collected and entered into the NELA database have driven changes in care for patients undergoing emergency laparotomy at local and national levels. These changes have resulted in significantly improved outcomes with reduced mortality rates, reduced length of stay, and improvements in other measures (see Tables 57.1 and 57.2). This is particularly true of areas of care that are dependent on the practice of individual clinicians, where there is no additional financial cost to making a change.

The Enhanced Peri-Operative Care for High-Risk Patients (EPOCH)[16] study evaluated a QI intervention to implement an evidence-based bundle of care. They used NELA data to evaluate process and outcome measures and took ethnographic data from some participating hospitals. The process evaluation of the study[17] revealed that clinicians leading improvement were often working in very challenging contexts. Engaging colleagues and challenging and changing clinician behavior was seen to be important but often very difficult. Time and resource constraints within an organization were also highlighted as a key barrier.

Through the 7 years of the audit, "case ascertainment" has risen as a proportion of the total number of emergency laparotomy cases. This suggests that despite the many challenges to delivering emergency surgical care, data collection for the audit is sustainable and, in most hospitals, has become routine. The use of tariffs to incentivize delivery of better care has helped improve engagement from some stakeholders who had previously not engaged with NELA.

The NELA data set is reviewed regularly to reduce the burden of data collection. Some items within the data set are optional; these are not benchmarked nationally but are used for local improvement initiatives (e.g., sepsis data). The NELA data capture platform has been used to collect data for complimentary research studies (Flo-ela,[8] the Emergency Laparotomy Collaborative,[18] ALPINE[19]) and has a locally adaptable data collection area, which some hospitals have used to collect data on ventilation and postoperative pain to inform their local improvement work. The work developed in NELA has also helped inform international guidelines to improve care for patients undergoing emergency laparotomy.[20]

Limitations

The majority of the NELA data set is potentially available from other NHS databases or electronic patient records (EPRs), yet data collection remains dependent on entry by clinical teams. NELA links directly to routine NHS databases but only after the end of the audit data collection year because of information governance and financial constraints. Hence there is some "tension" between the desire for near-real-time reporting and linkage with other data sources to reduce burden of data collection. More frequent data flows between routine data sets, or unified NHS EPRs, would potentially reduce the burden of data collection for clinical teams.

The quality of analysis generated by the NELA data set is dependent on the quality of the data that is entered. "Time stamp" data (e.g., date and time of computed tomography [CT] scan report) have been harder to capture than datapoints requiring yes/no answers. This has limited the ability of NELA to provide high-quality data on some areas of care.

Other areas of care have been more resistant to change, especially organizational elements and those related to how the emergency surgical service "fits" in with other hospital activity, such as access to operating rooms.

NELA's data set has, to date, predominantly concentrated on the immediate perioperative pathway, reflecting the emphasis of published standards available at the time of NELA's commissioning. NELA data has highlighted ongoing concerns over provision of care in the following areas:

- The "front of house" pathway, from admission to the point at which the decision is made for surgery
- Management of patients with sepsis and suspected sepsis
- Timely access to operating rooms, especially for the most urgent patients

Emergency laparotomy patients represent a heterogenous population delivered by a wide range of providers (i.e., small district hospital vs. large tertiary referral centers). A continuous national audit and its associated data set is a relatively blunt tool. It is likely that smaller sprint audits, with bespoke data sets that advance local healthcare provision, can better drive improvement in these areas.

A further limitation is the cost associated with external collaborators wishing to access the data for secondary research. There are understandably rigorous processes in place to give teams the opportunity to apply for use of this data. These include assessing the validity of the request, ensuring that legal information governance requirements have been met, and providing data processing by the NELA project team. The costs for local teams can be a significant barrier in preventing the wider use of NELA data.

Improvements are still needed nationally to increase access to healthcare professionals in the multidisciplinary team like physiotherapists and dieticians. Inclusion of patient-reported outcome measures and pain management metrics are being explored, as are enhanced recovery programs for emergency surgery.

Conclusion

By using data for both quality assurance and QI, NELA has resulted in national improvements in mortality and other outcomes. Recent adaptions to more bespoke, timely, and granular data outputs have facilitated local QI. NELA will continue to evolve and change its recorded metric and outputs to reflect the changing nature of the challenge of providing care for this heterogeneous and high-risk group of patients.

References

1. RCoA. Fourth patient report of the National Emergency Laparotomy Audit (NELA) project team; 2018. https://www.nela.org.uk/downloads/The%20Fourth%20Patient%20Report%20of%20the%20National%20Emergency%20Laparotomy%20Audit%202018%20-%20Full%20Patient%20Report.pdf. Accessed November 9, 2021.
2. Saunders DI, Murray D, Pichel AC, Varley S, Peden CJ. Variations in mortality after emergency laparotomy: the first report of the UK emergency laparotomy network. *Br J Anaesth*. 2012;109(3):368–375. https://doi.org/10.1093/bja/aes165.
3. Symons NR, Moorthy K, Almoudaris AM, et al. Mortality in high-risk emergency general surgical admissions. *Br J Surg*. 2013;100(10):1318–1325. https://doi.org/10.1002/bjs.9208.
4. Al-Temimi MH, Griffee M, Enniss TM, et al. When is death inevitable after emergency laparotomy? Analysis of the American College of Surgeons National Surgical Quality Improvement Program database. *J Am Coll Surg*. 2012.
5. Royal College of Surgeons of England. Emergency surgery. Standards for unscheduled surgery. https://www.rcseng.ac.uk/library-and-publications/rcs-publications/docs/emergency-surgery-standards-for-unscheduled-care/. Accessed November 9, 2021.
6. The Royal College of Surgeons. *The high risk surgical patient*. Raising the standard; 2018.
7. Oliver CM, Hare S. What do perioperative national clinical audits tell us? The evolving role of national audits in changing practice and improving outcomes. *BJA Education*. 2019;19(10):334–341. https://doi.org/10.1016/j.bjae.2019.05.004.
8. FLOELA. Welcome—FLuid Optimisation in Emergency LAparotomy Trial [Internet]; 2021. https://floela.org/.
9. Eugene N, Oliver CM, Bassett MG, et al. Development and internal validation of a novel risk adjustment model for adult patients undergoing emergency laparotomy surgery: the National Emergency Laparotomy Audit risk model. *Br J Anaesth*. 2018;121(4):739–748. https://doi.org/10.1016/j.bja.2018.06.026.
10. Abstracts. *Anaesthesia*. 2020;75(S2):9–98. DOI: https://doi.org/10.1111/anae.14953.
11. Richards SK, Cook TM, Dalton SJ, Peden CJ, Howes TE. The 'Bath Boarding Card': a novel tool for improving pre-operative care for emergency laparotomy patients. *Anaesthesia*. 2016;71(8):974–976.
12. Abstracts. *Anaesthesia*. 2019;74:9–79. DOI: https://doi.org/10.1111/anae.14540.
13. National Emergency Laparotomy Audit. Reports; 2021. https://www.nela.org.uk/reports.
14. *The Independent. UK hospital has 40 per cent death rate after abdominal ops*. https://www.independent.co.uk/life-style/health-and-families/health-news/uk-hospital-has-40-cent-death-rate-after-abdominal-ops-8160924.html.
15. BBC News. Bowel surgery death rate warning; 2021. https://www.bbc.co.uk/news/health-33308262.
16. Peden CJ, Stephens T, Martin G, et al. Enhanced Peri-Operative Care for High-risk patients (EPOCH) trial group. *Lancet*. 2019.
17. Stephens TJ, Peden CJ, Pearse RM, et al. Improving care at scale: process evaluation of a multi-component quality improvement intervention to reduce mortality after emergency abdominal surgery (EPOCH trial). *Implement Sci*. 2018;13:142.
18. Aggarwal G, Peden CJ, Mohammed MA, et al. Emergency Laparotomy Collaborative. *JAMA Surg*. 2019;20:e190145.
19. ALPINE: Adoption of Lung Protective ventilation IN patients undergoing Emergency laparotomy. http://www.uk-plan.net/ALPINE. Accessed November 9, 2021.
20. Peden CJ, Aggarwal G, Aitken RJ, et al. Guidelines for Perioperative Care for Emergency Laparotomy Enhanced Recovery After Surgery (ERAS). Society Recommendations: part. 1–4.

CHAPTER 58

Provider Resilience and Caring for the Carer

Geeta Aggarwal, MBBS, MRCP, FRCA ■ Nial Quiney, MBBS, FRCA

KEY POINTS

- Resilience is needed, both individually and for an organization.
- To improve staff resilience, promote a culture of wellness in the organization and include executive buy-in.
- Developing data on risk of burnout in staff, using validated inventories, can help.
- A community that enhances support networks is vital.
- Self-awareness and mindfulness training should be provided to all healthcare workers.

Background

The term *resilience* can be defined as "the ability of an individual (or a system) to provide adaptations that are needed to produce good outcomes, both when the conditions are favorable and when they are not."[1] A resilient person can bounce back from any adversity and cope with challenging situations, both in and out of work, with ease.

Media stories on the topic of mental health and resilience are becoming more common. Olympic athletes withdrawing from games because of mental health problems,[2] celebrities committing suicide, and the effects of the COVID-19 pandemic on mental health around the world have all been reported.[3,4] Occupations such as fire fighters, police officers, military teams, and healthcare workers require a high degree of resilience. Resilience is required not only in the individual but also in the organization. For example, it is thought that health care can be made safer not only by addressing unanticipated events but also through a culture of improved resilience in the workforce.[1] In health care, adaptability and resilience are key to enhancing the quality of care delivered and the sustainability of the workforce.[1,5,6]

Burnout, Resilience, and the Quality and Safety of Health Care

Health care is a physically, intellectually, and emotionally demanding profession, so healthcare workers require a high level of resilience.[5,6] Healthcare workers are exposed to high-pressure, stressful situations repeatedly and, as a result, burnout can ensue. Low morale, increased disengagement, and decreased empathy both decrease patient safety, productivity, and the quality of patient care and increase the number of errors.[5-7]

The quality of health care, healthcare costs, and workforce wellbeing are all now found to be critically linked, and changes in one area will affect others.[8]

Psychological safety is a very important aspect of burnout and resilience. Staff need to feel safe in their place of work. An open and transparent culture, where people feel that they can ask for help, admit mistakes, and not be punished for raising concerns, needs to be supported.[1] Cultivating personal and organizational resilience by reducing burnout risk and improving the working environment is important for any perioperative clinician, department, or organization to thrive.

Resilience can be taught, both to an individual and to an organization, but it is important that individuals recognize stress and understand their own responses to stress. Many of us ignore the signs of stress, such as irritability, fatigue, and the feeling of being overwhelmed with difficulty concentrating,[9] in the hope that these issues will go away or get better with baseline adaptation skills.[8] This, in turn, increases the risk of cardiovascular disease, suicide, clinical depression, and substance abuse. Stress can lead to cognitive error and moral distress.

Creating a Culture of Resilience, Wellness, and "Joy in Work"

Promoting a culture of wellness in the organization improves resilience and a better quality of care. A white paper from the Institute of Healthcare Improvement (IHI) titled *Joy In Work*[7] reviews and outlines ways of improving the "joy in work."

The paper uses quality improvement methodology to construct a framework of cultural wellness. The nine components are:

1. Physical and psychological safety
2. Meaning and purpose
3. Autonomy and choice
4. Recognition and reward
5. Participative management
6. Teamwork and working together
7. Daily improvement
8. Wellness and resilience
9. Real-time measurement

There are also a few key actions to promote resilience:

- Obtain executive buy-in for a commitment to embrace cultural wellness.
- Add cultural wellness to the organization's strategic aims (this can take time to achieve).
- Appoint a lead person to promote wellness and resilience.
- Identify priorities and help staff to articulate ideas and solutions.
- Create a measure of wellness and the risk of burnout. There are many simple questionnaires that can be carried out to assess the risk of burnout and to obtain a baseline. The Oldenburg Burnout Inventory and the Maslach Burnout Inventory are examples of surveys that can be performed.[10,11]

Many interventions have been described to improve cultural wellness. Easy wins revolve around flexibility of work and on-call arrangements. Involving healthcare providers to identify their specific "stones in my shoes" issues is an important technique to identify potentially useful strategies for different environments. Involving individuals in developing solutions also starts to provide them with a sense of control over their work environment, leading to greater job satisfaction.

Forums for prioritizing and planning are useful and will deliver change more readily than "corridor conversations." Peer support, especially after adverse events, and recognition of outstanding contributions should be promoted. Communication across all team members should also be encouraged with multidisciplinary working and more specific tools, such as Schwartz rounds and Balint groups.[8,12]

Development of a Local Intervention

Some of the interventions described earlier were used in the Anaesthetic Department at Royal Surrey County Hospital, UK before the COVID-19 pandemic. The Wellbeing in Work Initiative (WinWin) project was set up with teaser posters put across the department to try to get staff interested (Fig. 58.1). Data were collected across all staff groups. Two means of data collection were

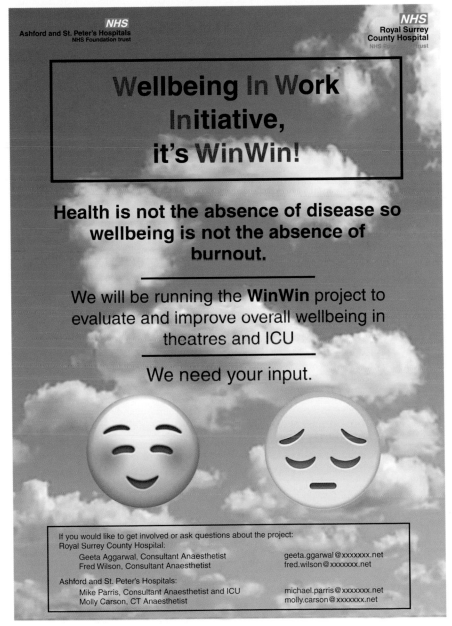

Fig. 58.1 Launch of Wellbeing In Work Initiative. *ICU,* Intensive care unit.

used. First, boxes were placed outside the operating room complex exit with a pot of small plastic discs. One box had a happy face icon and the other a sad face icon. This was done to obtain coarse data on how people felt at the end of the day. Second, the Oldenburg Inventory was perfomed[10] with extra demographic data and number of years of working in the department collected. A further question was added: "Would you recommend the department as a place to work?" This was marked out of 10, with 10 being most likely to recommend the department as a place of work.

On the basis of ideas collected and feedback, rest areas were refurbished and discussions held with staff on the importance of taking regular breaks to feel refreshed because staff rest emerged as an important issue. A sub project called "ScrubHero" was initiated (Fig. 58.2). This was a recognition program, where every week peers voted for their colleagues if that person had gone "above and beyond the call of duty" that week. Local companies donated prizes for this, and the winner each week was commended both within the department and on social media (Fig. 58.3). Allowing staff to publicly recognize colleagues when they had worked hard encouraged them and others to be more engaged in the workplace.

The IHI white paper describes a conversation guide as to how leaders should ask colleagues at all levels "What matters to you?" alongside asking "What's the matter?" to better understand the barriers to working well and to enjoyment of work.[7] Staff who do not feel that they can make a difference to their workplace and do not feel listened to are more prone to burnout. The final aspect of the WinWin project was developing "What matters to you?" forums. Questions were set for staff who came individually to speak, as set out in the *Joy in Work* paper:

- What makes a good day for you?
- What makes you proud to work here?
- When we are at our best, what does that look like?

The aim was to learn from staff and listen without time pressure, something that can be very challenging in a busy healthcare environment. It was not a forum for sorting out problems or solutions.

Discussion

The current state of health care, including pressures of the COVID-19 pandemic, has threatened the mental health and stability of providers, and this appears not to be confined to one hospital system or country, but to be a huge issue internationally. Burnout of staff in health care is endemic; staff are withdrawing from health care, leaving thousands of gaps across the workforce, and urgent work needs to be done to stop this.

Two important issues have been identified for preventing burnout and retaining staff by Epstein and Krasner.[8] The first is that physicians are increasingly isolated in their work. This is because of the physical and social distancing required during the pandemic, as well as emotional isolation because of having less time to listen and to talk to each other about problems and to develop personal connections. There is a need and a real benefit in developing a community to enhance support networks.[8] The second aspect is that physicians do not always give themselves permission to look after themselves. They find it difficult to respond to their own needs.[8] Self-awareness, resilience, and mindfulness training are lacking, both individually and within the organization. When issues are shared, it creates a feeling of togetherness, regardless of whether a solution is found for that problem. When staff feel that they can feedback, without retribution and blame, and feel listened to, trust is built and psychological safety increases.[13]

In summary, physicians who care for themselves can care better for others and are less likely to leave their practice early. Investing in resilience is likely to develop an organization with better quality of care and less error.

NHS
Ashford and St. Peter's Hospitals
NHS Foundation trust

Royal Surrey County Hospital NHS
NHS Foundation trust

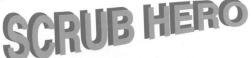

SCRUB HERO

Starts 17th September

We want to recognise and celebrate those using heroes. Has someone gone above and beyond to help a patient? Has someone gone out of their way to brighten your day?

Any number of staff who work in theatres or critical care can be nominated.

There will be a winning #ScrubHero every day for the first week and thereafter once a week

#ScrubHero nomination forms can be found in the main theatre department and intensive care unit coffee rooms.

Please fill out a nomination form with:

- Today's date
- Who you are nominating
- Why you are nominating them

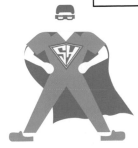
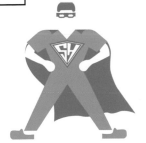

**Brought to you by the
Wellbeing in Work Initiative**

Fig. 58.2 ScrubHero poster.

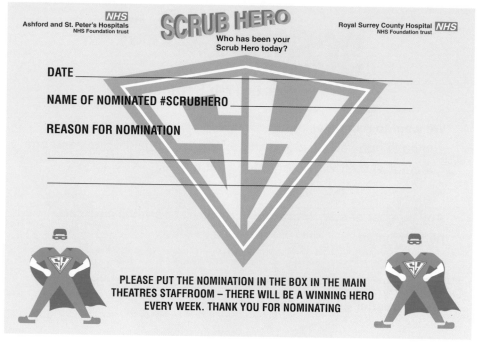

Fig. 58.3 Nomination form for ScrubHero.

References

1. Smith AF, Plunkett E. People, systems and safety: resilience and excellence in healthcare practice. *Anaesthesia.* 2019;74(4):508–517.
2. The Conversation. Tokyo 2020: Simone Biles' withdrawal is a sign of resilience and strength. https://theconversation.com/tokyo-2020-simone-biles-withdrawal-is-a-sign-of-resilience-and-strength-165287.
3. Covid-19: two fifths of doctors say pandemic has worsened their mental health. *BMJ.* 2020;371:m4148. https://www.bmj.com/content/371/bmj.m4148.
4. Panchal N, Kamal R, Cox C, Garfield R. The Implications of Covid-19 for mental health and substance use; 2021. https://www.kff.org/coronavirus-covid-19/issue-brief/the-implications-of-covid-19-for-mental-health-and-substance-use/.
5. West CP, Dyrbye LN, Erwin J, Shanafelt TD. Interventions to prevent and reduce physician burnout: a systematic review and meta-analysis. *Lancet.* 2016;388:2272–2281.
6. Salyers MP, Bonfils KA, Luther L, et al. The relationship between professional burnout and quality and safety in healthcare: a meta-analysis. *J Gen Intern Med.* 2017;32:475–482.
7. Perlo J, Balik B, Swensen S, et al. IHI Framework for Improving Joy in Work. IHI White Paper. Cambridge, MA: Institute for Healthcare Improvement; 2017. http://www.ihi.org/resources/Pages/IHIWhitePapers/Framework-Improving-Joy-in-Work.aspx.
8. Epstein RM, Krasner MS. Physician resilience: what it means, why it matters and how to promote it. *Acad Med.* 2013;88:301–303.
9. NHS. Stress. https://www.nhs.uk/mental-health/feelings-symptoms-behaviours/feelings-and-symptoms/stress/.

10. Oldenburg burnout inventory. http://www.goodmedicine.org.uk/sites/default/files/assessment%2C%20burnout%2C%20olbi.pdf.
11. Maslach C, Jackson SE, Leiter MP. Maslach burnout inventory: third edition. In: Zalaquett CP, Wood RKJ, eds. Evaluating Stress: A Book of Resources. Scarecrow Education; 1997:191–218.
12. Pepper JR, Jaggar SI, Mason MJ, et al. Schwartz Rounds: reviving compassion in modern healthcare. *J R Soc Med.* 2012;105(3):94–95.
13. Martin A. The Changing Nature of Leadership. Center for Creative Leadership; 2007. https://files.eric.ed.gov/fulltext/ED488741.pdf.

CHAPTER 59

Nursing and Perioperative Quality Improvement

Angie Balfour, RN, MSc

KEY POINTS

- Evidence-based medicine, quality improvement (QI), and clinical research are three cornerstones of perioperative nursing.
- Nurse education and empowerment is crucial to ensure best practice.
- Multidisciplinary teamwork is essential for optimal patient care.
- Communication is key among all perioperative clinicians to ensure safe and patient-centered care.
- Nurses are central to ensuring personalization of perioperative care.

Introduction

The term "perioperative medicine" (POM) is often used to describe the patient-centered, multidisciplinary, and integrated clinical care of patients from the moment of contemplation of surgery until full recovery has been achieved. Perioperative care has changed a great deal over the last two decades, in large part because of evidence-based initiatives such as "enhanced recovery after surgery" (ERAS) programs,[1] minimally invasive surgery,[2] and continuous developments in opioid-sparing techniques and regional blockade.[3] Nurses have been at the vanguard of these positive changes.

What Is a Perioperative Nurse?

The definition of POM varies and often focuses on the intraoperative period or the operating room (OR) as opposed to the continuum of surgical care described by Dean et al.[4] The role of the perioperative nurse has clearly adapted over the last few decades. In 1978 the definition of perioperative nursing published by the AORN House of Delegates stated, "The perioperative role of the operating room nurse consists of nursing activities performed by the professional operating room nurse during the preoperative, intraoperative, and postoperative phases of the patient's surgical experience."[5] In the mid 80s, however, the focus shifted toward perioperative nursing practice being associated with the intraoperative setting, and the key roles of circulator, scrub, and recovery room nurses were described.

As a result of this shift in the definition of perioperative nursing, the literature examining nursing care seems to focus more on care in the OR setting. Marsh et al.[6] conducted a survey among OR nurses examining perioperative nursing care and highlighted that there are instances of so-called "missed perioperative nursing care" elements. Most importantly, poor communication and coproduction between the team members was noted, two cornerstones of high-quality perioperative nursing care.[7,8] More recently, the literature has begun to define the role of the perioperative nurse as a more holistic one, occurring before, during, and after surgery. Anaba et al.[9] describe the role of the perioperative nurse in a tertiary hospital as including providing preoperative education, reducing patient anxiety throughout the perioperative journey, assisting during surgery, and delivering nursing care postoperatively.

Sadly, because the role of perioperative nurse is not well defined in the literature, this also becomes the case in nurse education programs. Many nursing schools do not include perioperative nursing as a specialty. Kapaale et al.[10] highlight current challenges in ensuring sufficient nursing workforce entering perioperative nursing. A lack of exposure often results in newly qualified nurses being unaware of the value of a career in perioperative nursing.

What Is the Role of the Nurse in Perioperative Quality Improvement?

Nursing engagement and input are critical to successful perioperative quality improvement (QI) because nurses are highly aware of the continuum of care for patients. Within this context, rigorous work to identify the root causes of poor-quality care notes that nurses routinely observe contributing defects in human factors, such as lack of leadership and communication.[11] These observations have fueled efforts to augment human factors training for nurses and other perioperative clinicians (Fig. 59.1).

Perioperative nurses use three essential components in everyday practice: evidence-based practice (EBP), QI, and nursing research (NR).[12] Perioperative nurses must monitor processes and

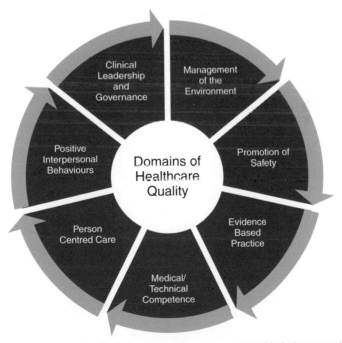

Fig. 59.1 The multiple domains of quality that a perioperative nurse must consider in the preparation for surgery, during surgery, and in postoperative care. (From Oldland E, Botti M, Hutchinson A, Redley B. A framework of nurses' responsibilities for quality health care—exploration of content validity. *Collegian*. 2020;27[2]:150–153.)

outcomes, review available data, and share relevant research. Perioperative nurses must be empowered to adapt and adjust their care practices in accordance with best evidence. Nurses lead care pathway change and QI efforts that best achieve cooperation, involvement, and empowerment of patients.[13] One frustration among many perioperative nurses is their lack of involvement in clinical change decisions that may deleteriously affect patient care. As key knowledge workers and care givers for patients, nursing insights provide needed data from patients regarding best care. For example, as "throughput" of patients in the perioperative space continues to grow in importance for health systems, many nurses have felt the patient has suffered at times with poor education and a lack of bespoke care. Postoperatively, patients are now expected to mobilize and eat much more quickly than before, and QI nursing has assured these changes have been feasible for patients.[14–16]

Following nurse-led QI and process change, perioperative nurses must require educational programs for nurse training and in-house induction programs. Rigorous QI work has noted the critical role of nurse education for successful EBP implementation.[17,18]

References

1. Thacker J. Overview of enhanced recovery after surgery. *Surg Clin North Am.* 2018;98(6):1109–1117.
2. Keller DS, et al. A new perspective on the value of minimally invasive colorectal surgery-payer, provider, and patient benefits. *Surg Endosc.* 2017;31(7):2846–2853.
3. Faculty of Pain and Medicine at the Royal College of Anaesthetists. Surgery and opioids: Best Practice Guidelines 2021. https://fpm.ac.uk/surgery-and-opioids-best-practice-guidelines-2021. Accessed June 24, 2021.
4. Dean HF, Carter F, Francis NK. Modern perioperative medicine—past, present, and future. *Innovative surgical sciences.* 2019;4(4):123–131.
5. AORN House of Delegates. Operating room nursing: perioperative role. *AORN J.* 1978;27:1156–1178.
6. Marsh V, et al. Nurses' perceptions of the extent and type of missed perioperative nursing care. *AORN J.* 2020;112(3):237–247.
7. Kehlet H. Enhanced postoperative recovery: good from afar, but far from good? *Anaesthesia.* 2020;75(S1): e54–e61.
8. Ljungqvist O, et al. Opportunities and challenges for the next phase of enhanced recovery after surgery: a review. *JAMA Surg.* 2021;156(8):775–784.
9. Anaba P, Anaba EA, Abuosi AA. Patient satisfaction with perioperative nursing care in a tertiary hospital in Ghana. *Int J Health Care Qual Assur.* 2020. Epub ahead of print.
10. Kapaale CC. Understanding value as a key concept in sustaining the perioperative nursing workforce. *AORN J.* 2018;107(3):345–354.
11. Peñataro-Pintado E, et al. Perioperative nurses' experiences in relation to surgical patient safety: a qualitative study. *Nurs Inq.* 2021;28(2), e12390-n/a.
12. Baker JD. Nursing research, quality improvement, and evidence-based practice: the key to perioperative nursing practice. *AORN J.* 2017;105(1):3–5.
13. Grocott MPW. Pathway redesign: putting patients ahead of professionals. *Clin Med (Lond).* 2019;19 (6):468–472.
14. Levy N, Mills P, Mythen M. Is the pursuit of DREAMing (drinking, eating and mobilising) the ultimate goal of anaesthesia? *Anaesthesia.* 2016;71(9):1008–1012.
15. Jeff A, Taylor C. Ward nurses' experience of enhanced recovery after surgery: a grounded theory approach. *Gastrointest Nurs.* 2014;12(4):23–31.
16. Ilott I, et al. How do nurses, midwives and health visitors contribute to protocol-based care? A synthesis of the UK literature. *Int J Nurs Stud.* 2010;47(6):770–780.
17. Foss M. Enhanced recovery after surgery and implications for nurse education. *Nurs Stand.* 2011; 25(45):35–39.
18. Byrne BE, et al. A protocol is not enough: enhanced recovery program-based care and clinician adherence associated with shorter stay after colorectal surgery. *World J Surg.* 2021;45(2):347–355.

CHAPTER 60

Certified Registered Nurse Anesthetists and Perioperative Medicine

Desiree Chappell, MSNA, CRNA ■ Jennifer Harpe-Bates, DNAP, APRN, CRNA ■
Wendy Odell, DNP, CRNA

KEY POINTS

- Certified registered nurse anesthetists (CRNAs) are well positioned within the perioperative care model to provide high-quality care throughout the surgical continuum.
- Many areas of practice within the profession of nurse anesthesia, including background, training, and personal care delivery, align with the delivery needs of perioperative medicine.
- The CRNA's perspective enables them to be effective leaders, champions, and active participants in the organization, planning, and delivery of perioperative medicine.

The Certified Registered Nurse Anesthetist Lens

The concept of "upstream thinking" is ingrained in nurses early in their education. Nurses attempt to avoid the downstream fallout of a particular condition by focusing on the origin of a pathophysiological problem and the relevant social concerns and not just reacting to the presenting illness. This concept necessarily involves and addresses health inequalities and population health, which, as presented in an earlier chapter, overlaps with perioperative medicine (POM). The foundational education and experience of certified registered nurse anesthetists (CRNAs) is rooted in this "upstream thinking" (i.e., not "reacting" but being "proactive" in caregiving). On the path to becoming a CRNA, many nurses witness postoperative complications first-hand, such as comforting a disoriented elderly patient, attempting to ease the intractable nausea and vomiting of a young woman, and denying a hungry patient food while awaiting bowel sounds to return. However, on becoming a CRNA, nurses are empowered to make decisions that directly impact those outcomes that they seemingly had no control over as a nurse. The problem was upstream. Now as a CRNA the nurse is working upstream, positioned to make an impact.

An additional aspect of CRNA training, rooted in the nursing background, is developing the ability and desire to provide patient education and to use empathetic communication with patients and colleagues. CRNAs enter anesthesia understanding the importance of multidisciplinary teamwork in patient care. This team-based experience creates an ideal opportunity for CRNAs to engage in interdepartmental education, helping healthcare teams recognize the importance that a multidisciplinary contribution brings to patient healing and recovery.

CRNAs can act as touchpoints in multiple phases of care as they monitor the evolution of the patient's condition across the surgical continuum. Many CRNAs lead or staff preadmission clinics, perform preoperative evaluations, deliver intraoperative care, collaborate care in the postanesthesia care unit, and often round on patients postoperatively. With this vantage point, CRNAs possess the ability to bridge disparate groups of clinicians brought together in perioperative care models. The value of the CRNA role in POM can be overlooked because of their clinical workload, but their work inside and outside of the operating room (OR) links physicians and nursing.

Implementation of Perioperative Medicine: The CRNA Perspective

Previous chapters offer an in-depth discussion and multiple examples of the "what, whys, and hows" of POM. Although there is no silver bullet or "secret sauce" to success, countless enhanced recovery after surgery (ERAS) programs and perioperative pathways are based on following the general principles of enhanced recovery and using implementation science and quality improvement (QI) to put these pathways into practice. The intent of this chapter is to highlight the CRNA's ability to adopt such principles and operationalize them. The CRNA's perspective enables them to be effective leaders, champions, and active participants in the organization, planning, and delivery of POM. This chapter also aims to inspire and empower fellow CRNA colleagues and all providers in the perioperative space to examine their practice and to ask these key questions:

- "Do I know my own outcomes?"
- "Can my practice be enhanced through perioperative medicine models?"
- "Can I, as a (insert provider type), use my training and experience to be the catalyst for better patient care?"

The following are three real-world examples of CRNA providers and their contribution to POM.

Example 1: "Being Part of the Bigger Picture"

A small team of providers (an anesthesiologist, general surgeon, advanced practice nurse, and a CRNA) developed, implemented, and disseminated the adoption of an ERAS initiative in a large community facility in 2015.

BACKGROUND

Within the hospital facility, routine postoperative rounds were performed by CRNAs approximately 24 hours after surgery. Commonly noted were differing states of recovery between different surgeons and patient types. Because of a lack of data, true quantitative outcomes were unknown, though it was assumed there was room for improvement. At the time, ERAS programs were reported to improve recovery by reducing length of stay (LOS), complications, and readmission rates, ultimately improving the value of care delivered by the hospital as a whole. Inspired by the work in the National Healthcare System of Great Britain (NHS)[1] and Henrik Kehlet,[2] an ERAS team was formed, organically derived from a small group of interested clinicians and driven by the Department of Anesthesiology Medical Director. The team reviewed the available research and evaluated its potential effectiveness for the patient population of the facility, located in Kentucky, ranked 44th in the United States for overall health of the population.[3]

METHODS

A standardized service line protocol was developed for colorectal patients. It included the major tenets of ERAS: preadmission testing (PAT) education, preoperative carbohydrate loading, nothing by mouth (NPO) for clear fluids 2 hours before surgery, multimodal pain management, intraoperative goal-directed fluid therapy, routine surgical site infection prevention, immediate postoperative regional anesthesia, and postoperative "DrEaMing" (patients no longer had lines or drains and were encouraged to "**Dr**ink **Ea**t and **M**obilize" within 24 hours of surgery).

The protocol was disseminated through printed materials, educational sessions, group meetings and one-on-one conversations. The program was highlighted by the hospital, and provider engagement was prioritized by designing internal marketing material for the clinicians and external patient-facing ERAS packets. Providers were empowered to follow the protocols, knowing their decisions would be supported based on those best practice guidelines. The hospital provided metrics of success, such as LOS data, readmission rates, discharge disposition, intensive care unit (ICU) admissions, blood bank costs, and pharmacy costs.

RESULTS

The ERAS program implementation was deemed a success by the hospital, providers, and patients. Anecdotally, through a sharing of patient experiences, postoperative cognitive delirium was reduced, and patient satisfaction improved. Compared with the previous year, there were significant improvements, including a reduction of LOS by half, reduction of readmission rates, increased disposition to home versus skilled nursing facilities (SNFs), reduction of surgical ICU admissions, and reduction in blood transfusions.

DISCUSSION

Organic formation and implementation of an ERAS initiative can work in a large-sized facility. The multidisciplinary approach was imperative to the success of the program. The unique perspective of each individual coming together to form a team ensured that all providers were considered in the workflows and process of implementation. Additionally, the team realized the need for teaching the whys of an intervention and not just order execution. The CRNA role was an asset on many levels, specifically when it came to integrating new protocols into practice, liaising between clinician groups, educating providers, advocating for the importance of communication, and encouraging overall provider empowerment. As stated earlier, CRNAs are uniquely suited to bridge the gap between physician and nursing clinical leaders and staff. The program worked through collaboration, engagement, education, and empowerment of all the providers throughout the perioperative continuum.

Example 2: "Drive to Excellence"

As part of a Doctoral of Nurse Anesthesia Practice program, a CRNA-led, acute pain management initiative was developed.

BACKGROUND

Providing a regional anesthesia component in the anesthesia plan of care for abdominal procedures addresses the need to reduce the overall opioid requirements of surgical patients throughout the continuum of care and to optimize pain control, which is a basic tenet of ERAS programs and POM models. An effective means of blocking pain to the abdominal wall, providing relief for abdominal procedures, is the use of the regional transversus abdominis plane (TAP) block. It has been demonstrated that the administration of TAP blocks decreases pain scores, reduces the incidence of postoperative nausea and vomiting, and reduces postoperative oral opioid consumption.[4]

METHODS

The project was designed to implement an educational program for TAP blocks for abdominal surgeries, as the regional component of a multifaceted anesthesia plan. The implementation of TAP blocks would be accomplished by the education of all stakeholders; however, foremost was the education of the surgeons via one-on-one communication regarding the benefits and risks of TAP blocks for their patients' postoperative pain control. Education of the perioperative staff included patient inclusion, TAP block process, and potential complications. The scope of the project also included the evaluation of CRNA practice regarding TAP blocks.

RESULTS

The desired outcome measure was the number of TAP blocks performed over time to gauge the project implementation. The electronic health record (EHR) was searched to obtain the number of TAP blocks performed monthly, starting with 2017. The first TAP blocks for the practice started in June of 2017 with three blocks during that month. Over the 7 months of 2017, the average monthly performance of TAP blocks was 27. With increasing education on TAP blocks for patients and healthcare staff, the average number of TAP blocks performed grew to 56 per month for 2018. For the first 6 months of 2019, the average number of monthly TAP blocks performed was 69, a 156% increase from 2017 to 2019 (Fig. 60.1).

The results of the TAP block survey revealed that a majority of the CRNAs had been practicing less than 5 years. Most of the CRNAs demonstrated proficiency in TAP blocks and felt comfortable performing the block and agreed on the need for reduction of opioid requirements. Before working with the group, 56% had not performed any TAP blocks (Table 60.1).

DISCUSSION

The implementation of a CRNA-led TAP block program through education of anesthesia staff, surgeons, patients, and perioperative staff resulted in a significant increase in the number of blocks performed. The education of anesthesia staff produced a 156% increase in placement of TAP blocks from 2017 to 2019. The development of a TAP block team was valuable for education and reassurance while learning the block. The TAP block program resulted in a positive practice change for anesthesia providers and will lead to other regional blocks being offered to patients to reduce overall opioid requirements. This CRNA-led project can be used as a model to introduce TAP blocks in any anesthesia practice setting, private or academic.

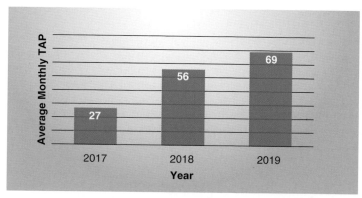

Fig. 60.1 Average number of transversus abdominis plane (*TAP*) blocks performed monthly, 2017 to 2019.

TABLE 60.1 ■ **CRNA TAP Block Survey Results**

CRNA TAP Block Survey	Survey Responses
How long have you been a CRNA?	☐ 15 years = 5 ☐ 10–15 years = 2 ☐ 5–10 years = 4 ☐ < 5 years = 12 ☐ < 1 year = 2
Have you performed TAP blocks before working here?	Yes = 44% No = 56%
I am comfortable performing TAP blocks.	88 % were comfortable performing TAP blocks
TAP blocks reduce the overall opioid requirements for most patients.	96% agreed TAP blocks reduce opioid requirements
I enjoy performing TAP blocks.	92% enjoyed performing TAP blocks
The PACU staff appreciate the patient having TAP blocks.	100% agreed the PACU staff appreciated the block.

CRNA, Certified registered nurse anesthetists; *PACU*, postanesthesia care unit; *TAP*, transversus abdominis plane.

Example 3: "Lead by Leading"

An anesthesia business executive recognized the impact of evidence-based anesthesia delivery and initiated enhanced recovery models throughout a national anesthesia management company footprint.

BACKGROUND

Having practiced in rural hospitals where opioid and methamphetamine abuse was epidemic and poverty-driven behaviors left patients unoptimized and at higher acuity risk, a CRNA leader championed enhanced strategies for recovery optimization in rural clinical settings. After leaving clinical practice, the CRNA leader pivoted into clinical operational leadership as the chief anesthetist officer (CAO) with a national anesthesia management company. Leading a spectrum of anesthesia teams with disparate practice patterns, the CAO motivated clinical teams to adopt enhanced recovery techniques and standardized practice to impact anesthesia delivery and optimize surgical outcomes.

METHOD

The CAO initially focused on rural teams within the larger anesthesia group that typically had limited resources. She outsourced educational companies to teach teams the importance of enhanced recovery, including on-site acute regional anesthesia training. A toolkit was developed for CRNAs to use in partnership with hospital departments, including pharmacy, physical therapy, and nursing services. This toolkit included protocols, sample order sets, educational materials, and supply acquisition and set-up processes. A data collection system was established to report metrics and outcomes to hospital surgical services and C-suite administration.

RESULTS

Of the rural facilities who implemented the toolkit, narcotic usage during the first 24 hours of surgery was eliminated to zero in over 70% of patients undergoing total joint replacement. LOS decreased to approximately 36 hours, outpacing Medicare's authorization to rehabilitation care transfers.

DISCUSSION

The successful toolkit was replicated in over 8 rural Texas facilities during a 2-year period. The CAO went on to partner with the anesthesia company's physician leadership to drive enhanced recovery education and program implementation throughout medium-large facilities across their national footprint. As of today, 100% of affiliated facilities have enhanced recovery protocols implemented in at least one service line.

Conclusion

CRNAs are well positioned to lead in the space of POM. This clinician group possesses an in-depth understanding of the intraoperative phase and interacts across much of the continuum. As with any culture change and initiative, challenges and barriers exist. Major barriers to CRNA involvement in POM are shown in Box 60.1.

CRNAs are well positioned in the healthcare system to work collaboratively and collegially with the POM multidisciplinary team. They can also be change agents during this formative time in health care.

One person can make a difference, and everyone should try

—JOHN F. KENNEDY

BOX 60.1 ■ CRNA Barriers to POM Involvement

1. A knowledge gap as to what POM is and how CRNAs fit into the broader picture.
2. How CRNAs can best use their talents, skillsets, and expertise to influence and lead clinical change
3. The business of anesthesia related to the impact of POM is unclear to many CRNAs
4. CRNAs do not realize the inherent value and unique perspective they offer as a provider group

---

To overcome these and other challenges, CRNAs should lean into their background and experience. In response to the aforementioned questions, CRNAs need to find answers outside of the operating room:

1. "Do I know my own outcomes?" If not, ask your chief CRNA or medical director. If the answer is still unclear, talk to the surgeon or nurse navigator for a specific service line, and if roadblocks persist, ask the director of quality.
2. "Can my practice be enhanced through perioperative medicine models?" If you or your colleagues are unsure of what POM is, do a quick literature review and educate yourself about the business of anesthesia and value-based care.
3. "Can I, as a (insert provider type), use my training and experience to be the catalyst for better patient care?" Refer to previous examples of CRNA leaders and find your voice to influence change.

CRNA, Certified registered nurse anesthetists; *POM,* perioperative medicine.

References

1. Enhanced Recovery Partnership Programme. Delivering enhanced recovery: helping patients to get better sooner after surgery. London, UK: Department of Health and Social Care; 2010. https://www.gov.uk/government/publications/enhanced-recovery-partnership-programme. Accessed September 12, 2021.
2. Kehlet H. Multimodal approach to control postoperative pathophysiology and rehabilitation. *Br J Anaesth.* 1997;78(5):606–617.
3. United Health Foundation. *America's Health Rankings composite measure*; 2015. AmericasHealthRankings.org.
4. Erdogan MA, Ozgul U, Uçar M, et al. Effect of transversus abdominis plane block in combination with general anesthesia on perioperative opioid consumption, hemodynamics, and recovery in living liver donors: the prospective, double-blinded, randomized study. *Clin Transplant.* 2017;31, e12931.

CHAPTER 61

Environmental Sustainability and Perioperative Quality Improvement

Emily H. Johnson, MD, MS ■ Benjamin H. Cloyd, MD, MIPH

KEY POINTS

- Sustainable quality improvement (QI) aims to deliver care that maximizes positive health outcomes through best use of environmental, social, and financial resources.
- Average global temperatures on earth are rising because of human activity.
- The US healthcare industry produces 8% to 10% of US greenhouse gases, at a rate of 1.51 tCO_2/capita, which is about twice as high as other nations with advanced healthcare systems.
- Perioperative spaces produce a disproportionate share of waste and emissions within hospitals, with evidence indicating the average surgical case produces about 200 kg of CO_2, equivalent to driving about 500 miles in an average vehicle.
- Readily achievable objectives, such as anesthetic gas optimization, efficient energy use, and device life prolongation, can significantly reduce the impact of perioperative care on the environment now.

Introduction

Quality improvement (QI) seeks to increase the value of health care by achieving the best outcomes through the best use of resources. Traditionally, this has been limited to financial and social resources. By expanding the definition of "available resources" to include environmental considerations, QI strategies offer a framework for approaching issues of environmental sustainability. Just as QI is currently used to target efficiency, cost, or patient safety, we can target greenhouse gas (GHG) emissions or waste as guiding goals to improve the value of health care. Thus the aim of *sustainable* QI is to deliver care in a way that maximizes positive health outcomes through best use of environmental, social, and financial resources, as illustrated in Fig. 61.1.[1]

Environmental Sustainability

Environmental sustainability can be defined as meeting current needs without compromising the ability of future generations to meet their own. This definition is broad and seeks to encompass all resources necessary for human thriving, including water, land, biodiversity, a stable climate, and others, which are collectively referred to as the planetary boundaries.

$$Value = \frac{Outcomes\ for\ patients\ \&\ populations}{Environmental + Social + Financial\ Impacts}$$
$$('Triple\ Bottom\ Line')$$

Fig. 61.1 Sustainable quality improvement. A formula for value within a sustainable quality improvement framework.

Climate Change

Climate change refers to change in average temperatures, precipitation and wind patterns because of rising atmospheric concentrations of GHGs, especially carbon dioxide (CO_2). GHGs exist naturally but are also generated by human activities. Atmospheric CO_2 levels have increased by 40% since preindustrial times and are presently at the highest concentrations reached in 800,000 years.[2] Because of these changes, there is virtual certainty that average temperatures on earth are rising and that this increase is because of human activity, primarily from burning fossil fuels. The downstream effects of higher GHG concentrations include intensified hurricanes, heat waves, droughts, precipitation, flooding, and sea level rise. Climate change is only one planetary boundary through which human impact is unsustainable, but currently it is the most urgent threat and will be the focus of this chapter on sustainability.

CLIMATE CHANGE AND HUMAN HEALTH

There is strong, growing evidence that climate change harms health. Through temperature-related illness, changes to air quality and respiratory illness, infectious disease-like vector and waterborne pathogens, extreme weather-related injury, malnutrition and food insecurity, and mental health disorders, climate change is already having profound effects on health worldwide.[3]

CLIMATE CHANGE AND HEALTH CARE

Like all industries, the US healthcare sector contributes to climate change. Health care in the United States produces 8% to 10% of US GHGs,[4] at 1.51 tCO_2/capita, which is about twice as high as many other nations with advanced healthcare systems like the UK (0.64 tCO_2/capita) and Canada (0.83 tCO_2/capita).[5] Through direct and indirect emissions, US health care is responsible for a significant burden of air pollution and public health damages from acidification, smog formation, respiratory disease from particulate matter, ozone depletion, and carcinogenic air toxins, estimated at 470,000 disability-adjusted life years lost annually.[6]

CLIMATE CHANGE AND PERIOPERATIVE SPACES

Perioperative spaces produce a disproportionate share of waste and emissions within hospitals because of anesthetic gas use, electricity requirements, and the perioperative supply chain. Inhaled anesthetic gases are potent GHGs responsible for 30% to 70% of a surgical procedure's total emissions and approximately 1% of all US healthcare emissions annually.[7,8] Operating rooms (ORs) are more energy intensive than other areas of a hospital, by square foot, because of the electricity intensity of lighting, ventilation, temperature, and sterilization needs. Finally, the perioperative supply chain, which includes all the reusable and disposable instruments, protective equipment, and devices necessary to perform procedures safely, contributes significantly to perioperative emissions. The clearest picture on current emission in surgery to date is a 2017 study from MacNeill et al., which compared perioperative spaces in three countries (UK, Canada, and the US).[9] Totaling direct and indirect emission sources, the average surgical case produces between 146 and 232 kg of CO_2 equivalents, comparable to driving more than 350 miles in an average vehicle (Fig. 61.2).

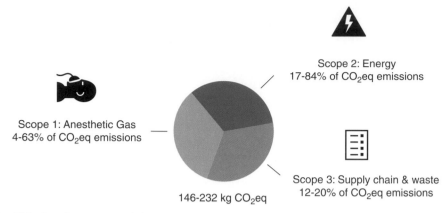

Fig. 61.2 Greenhouse gas emissions in perioperative spaces. The contribution of each greenhouse gas protocol scope to total perioperative emissions. Contributions from each scope varied between hospitals depending on the source of electricity (i.e., coal, renewable) and inhaled anesthetic gas usage.

MEASURING EMISSIONS

The first step to reducing emissions is to recognize and measure current emissions. The Greenhouse Gas Protocol is a formal accounting system used around the world in all industries to measure and report carbon emissions. Application of this framework is explored in Table 61.1.

Measures and Approaches

Here we describe several potential areas of focus for perioperative departments seeking to employ sustainable QI approaches to reduce environmental impact.

ANESTHETIC GASES

Problem

Inhaled anesthetic gases, unique to surgery, are potent GHGs and a major source of emissions in perioperative spaces. The GWP-20 (or the global warming potential of a gas over 20 years) for inhaled gases is provided in Table 61.2. Desflurane and isoflurane have thousands of times greater global warming potential than CO_2 by weight. These inhaled gases undergo very little metabolism and, in most cases, are vented directly into the atmosphere unchanged as waste gases.

TABLE 61.1 ■ Greenhouse Gas Protocol

Scope	Definition	Perioperative Application
Scope 1	Direct emissions from an organization	Anesthetic gases
Scope 2	Indirect emissions because of electricity consumption	Electricity use for heating, ventilation, air conditioning, lighting
Scope 3	All other indirect emissions occurring as a consequence of organization activities	Perioperative supply chain, waste disposal

TABLE 61.2 ■ **Comparing Inhaled Anesthetic Gases**[10,11]

Inhaled Gas	GWP_{20}[a]	CO_2eq/MAC-hour[b]
Carbon dioxide (reference)	1	-
Sevoflurane	349	8 miles
Isoflurane	1401	15 miles
Desflurane	3714	378 miles
Nitrous oxide	289	112 miles

[a]GWP_{20} indicates the 20-year global warming potential.
[b]CO_2eq/MAC-hour means the emissions of CO_2 equivalents per minute alveolar concentration hour of inhale anesthetic gas use, expressed in miles driven by standard vehicle (23.9 miles/gallon).

Opportunities

Recommendations for limiting this impact include reducing fresh gas flows to the lowest rate necessary for a given gas and situation and reserving desflurane and nitrous oxide to cases where they would reduce morbidity and mortality over other anesthetic choices. Additionally, hospitals can consider waste anesthetic gas capture technologies, some of which can be retrofitted to existing hospital scavenging and exhaust systems. In an effort to analyze the environmental impact of unexplained anesthesia practice variability, the QI arm of the Multicenter Perioperative Outcomes Group (MPOG) has created new "sustainability" quality metrics. SUS-01 is a sustainability metric for fresh gas flow that measures the percent of cases where mean gas flow of inhaled anesthetic gases is less than or equal to 3 L per minute.[12]

HEATING, VENTILATION, AND AIR CONDITIONING

Problem

Regulatory standards require ORs to meet strict temperature, humidity, and ventilation standards, which increase energy use.[13] Energy use in ORs is 3 to 6 times greater per unit area compared with any other space in a hospital; heating, ventilation, and air conditioning (HVAC) demands make up more than 90% of this energy consumption.

Opportunities

ORs are frequently unoccupied, but often HVAC systems run around the clock. Setback systems and occupancy sensors can reduce air exchange rates when rooms are unoccupied and reduce energy consumption.[14] With occupancy setbacks for air exchange rates, hospitals can achieve significant savings, in excess of $2000 USD per OR per year.[15] Along with converting to light-emitting diode (LED) lights, these solutions require minimal upfront investment and produce significant, realized savings and emissions reductions without impacting staff responsibilities or patient care.

SINGLE-USE DEVICES

Problem

Single-use products are an important source of perioperative energy use and pollution, generating more than 10 kg of physical waste per patient per day. When considering the resources required to produce, package, transport, and dispose of these products, single-use products represent a significant source of emissions. A study of cataract surgery in the UK demonstrated that the manufacturing of disposable materials accounts for more than 50% of the total carbon emissions of the procedure.[16]

TABLE 61.3 ■ Opportunities to Reduce Emissions From Single-Use Devices and Equipment

Opportunities	Description
Reusable gowns and textiles	Reusable gowns use fewer resources, produce less waste, and have a reduced global warming potential compared with disposable gowns.[19]
Reusable hard cases for surgical instrumentation	Reduce dependence on "blue wrap" (polypropylene) in the sterilization process for reusable instruments
Surgical kit reformulation	Process of reviewing preference cards and/or auditing specific procedures and surgeons to determine where unneeded or excess items are being included

Opportunities

Reducing emissions from single-use devices in the supply chain can be accomplished through a variety of mechanisms, explored in Table 61.3. Additionally, emissions can be curbed through a return to reusable tools and devices. When properly decontaminated, reusable supplies carry no increased risk and offer a much lower environmental footprint in many cases.[17,18] For example, when comparing reusable and disposable laryngoscope blades and handles, the reusable options are associated with 25% the CO_2 emissions, 40% the cost, and 0.9% the carcinogen potential of single-use disposable versions, even after accounting for emissions and cost in the sterilization process.[19]

Reprocessing is a process through which single-use products are collected and sent to a third-party manufacturer to be properly decontaminated, sterilized, and repackaged.[20] In the United States, reprocessing is a Food and Drug Administration (FDA)–approved and regulated practice. Among other benefits, reprocessing reduces both the demand for new materials (i.e., mining metals, plastics) and creation of landfill waste. Reprocessed devices are less expensive than their new counterparts and associated with lower emissions.

BIOHAZARD WASTE MANAGEMENT

Problem

Another important area is biohazard waste management (i.e., red bag waste), which are materials contaminated by bodily fluids that must be separated from landfill bound waste and sent through a high-energy treatment process like autoclaving and incineration. Biohazard waste is associated with costs eight times higher per ton to dispose of than nonbiohazardous waste, and treatment processes are responsible for the production of GHGs and other pollutants.

Opportunities

Confusion around the definition of biohazard waste means that in most ORs, upwards of 90%, by weight, of items placed into biohazard bags do not meet criteria of "biohazardous waste." Performing a biohazard waste audit and regularly educating employees about the appropriate use of biohazard waste receptacles can reduce perioperative GHG emissions.

PERIOPERATIVE VALUE ANALYSIS

Problem

Perioperative supply chains are responsible for a large portion of emissions associated with ORs. Traditional valuations in perioperative spaces fail to consider the associated environmental emissions from resource extraction, manufacturing, packaging, transportation, utilization, and disposal management. An accurate accounting of cost should include the environmental emissions of these processes.

Opportunities

Perioperative departments must make decisions about which equipment and devices should be purchased and stored. Creating guiding principles and formal procedures for instrument value analysis can allow perioperative departments to incorporate environmental sustainability into decision-making processes. At our institution, a value analysis team is tasked with evaluating all new surgical instruments requested by surgeons, anesthesiologists, and staff in the institution. In recent years, the criteria to assess value has been expanded to include cost, quality, safety, innovation, and environmental sustainability. Evaluating environmental sustainability of new devices should be guided by a set of standards or principles, so it can be evaluated objectively against alternative devices. The gold standard for comparing the environmental impact between goods or services, especially GHG emissions, is a Life Cycle Analysis (LCA). This approach is used to evaluate multiple environmental impacts of a product throughout its life span ("cradle-to-grave") and is regulated by a series of international standards to ensure consistency across products and analysts. In recent years, there have been dozens of studies that apply LCA to medical equipment, services, and departments.[21,22] However, performing a complete LCA is tedious, time-consuming, and typically requires graduate-level training. An alternative approach is to establish a set of simple guidelines with binary outcomes. Kaiser Permanente has developed Environmentally Preferable Purchasing Principles, which outline a series of specific guidelines regarding chemicals and waste for suppliers or manufacturers to meet, provided in Table 61.4. In many cases, perioperative departments can work with suppliers or a group purchasing organization (GPO) to collect this information for each product. For example,

---

TABLE 61.4 ■ **Kaiser Permanente Environmentally Preferable Purchasing Standards**

Chemical Criteria	• All homogenous electronic parts are compliant with all European Union Restriction of Hazardous Substances (EU RoHS) Directive's restricted limits. • All homogenous materials contain less than 1000 ppm of intentionally added Bisphenol A and related structural/functional analogs. • Does not contain polyvinyl chloride (PVC). • All homogenous materials contain less than 1000 ppm of bromine and chlorine-based components. • All homogenous materials contain less than 1000 ppm of phthalates. • Does not contain intentionally added chemicals listed by the State of California to cause cancer, birth defects, or reproductive harm that require warning or are prohibited from release to the environment under the California Safe Drinking Water and Toxic Enforcement Act of 1986. • Does not contain intentionally added antimicrobial/antibacterial agents to reduce surface pathogens. • All homogenous materials contain less than 1000 ppm of persistent, bio-accumulative toxins (PBTs). • All nonelectronic homogenous materials contain less than 1000 ppm of any chemical or chemical compound for which a functional use is to resist or inhibit the spread of fire, including but not limited to phosphorous-based and nitrogen-based chemicals. • Does not contain mercury, lead, cadmium, or organotin compounds. • Products do not contain stain- or water-repellent treatment that contain a perfluorinated compound.
Waste Criteria	• Product is not regulated as a state or federal hazardous waste when used for its purpose. • Product contains more than 10% postconsumer recycled content. • Product is recyclable. • Primary packaging contains more than 10% postconsumer recycled content. • Secondary packaging contains more than 30% postconsumer recycled content. • Packaging has received Forest Stewardship Council Certification. • Packaging is labeled with consumer-friendly recycling information. • Packaging is recyclable.

Vizient, a GPO, has incorporated most of Kaiser Permanente's parameters into their surgical supply catalogs to allow hospitals to prioritize products that meet various environmental attributes.

GETTING STARTED IN YOUR HOSPITAL

When considering your own organization, it may feel overwhelming to get started. There remain many opportunities to create perioperative spaces that are more environmentally sustainable, and here we provide recommendations to guide these efforts. First, determine what, if any, sustainability initiatives already exist in your hospital. Second, build a multidisciplinary team, including nurses, surgeons, anesthesiologists, surgical technicians, hospital cleaning staff, hospital administrators, and engineers, who can work collaboratively and identify diverse opportunities for improvement. Next, perform an audit of current clinical practices to determine where QI projects can produce the most benefit. The Surgical Providers Assessment and Response to Climate Change (SPARC2) Tool provides guidance on conducting an audit.[23] Focus should be placed on solutions that are high impact, low energy, and cost effective. These accomplishments serve the dual purpose of quickly reducing emissions and garnering interest among colleagues for wider organization involvement and impact. Finally, we recommend this team regularly communicate with hospital leadership to help generate a culture of sustainability in clinical spaces.

Discussion

There is growing recognition of the need to optimize the environmental impact of health care. Perioperative spaces have many opportunities to reduce carbon emissions and waste without compromising quality or patient safety, as detailed in this chapter.

There remain several opportunities for sustainability optimization. First, better methods are needed to account for environmental emissions associated with the production and use of medical devices and products in perioperative spaces. LCA is the gold standard for evaluating environmental impact of a good or service, but currently life cycle inventory databases contain very limited information about healthcare products. Expanding available information about perioperative equipment will provide objective data about environmental impact to guide supply chain value analysis.

Second, there must be more opportunities to link environmental impact reduction with financial incentive. An obvious model for this is through state-based quality collaboratives, such as the Michigan Surgery Quality Collaborative, which link quality metrics with reimbursement through Blue-Cross Blue Shield. As previously described, MPOG has already created one such quality metric for anesthesiologists, which measures inhaled anesthetic gas flow rates. Similar metrics can and should be created for surgeons related to instrument procurement, waste production, and electricity use.

Finally, hospital leadership needs to identify and empower stakeholders from the diverse groups working in the hospital. Identifying and empowering a multidisciplinary team will allow a variety of sustainability problems to be addressed from multiple angles.

Although the focus of this chapter has largely been on GHG emission reduction, environmental sustainability is much broader and involves optimizing our use of resources, including the chemicals we drain into our water systems, plastic waste we place in municipal landfills, and toxic pollution we release into the air. As GHG emissions trend downward, we must think holistically about creating more efficient and circular processes in perioperative spaces.

Even with significant intervention, healthcare and perioperative spaces will continue to be resource intensive. This is considered necessary to provide safe and effective surgical services. Just as we use measures of value to help make decisions in perioperative spaces in the form of cost or innovation, there should be a balance between our commitment to serving individual lives and the impact that emissions from those actions have on a broader community. Importantly, we should recognize that it is possible to provide more environmentally sustainable care without sacrificing high standards of quality and safety.

References

1. Mortimer F, Isherwood J, Wilkinson A, Vaux E. Sustainability in quality improvement: redefining value. *Future Healthc J.* 2018;5(2):88.
2. Lindsey R. *Climate Change: Atmospheric Carbon Dioxide.* Copenhagen, Denmark: National Oceanic and Atmospheric Administration; 2020.
3. Crimmins A, Balbus J, Gamble JL, et al. Executive Summary. In: *The Impacts of Climate Change on Human Health in the United States: A Scientific Assessment.* Washington, DC: U.S. Global Change Research Program; 2016:1–24.
4. Chung JW, Meltzer DO. Estimate of the carbon footprint of the US health care sector. *JAMA.* 2009;302 (18):1970–1972.
5. Pichler P-P, Jaccard IS, Weisz U, Weisz H. International comparison of health care carbon footprints. *Environ Res Lett.* 2019;14(6), 064004.
6. Eckelman MJ, Sherman J. Environmental impacts of the U.S. health care system and effects on public health. *PLoS One.* 2016;11(6). e0157014.
7. Sherman JD, Schonberger RB, Eckelman M. Estimate of carbon dioxide equivalents of inhaled anesthetics in the United States. Proceedings of the American Society of Anesthesiologists Annual Meeting; 2014.
8. Thiel CL, Eckelman M, Guido R, et al. Environmental impacts of surgical procedures: life cycle assessment of hysterectomy in the United States. *Environ Sci Technol.* 2015;49(3):1779–1786.
9. MacNeill AJ, Lillywhite R, Brown CJ. The impact of surgery on global climate: a carbon footprinting study of operating theatres in three health systems. *Lancet Planet Health.* 2017;1(9):e381–e388.
10. Ryan SM, Nielsen CJ. Global warming potential of inhaled anesthetics: application to clinical use. *Anesth Analg.* 2010;111(1):92–98.
11. Sherman J, Feldman J, Berry JM. Reducing inhaled anesthetic waste and pollution. *Anesthesiology News.* 2017;04–17.
12. Sustainability Quality Metric (SUS-01). Multicenter Perioperative Outcomes Group (MPOG); May 2021.
13. Ventilation in health care facilities. In: ASHRAE ASoHCEA, ed. *Standard 170–2017,* 2017.
14. Love C. *Operating Room HVAC Setback Strategies.* Chicago, IL: The American Society for Healthcare Engineering; 2011.
15. Practice Greenhealth. 2019 Sustainability Benchmark Data; 2019.
16. Thiel CL, Schehlein E, Ravilla T, et al. Cataract surgery and environmental sustainability: waste and life-cycle assessment of phacoemulsification at a private healthcare facility. *J Cataract Refract Surg.* 2017;43 (11):1391–1398.
17. Rutala WA, Weber DJ. Disinfection and sterilization: an overview. *Am J Infect Control.* 2013;41(5):S2–S5.
18. Siu J, Hill AG, MacCormick AD. Systematic review of reusable versus disposable laparoscopic instruments: costs and safety. *ANZ J Surg.* 2017;87(1–2):28–33.
19. Sherman JD, Raibley IV LA, Eckelman MJ. Life cycle assessment and costing methods for device procurement: comparing reusable and single-use disposable laryngoscopes. *Anesth Analg.* 2018;127(2):434–443.
20. Office USGA. *Reprocessed Single-use Medical Devices: FDA Oversight Has Increased, and Available Information Does Not Indicate that Use Presents an Elevated Health Risk: Report to the Committee on Oversight and Government Reform, House of Representatives.* US Government Accountability Office; 2008.
21. Donahue LM, Hilton S, Bell SG, Williams BC, Keoleian GA. A comparative carbon footprint analysis of disposable and reusable vaginal specula. *Am J Obstet Gynecol.* 2020.
22. Ibbotson S, Dettmer T, Kara S, Herrmann C. Eco-efficiency of disposable and reusable surgical instruments—a scissors case. *Int J Life Cycle Assess.* 2013;18(5):1137–1148.
23. Ewbank C, Stewart B, Bruns B, et al. Introduction of the Surgical Providers Assessment and Response to Climate Change (SPARC2) Tool: one small step toward reducing the carbon footprint of surgical care. *Ann Surg.* 2021;273(4):e135–e137.

Further Reading

Chen, et al. The triple bottom line and stabilization wedges; a framework for perioperative sustainability. *Anesth Analg.* 2021. In press.

CHAPTER 62

Gaining and Keeping C-Suite Support for Perioperative Quality Improvement Initiatives

Thomas E. Jackiewicz, MPH ■ Susan LaFollette Arnold, BS

KEY POINTS

- Understanding the chief executive officer (CEO) mindset and what they worry about helps teams frame performance improvement initiatives in ways that will resonate.
- Proposed quality improvement projects should ideally have direct ties to an organization's strategic plan or key strategic initiatives.
- Teams should be candid about "known unknowns" and have plans in place for addressing them.
- Successful projects include timelines, with milestones and data, to demonstrate progress.
- Be prepared for resistance and challenges to your ideas and proposals.

A Personal Perspective

I am honored to contribute the final chapter of this book and share the chief executive officer (CEO) perspective on quality improvement (QI) for perioperative medicine. Throughout my career, I have had the opportunity to observe performance improvement from the bottom up and the top down. During my career progression through financial leadership to my last 12 years as a CEO of top health systems, I have seen unlikely QI initiatives succeed, whereas simpler and much-needed projects fell apart.

This chapter provides suggestions and tips on how to understand the C-suite mindset and increase the likelihood that a QI project will receive the support and resources it needs to succeed.

Walk in Our Shoes: Understanding the CEO Role

I have spent over 30 years of my career working within academic health systems. I have worked closely with many CEOs during that time, but it was not until I became one that I understood the magnitude of the role and its daily demands. A study published in the *Harvard Business Review* tracked the time allocations of 27 CEOs and determined that these leaders had 37 meetings of various lengths each week, meaning that 72% of their total work time is spent at meetings.[1] The authors conclude that more than anyone else in an organization, CEOs regularly confront the shortage of one resource: time. I can confirm their conclusion and also support the viewpoint that the COVID-19 crisis made it even clearer that CEOs must be intentional about how they use their time.[2]

CEOs are ultimately accountable for everything throughout the organization. Even the best delegators have to engage with many constituencies to ensure they remain informed and engaged. Packed schedules are a constant reminder of the volume of things that need attention, from taking care of people to keeping the organization healthy and growing. Although the CEO may appear to be a victim of busy schedules, they are also keenly aware that how they spend their time communicates their priorities throughout the organization.

CEOs wield great influence and authority but also face pressures and constraints that may be less noticeable or understood outside of the C-suite. CEOs continually focus on strategy—the overarching strategic direction of the organization and the performance and alignment of all of the components within the organization. When that organization is a highly complex healthcare institution, setting priorities and maintaining clarity of direction can easily become complicated and politicized.

Saying yes or no to a performance improvement initiative from the CEO perspective is much more than assessing a project's individual merits and securing funding. Instead, CEOs must think carefully about how and when to exert their leverage and political capital in support of a project. They must look at the risk-reward equation for how an initiative might impact other items under consideration or in the pipeline and the reactions of stakeholders attached to those projects.

What Keeps Healthcare CEOs Awake at Night

Given the scope and consequential nature of what CEOs tackle on any given day, leaving it all behind at the end of a long work day is not a simple disconnect. As QI teams think through what will capture and keep a CEO's attention, it is important to keep in mind the areas that CEOs tend to worry about the most. Why? Because CEOs are continually scanning the environment for fresh new thinking that could ease their concerns and produce real progress for their organization.

When I think about the list of top concerns that keep CEOs awake at night, I can come up with five things that worry me the most (Fig. 62.1):

1. **Culture.** Culture is not randomly at the top of my list. As CEOs focus on strategy, culture is always waiting in the wings as a potential destroyer of good strategy. "Culture eats strategy for lunch" resonates with people because it is true. Performance improvement initiatives must incorporate cultural considerations. Health care involves multiple team members, as do change initiatives. Successful presentations of QI projects to CEOs must demonstrate how the human element of leading people through change is incorporated and how resistance will be addressed.

2. **Patient Safety and Quality.** The good news is that patient safety and quality are top priorities for CEOs, more so than was the case a decade ago. The bad news is that because they are priorities, performance improvement projects related to safety and quality may be quite competitive. Teams that are organizing these efforts should not translate the ease with which they capture a CEO's attention into the assumption that their initiative will sail through unquestioned. Instead, teams should assume the competition will be tough and plan accordingly.

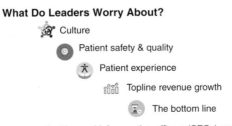

What Do Leaders Worry About?

Culture

Patient safety & quality

Patient experience

Topline revenue growth

The bottom line

Fig. 62.1   Top concerns that keep chief executive officers (CEOs) awake at night.

3. **Patient Experience**. QI projects have obvious ties to the patient experience—higher patient satisfaction, shorter lengths of stay, lower cost—all of which will initially capture a CEO's attention. When possible, ensure that components of the patient experience are measurable and that compelling data are captured and shared during the proposed QI project.

4. **Topline Revenue Growth**. Growth is right up there with strategy as a CEO priority that receives daily attention. C-suite healthcare leaders know that clinical success is the lifeblood of their organizations, and clinical growth is the natural offshoot of that success. QI teams should keep in mind that when using "this is the right thing to do" as a key selling point, it should be supplemented with information about potential growth opportunities.

5. **The Bottom Line**. CEOs know that growth and improvement will involve risk, including the financial risk of investing in initiatives that may fail to produce expected results. QI teams should keep in mind that when CEOs sign off on a project, they are signaling a personal commitment of resources that come from the organization's bottom line. That commitment should not be taken lightly and instead should drive judicious use of resources.

What CEOs Want to See in a Performance Improvement Initiative Proposal

With the backdrop of packed CEO schedules and CEOs' deserved reputation for short attention spans, QI teams must prepare carefully for their CEO meetings. To increase the likelihood that a proposal receives a thorough and fair review and discussion, a high-quality document must be prepared and the team should practice how it will be presented.

1. **Create a proposal that covers the basics concisely but comprehensively.** The following components should be included in the document. To ensure that the main points garner attention, consider using a simple primary document and putting details in the appendices.
   - **Statement of the challenge.** Build a story or narrative that tells why this is the right thing to do and why now is the right time to do it. Be clear about the root causes and issues that require change and include data to back up key points.
   - **Goals/objectives.** Clearly state the initiative's goals (outcomes to be achieved) and objectives (specific actions that will occur to achieve the goal). Factor in the CEO's focus on strategy and ensure that the goals connect to the organization's strategic plan or strategic priorities. Provide specifics about what clinical teams will be asked to change in their workflows.
   - **Timeline.** Provide a timeline for the project with major milestones noted. Be honest about the potential for delays and unknowns.
   - **Monitoring and measuring progress.** Identify measures that will be used to determine achievement of milestones and the success of the initiative. Be candid about where people may passively or actively resist change and how that resistance can be managed to maintain progress.
   - **Team.** Specify who will lead the initiative and who will be in supporting roles. If C-suite leaders are needed to complete tasks or fulfill unofficial roles (e.g., communicating with hesitant physicians), state those expectations clearly.
   - **Resource requirements.** Delineate what resources and skills will be required by the project, including external support, if needed. Remember to specify the cost of doing nothing in both financial and nonfinancial terms.
   - **Desired outcomes.** Be clear about projected outcomes, particularly for patients, but also make the business case for the project by specifying other anticipated benefits, such as growth opportunities and efficiencies that lower costs.

2. **Practice the presentation rather than winging it.** Teams should prepare carefully for their CEO presentation. Efficiency with getting major points across and time management are key.

   ■ **Focus on essentials.** Keep the presentation concise with three to five key points. The main document should be lean with appendices that provide additional detail.

   ■ **Consider presenting recommendations first and then sharing evidence and details later.** CEOs routinely get called out of meetings to handle pressing matters. By leading with the most important information (the project's recommendations), rather than long lists of data and evidence, teams will be better positioned to capture CEO attention.

   ■ **Allow plenty of time for questions and discussion.** Leave at least half of the allotted time for discussion and questions rather than spending the majority of time presenting materials to the CEO.[3]

3. **Be positive but realistic.** Remember that CEOs have witnessed failed performance improvement projects. They understand that change can be extremely difficult, especially among clinical staff who may view their work as a calling as much as a profession. Acknowledging potential challenges and preparing for them may help avert derailed initiatives.

Eight Tips for Successful CEO Meetings

Given the research that shows CEOs in roughly 37 meetings each week, QI teams should consider these tips for making meetings meaningful, memorable, and ending with momentum.

1. **Use visuals but keep them simple.** CEOs regularly experience death by PowerPoint. Avoid using crowded, complicated slides in favor of simple visuals that enhance rather than detract from what the team is saying.

2. **Do not overpromise.** Be candid about what the team does not know and potential pitfalls. If possible, speculate about actions that may be needed to get activities back on track after a setback.

3. **Avoid clinical jargon and excessively complex language.** All CEOs, even if they are clinicians, appreciate a presentation with clean, easily understood language.

4. **Prepare for questions.** Assume that CEOs will have tough questions and be prepared for them (think Shark Tank). Do not assume their questions are a negative. In fact, they may indicate quite the opposite.

5. **Do not pretend to have all of the answers.** If the team is unable to answer a question, simply promise to get back to the CEO with more details. Do not make excuses or try to spin an answer.

6. **Be open to suggestions.** Most CEOs have experienced performance improvement successes and failures and have lessons learned from those experiences. Listen to their ideas with an open mind.

7. **Be clear about what is needed from the executive as next steps.** Do not assume that the executive will initiate next steps. Be ready to tell them what is needed.

8. **Passion and enthusiasm alone will not win the day, but the absence of them can impact success.** Performance improvement is not easy work. CEOs want to see energy and enthusiasm in presentations and evidence of confidence to drive the project through to completion.

Once all of the initial hurdles to gaining CEO support have been navigated and projects have the green light, teams should plan regular check-in calls with CEOs or their designees to keep them apprised of the initiative. These interactions should be approached with the same candor and honesty used earlier with the CEO and leave plenty of time for meaningful discussion to ensure the executive has what they need to continue to be confident in the project.

My last piece of advice to QI teams planning a perioperative initiative is to prepare for criticism, which is an inevitable part of every change management process. Peers and colleagues will criticize the necessity of change, the type of change being enacted, and the pace of change, among other things. They will resist both small and large elements of change in ways that can feel quite personal. Successful teams will prepare for these inevitabilities and work through them as a unified front that is focused, committed, and driven to see their initiative succeed.

To all of you who are pushing forward with perioperative QI initiatives, I wish you well and thank you for all you do to provide the best possible care for patients, now and in the future.

References

1. Porter ME, Norhia N. How CEOs manage time. Harvard Business Review. 2018. https://hbr.org/2018/07/how-ceos-manage-time.
2. Dewar C, Keller S, Sneader K, Strovink K. The CEO moment: leadership for a new era. McKinsey & Company; 2020. https://www.mckinsey.com/featured-insights/leadership/the-ceo-moment-leadership-for-a-new-era.
3. Nawaz S. How to blow a presentation to the C-suite. Harvard Business Review. 2018. https://hbr.org/2018/10/how-to-blow-a-presentation-to-the-c-suite.

Suggested Reading

1. Bossidy L. What your leader expects of you. Harvard Business Review. 2007. https://hbr.org/2007/04/whatyour-leader-expects-of-you.
2. Charan R. The discipline of listening. Harvard Business Review. 2012. https://hbr.org/2012/06/thediscipline-of-listening.
3. Lee TH. Turning doctors into leaders. Harvard Business Review. 2010. https://hbr.org/2010/04/turningdoctors-into-leaders.

INDEX

Note: Page numbers followed by *f* indicate figures, *t* indicate tables, and *b* indicate boxes.